Transdermal Controlled
Systemic Medications

DRUGS AND THE PHARMACEUTICAL SCIENCES

A Series of Textbooks and Monographs

Edited by

James Swarbrick

School of Pharmacy
University of North Carolina
Chapel Hill, North Carolina

Transdermal Controlled Systemic Medications

edited by

YIE W. CHIEN
Controlled Drug-Delivery Research Center
Rutgers–The State University
  of New Jersey
Piscataway, New Jersey

CRC Press
Taylor & Francis Group
an **informa** business
www.taylorandfrancisgroup.com

6000 Broken Sound Parkway, NW
Suite 300, Boca Raton, FL 33487
711 Third Avenue
New York, NY 10017
2 Park Square, Milton Park
Abingdon, Oxon OX14 4RN, UK

FIRST INDIAN REPRINT, 2015

Library of Congress Cataloging-in-Publication Data

Transdermal controlled systemic medications.

(Drugs and the pharmaceutical sciences ; v. 31)
Includes bibliographies and index.
1. Endermic medication. 2. Drugs--Controlled release.
3. Pharmaceutical technology. I. Chien, Yie W.
II. Series. [DNLM: 1. Administration, Cutaneous.
W1 DR893B v.31 / WB 340 T7722]
RM151.T74   1987   615'.67   87-13715
ISBN 0-8247-7760-3

MARCEL DEKKER, INC.
270 Madison Avenue, New York, New York   10016

Printed and bound in India by Bhavish Graphics.
FOR SALE IN SOUTH ASIA ONLY

Preface

This book presents a comprehensive and coherent treatment of the
science and technology associated with the development of transdermal
rate-controlled drug delivery systems. Development of a viable transdermal drug delivery (TDD) system with rate-controlled characteristics
requires both a fundamental understanding and optimization of physical
and biomedical sciences, including pharmaceutics, pharmacokinetics,
and pharmacodynamics. Therefore, transdermal controlled drug delivery technology is an expansive discipline encompassing areas of
interest germane to many biomedical and engineering principles.

    The purpose of this book is to provide a concise source of the
core knowledge related to transdermal controlled administration of
drugs, including fundamentals of skin permeation, development and
manufacturing of TDD systems, preclinical and clinical assessments
of transdermal controlled drug administration, as well as international
regulatory requirements for marketing approval. This core knowledge is important to all wishing to acquire a solid understanding of
how controlled-release technology can be utilized in the successful
development of TDD systems with programmable drug release characteristics. A viable TDD system can be developed successfully only
on the basis of a sound foundation of pharmacokinetic and pharmacodynamic principles. Only such a development permits one to achieve
the objectives of optimum bioavailability and maximum therapeutic
efficacy.

    This book consists of 18 chapters, including 13 developed from
the 20 lectures given by experts in the field at the 1985 International
Pharmaceutical R&D Symposium, "Advances in Transdermal Controlled

Drug Administration for Systemic Medications" at Rutgers University College of Pharmacy and five chapters contributed by specialists by special invitation. It is written for scientists and managers of diverse backgrounds who are interested in the conceptualization, development, and/or optimization of transdermal controlled drug administration or who are involved in the laboratory testing, production, clinical evaluations, or uses of TDD systems.

To provide the readers with a broad spectrum of scientific information in a concise, systematic manner, the 18 chapters in this book cover the historical perspective and recent advancements in transdermal systemic medication (Chapter 1), the development and preclinical and clinical assessments of TDD systems (Chapters 2–12), the engineering and manufacturing aspects of TDD systems (Chapters 13–15), as well as regulatory requirements for approval of TDD systems among international health authorities (Chapters 16–18).

With the cooperation of all the contributors and the able assistance of Ms. Marline Boslet, we have finally completed the proceedings of the symposium. We believe that this book offers a wealth of scientific documentation and technical information organized in a logical sequence and will be useful to everyone who is working on or interested in the research and development of transdermal controlled administration of drugs for systemic medications.

Yie W. Chien

Contributors

PAUL ADAMS   Department of Health and Social Security, London, England

VALERIE N. AHMUTY   Pharmaceutical Research and Development, Key Pharmaceuticals, Inc., Miami, Florida

RICHARD A. BERG   Department of Biochemistry, UMDNJ-Robert Wood Johnson Medical School, Piscataway, New Jersey

CAROL M. BIES*   Department of Clinical Pharmacology, Hahnemann University Hospital, and Hahnemann University School of Medicine, Philadelphia, Pennsylvania

DAVID J. BOVA   Product Development, Key Pharmaceuticals, Inc., Miami, Florida

DANIEL A. W. BUCKS   Departments of Pharmacy and Dermatology, University of California at San Francisco, San Francisco, California

----

Present affiliation:
*Nursing Staff Development, Lock Haven Hospital, Lock Haven, Pennsylvania.

WILLI CAWELLO   Department of Bio-mathematics, Schwarz GmbH, Monheim, West Germany

ROBERT R. CHASE*   Department of Clinical Pharmacology, Hahnemann University Hospital, and Hahnemann University School of Medicine, Philadelphia, Pennsylvania

YIE W. CHIEN   Controlled Drug-Delivery Research Center, Department of Pharmaceutics and Clinical Sciences, Rutgers—The State University of New Jersey, Piscataway, New Jersey

ROBERT L. CIRRITO   Technical Services, Key Pharmaceuticals, Inc., Miami, Florida

EUGENE R. COOPER†   Department of Drug Delivery, Alcon Laboratories, Inc., Fort Worth, Texas

GÜNTER CORDES   Technical Division, Schwarz GmbH, Monheim, West Germany

JOHN W. DOHNER   Engineering Department, Alza Corporation, Palo Alto, California

T. FAGAN   Department of Nursing, Hahnemann University Hospital, and Hahnemann University School of Medicine, Philadelphia, Pennsylvania

BONITA FALKNER   Division of Pediatric Nephrology, Hahnemann University Hospital, and Hahnemann University School of Medicine, Philadelphia, Pennsylvania

RICHARD H. GUY   Departments of Pharmacy and Pharmaceutical Chemistry, University of California at San Francisco, San Francisco, California

JOHATHAN HADGRAFT‡   Departments of Pharmacy and Pharmaceutical Chemistry, University of California at San Francisco, San Francisco, California

---

Present affiliations:
*Department of Orthopaedic Surgery and Rehabilitation, Hahnemann University Hospital, Philadelphia, Pennsylvania.
†Department of Pharmaceutics, Alcon Laboratories, Inc., Fort Worth, Texas.
‡Department of Pharmaceutical Chemistry, The Welsh School of Pharmacy, U.W.I.S.T., Cardiff, Wales, United Kingdom.

ROBERT S. HINZ   Department of Pharmacy, University of California at San Francisco, San Francisco, California

HANS RAINER HOFFMANN   Research and Development, LTS Lohmann Therapie-Systeme GmbH & Co. KG, Neuwied, West Germany

KAREN O'TOOLE HOLMES   Research and Development Documentation Office, Key Pharmaceuticals, Inc., Miami, Florida

YIH-CHAIN HUANG   Department of Pharmaceutics and Clinical Sciences, Controlled Drug-Delivery Research Center, College of Pharmacy, Rutgers-The State University of New Jersey, Piscataway, New Jersey

K. KASPER   Key Pharmaceuticals, Inc., Miami, Florida

CAROLINE LaPRADE   Research and Development, Key Pharmaceuticals, Inc., Miami, Florida

R. LaPRADE   Key Pharmaceuticals, Inc., Miami, Florida

DAVID T. LOWENTHAL*   Departments of Medicine and Pharmacology, Cardiovascular Institute, Hahnemann University Hospital, and Hahnemann University School of Medicine, Philadelphia, Pennsylvania

GUSTAV A. MAAG†   Research and Development, Key Pharmaceuticals, Inc., Miami, Florida

YOSHIHARU MACHIDA   Department of Pharmaceutics, Faculty of Pharmaceutical Sciences, Hoshi University, Shinagawa, Tokyo, Japan

JUAN A. MANTELLE   Research and Development, Key Pharmaceuticals, Inc., Miami, Florida

JOHN A. McCARTY   Research and Development, Key Pharmaceuticals, Inc., Miami, Florida

Present affiliations:
*Departments of Geriatrics and Adult Development, Medicine, and Pharmacology, The Mount Sinai Medical Center, New York, New York.
†Consultant, Miami Beach, Florida.

J. MIRANDA   Key Pharmaceuticals, Inc., Miami, Florida

FRANKIE A. MORTON   Research and Development, Key Pharmaceuticals, Inc., Miami, Florida

MARTIN C. MUSOLF   Technical Service and Development, Medical Products Business, Dow Corning Corporation, Midland, Michigan

TSUNEJI NAGAI   Department of Pharmaceutics, Faculty of Pharmaceutical Sciences, Hoshi University, Shinagawa, Tokyo, Japan

JAMES M. PACHENCE   Pachence Associates, Lawrenceville, New Jersey

ESTER PARAN*   Hahnemann University Hospital and Hahnemann University School of Medicine, Philadelphia, Pennsylvania

G. S. PERLMUTTER   Hahnemann University Hospital and Hahnemann University School of Medicine, Philadelphia, Pennsylvania

NATHANIEL REICHEK   Cardiovascular Section, Department of Medicine, Hospital of the University of Pennsylvania, Philadelphia, Pennsylvania

DŽENANA E. REZAKOVIĆ   Department of Medicine, University Hospital, and Faculty of Medicine, University of Zagreb, Zagreb, Yugoslavia

KATHLEEN V. ROSKOS   Department of Pharmaceutical Chemistry, University of California at San Francisco, San Francisco, California

STEVEN SABLOTSKY   Research and Development, Key Pharmaceuticals, Inc., Miami, Florida

VINOD P. SHAH   Science, Management Operations and Policy Branch, Division of Biopharmaceutics, Center for Drugs and Biologics, Food and Drug Administration, Rockville, Maryland

Present affiliation:
*Department of Medicine, Soroka Medical Center, Ben Gurion University of the Negev, Beersheba, Israel.

FREDERICK H. SILVER   Biomaterials Center, Department of Pathology, UMDNJ–Robert Wood Johnson Medical School, Piscataway, New Jersey

JEROME P. SKELLY   Division of Biopharmaceutics, Center for Drugs and Biologics, Food and Drug Administration, Rockville, Maryland

KAKUJI TOJO   Department of Pharmaceutics and Clinical Sciences, College of Pharmacy, Rutgers–The State University of New Jersey, Piscataway, New Jersey

KEVIN S. WEADOCK   Biomaterials Center, Department of Pathology, UMDNJ–Robert Wood Johnson Medical School, Piscataway, New Jersey

INGE WEISS   TTS Development, Schwarz GmbH, Monheim, West Germany

HANS-MICHAEL WOLFF   TTS Development, Schwarz GmbH, Monheim, West Germany

Contents

Transdermal Controlled Systemic Medications

1

Advances in Transdermal Systemic Medication

YIE W. CHIEN / *Rutgers—The State University of New Jersey,
Piscataway, New Jersey*

I. INTRODUCTION

Continuous intravenous administration at a programmed rate of infusion has been recognized as a superior mode of drug delivery not
only to bypass hepatic "first-pass" elimination, but also to maintain
a constant, prolonged, and therapeutically effective drug level in
the body. A closely monitored intravenous infusion can provide the
advantages of direct entry of drug into the systemic circulation and
control of circulating drug levels. However, this mode of drug delivery entails certain risks and, therefore, necessitates hospitalization
of the patients and close medical supervision of the medication.

Recently, there has been a growing recognition that the benefits
of intravenous drug infusion can be closely duplicated, without its
hazards, by using the intact skin as the port of drug administration
to provide continuous transdermal drug delivery into the systemic
circulation (1).

Several transdermal therapeutic systems have recently been developed for topical application on the intact skin surface aiming to
achieve systemic medication. This approach was exemplified first by
the development of scopolamine-releasing transdermal therapeutic
system (Transderm-Scop by Ciba) for 72-hr prophylaxis or treatment
of motion-induced nausea (2), and then by the successful marketing

of several nitroglycerin-releasing transdermal therapeutic systems
(Deponit by Pharma-Schwarz/Lohmann, Nitrodisc by Searle, Nitro-
Dur by Key, and Transderm-Nitro by Ciba), as well as an isosorbide
dinitrate-releasing transdermal therapeutic system (Frandol tape by
Toaeiyo, Yamanouchi) for once-a-day medication of angina pectoris
(3,4), and most recently by the regulatory approval of a clonidine-
releasing transdermal therapeutic system (Catapres-TTS by Boehringer Ingelheim) for weekly treatment of hypertension (4).

The intensity of interest in the potential biomedical applications
of rate-controlled transdermal drug administration is further demonstrated by a substantial increase in research and development
activities in many health care institutions aiming to develop patentable transdermal therapeutic systems to provide a continuous transdermal infusion of therapeutic agents for prolonged periods of time.
The drug candidates evaluated have ranged from antihypertensive,
antianginal, antihistamine, and anti-inflammatory agents to analgesic,
antiarthritic, steroidal, and contraceptive drugs.

This chapter discusses the logic behind the concept of using
intact skin as the port for continuous drug infusion as well as the
historic perspective and advances in the development of rate-controlled transdermal therapeutic systems.

II. THE SKIN: SITE OF TRANSDERMAL
DRUG ADMINISTRATION

The skin of an average adult body covers a surface area of approximately 2 square meters and receives about one-third of the blood
circulating through the body (5). It is one of the most readily
accessible organs of the human body. With a thickness of only a
few millimeters (2.97 ± 0.28 mm), the skin separates the vital organs
from the outside environment, serves as a protective barrier against
physical, chemical or microbial attacks, acts as a thermostat in maintaining body temperature, plays a role in the regulation of the blood
pressure, and protects the human body against the penetration of
ultraviolet rays.

Microscopically, the skin is a multilayered organ composed of many
histological layers. It is generally described in terms of three major
multilaminate layers: the epidermis, the dermis, and the hypodermis
(Fig. 1). The epidermis is further divided into five anatomical layers with the outermost layer of stratum corneum exposed to the
external environment.

The stratum corneum consists of many layers of compacted,
flattened, dehydrated, and keratinized cells. These cells are physiologically rather inactive and are continuously shed with constant

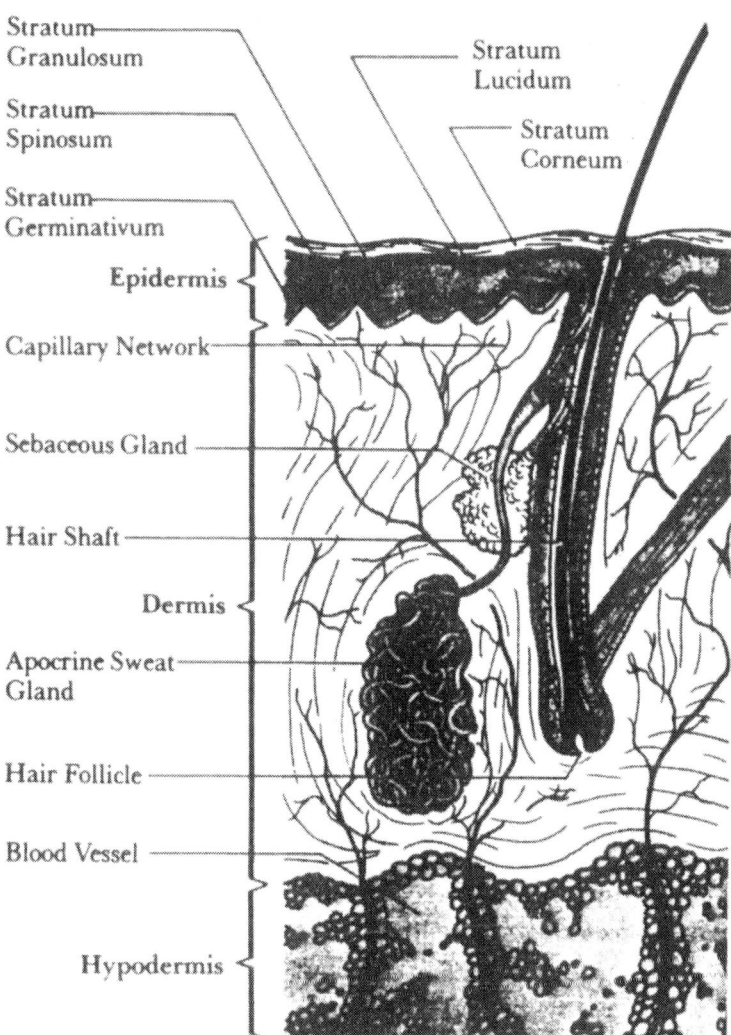

Figure 1   A cross-sectional view of human skin, showing various skin tissue layers and appendages.   (From Ref. 6.)

replacement from the underlying viable epidermal tissue (6). The stratum corneum has a water content of only 20% as compared to the normal physiological level of 70%, such as in the physiologically active stratum germinativum (which is the regenerative layer of the epidermis).

The human skin surface is known to contain, on the average, 10-70 hair follicles and 200-250 sweat ducts on every square centimeter of skin area. These skin appendages, however, actually occupy, grossly, only 0.1% of the total human skin surface. Even though foreign agents, especially water-soluble ones, may be able to penetrate the skin via these skin appendages faster than through the intact area of the stratum corneum, this transappendageal route of percutaneous absorption has provided a very limited contribution to the overall kinetic profile of transdermal permeation. Therefore, the transdermal permeation of most neutral molecules at steady state can be considered as, primarily, a process of passive diffusion through the intact stratum corneum in the interfollicular region. So, for a fundamental understanding of transdermal drug infusion (7), the organization of the skin can be represented by a simplified multi-layer model as shown in Figure 2.

For many decades, the skin has been commonly used as the site for the administration of dermatological drugs to achieve localized pharmacological action in the skin tissues. In such cases, the drug molecules are considered to diffuse to a target tissue in the proximity of drug application to produce their therapeutic effect before

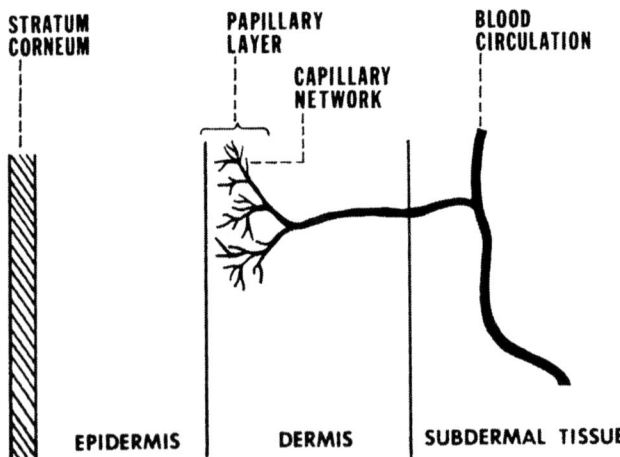

STRATUM CORNEUM   PAPILLARY LAYER   BLOOD CIRCULATION

CAPILLARY NETWORK

EPIDERMIS   DERMIS   SUBDERMAL TISSUE

Figure 2   A simplified model of the human skin for mechanistic analysis of skin permeation. (From Ref. 7.)

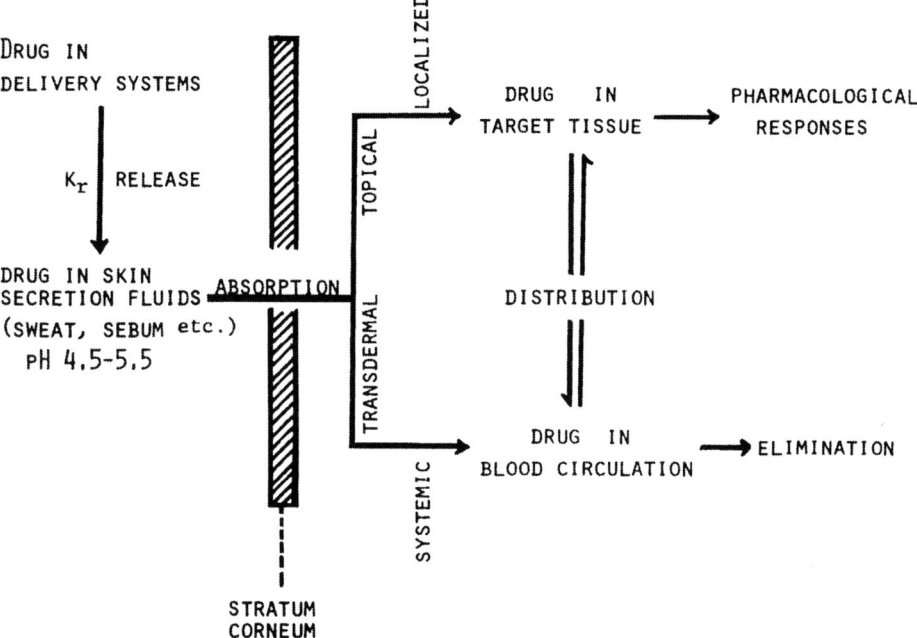

Figure 3   Schematic illustration of drug release and absorption across the skin tissues for localized therapeutic action in the tissues directly underneath the site of drug administration or for systemic medication in the tissues remote from the site of topical drug application. (From Ref. 7.)

being distributed to the blood circulation for elimination (Fig. 3). The use of hydrocortisone for dermatitis, benzoyl peroxide for acne, and neomycin for superficial infection (8) are the few examples of application.

As discussed earlier, there is increasing recognition that the skin can also serve as the port of administration for systemically active drugs (Fig. 3). In this case, the drug applied topically will be absorbed first into the blood circulation and then will be transported to target tissues, which could be rather remote from the site of drug application, to achieve its therapeutic purposes. Examples include the transdermal controlled delivery of nitroglycerin to the myocardium for the treatment of angina pectoris, of scopolamine to the vomiting center for the prevention of motion-induced sickness, and of estradiol to various estradiol-receptor sites for the medication of postmenopausal syndromes (9–11).

III. EARLY DEVELOPMENT OF TRANSDERMAL DRUG DELIVERY

The potential of using the intact skin as the port of drug administration to the human body has been recognized for several decades, as evidenced by the development of medicated plasters for administering medication through the skin to the underlying areas. By definition, the plaster is also a drug delivery system designed for external application. It is made of adhesive material and with proper balance of cohesive strengths, the adhesive is bonded to the backing support (Fig. 4). Such a proper balance also provides good bonding to the skin when a plaster is applied and permits a clean break from the skin surface when the plaster is removed. Historically, the medicated plaster can be viewed as the first development of the idea of transdermal drug delivery. It affords protection and support by its occlusive action, and it brings medication into close contact with the skin (12).

Little is known of the historical development of medicated plasters. However, their use can be traced back at least several hundred years to ancient China. Two representative Chinese medicated plasters, which are still available for medical practice in China, are shown in Figures 5 and 6. As indicated in Tables 1 and 2, these early generations of medicated plasters tend to contain multiple ingredients of herbal drugs and are intended for localized action in the tissues directly underneath the site of application (Fig. 7).

The medicated plaster is also very popular in Japan in over-the-counter pharmaceutical dosage forms and it is also called cataplasm (13). Salonpas is a typical example (Fig. 8). Although still composed of multiple ingredients, including six therapeutically effective agents (Table 3), the formulation has been so improved that Salonpas

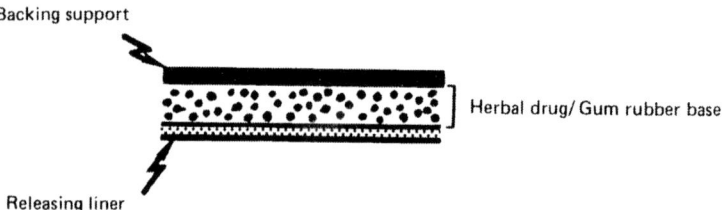

Backing support

Herbal drug/Gum rubber base

Releasing liner

Figure 4   Cross-sectional view of a medicated plaster, showing various major structural components.

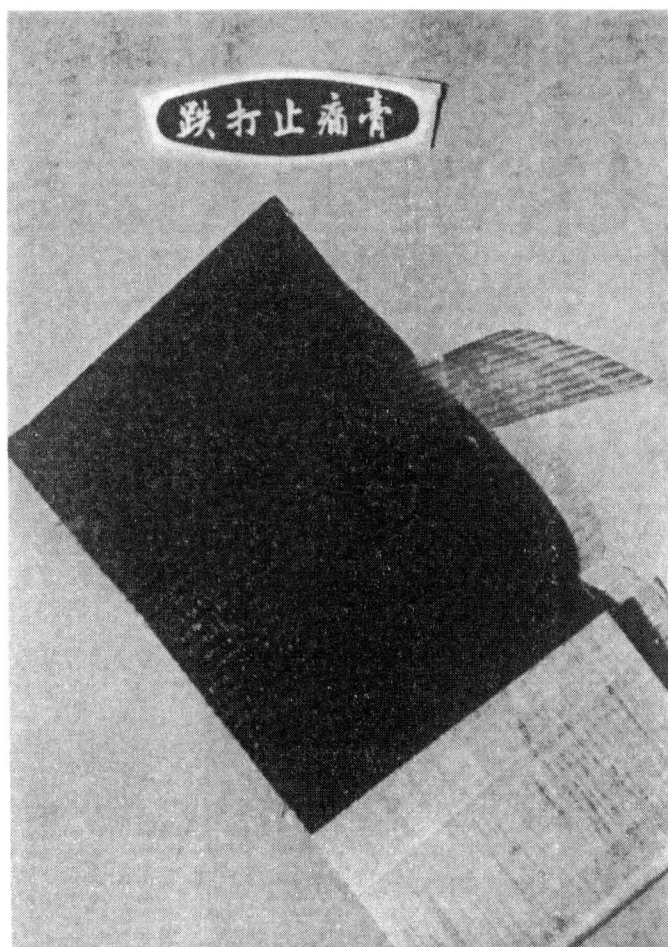

Figure 5 The Yang-Cheng medicated plaster, manufactured by the United Pharmaceutical Manufactory, Kwangchow, China, used on bruises and for its analgesic properties.

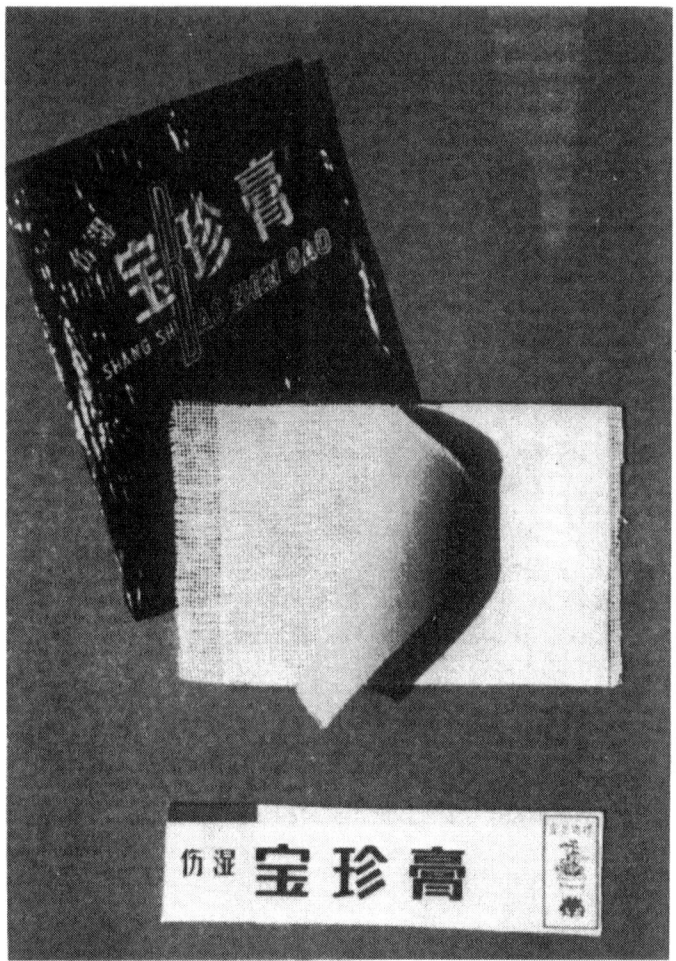

Figure 6 The Shang-Shi Bao Zhen Gao medicated plaster, manufactured by Shanghai Chinese Medicine Works, Shanghai, used for rheumatoid arthritis.

Table 1   Chinese Medicated Plaster for Bruises and
as Analgesic

Main ingredients	Content (%)
Fossilia ossis mastodi	10.42
Eupolyphagasinensis walker	10.42
Sanguis draconis	4.17
Catechu	6.25
Myrrha	6.25
Rhizoma drynariae	4.17
Radix dipsaci	4.17
Flos carthami	9.17
Rhizoma rhei	8.33
Herba taraxaci	8.33
Mentholum	20.00
Methylis salicylas	8.32

Description and action: This plaster is prepared
according to the dialectic therapeutics of traditional
Chinese medicine. The elements of the various drugs
and herbs, when applied to the skin, will penetrate
into the subcutaneous tissues to stimulate circulation
and produce a local analgesic effect. This plaster
helps to cure inflammation of muscles and to promote
the healing of bone fractures.
Indications: Bruises
Fractures
Sprains
Swelling and pains
Bad circulation of blood
Injuries and wounds
Rheumatic arthritis
Neuralgia
Limb languor
Directions: Cut a piece of desired size from the roll,
remove the cellophane and apply to the affected part.
Medicinal effect lasts 24 hr.

Table 2   Chinese Medicated Plaster for Trauma and
Rheumatic Pain

Ingredients	Content (%)
Musk	0.62
Extractum ruta	17.74
Menthol crystals	7.10
Camphor	7.10
Wintergreen oil	14.20
Extractum radix Asari, liquidum compositus	53.24

Actions: Scientifically prepared with various effective Chinese drugs such as musk and *Extractum
ruta*, this plaster is recognized as a specific
remedy for contusions, sprains, and rheumatic disorders, because its ingredients can rapidly infiltrate
into the hypodermis of the affected part, improve the
blood circulation, and promote hematopoiesis. Therefore, it achieves marked effects in the treatment of
neuralgia and soreness in bones and sinews.
Indications: Contusions
Sprains
Rheumatic neuralgia
Sore shoulders and backs
Lumbago
Pains in sinews and bones
Directions: Apply the plaster to the affected part
after cleaning and wiping the skin dry, or, even
better, after bath. Each sheet will be effective for
4-5 days.
Contraindications: Not recommended for pregnant
women.

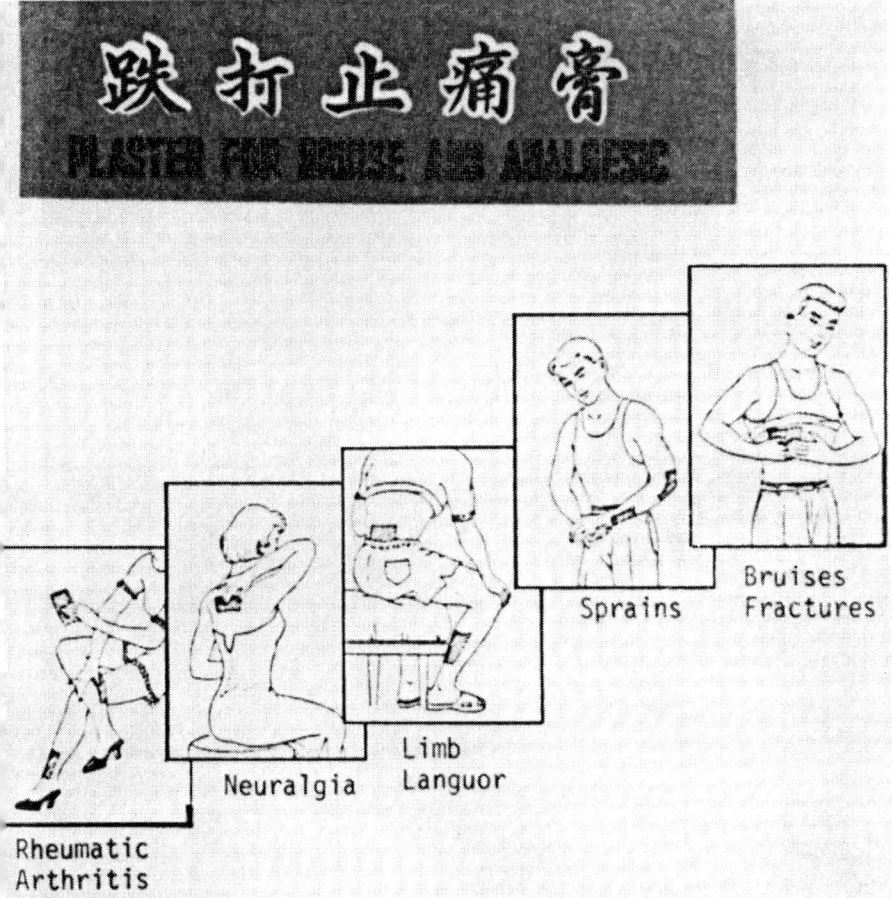

Figure 7   Diagrammatic illustration of the medical applications of Chinese medicated plasters for the treatment of bruises and various types of pain.

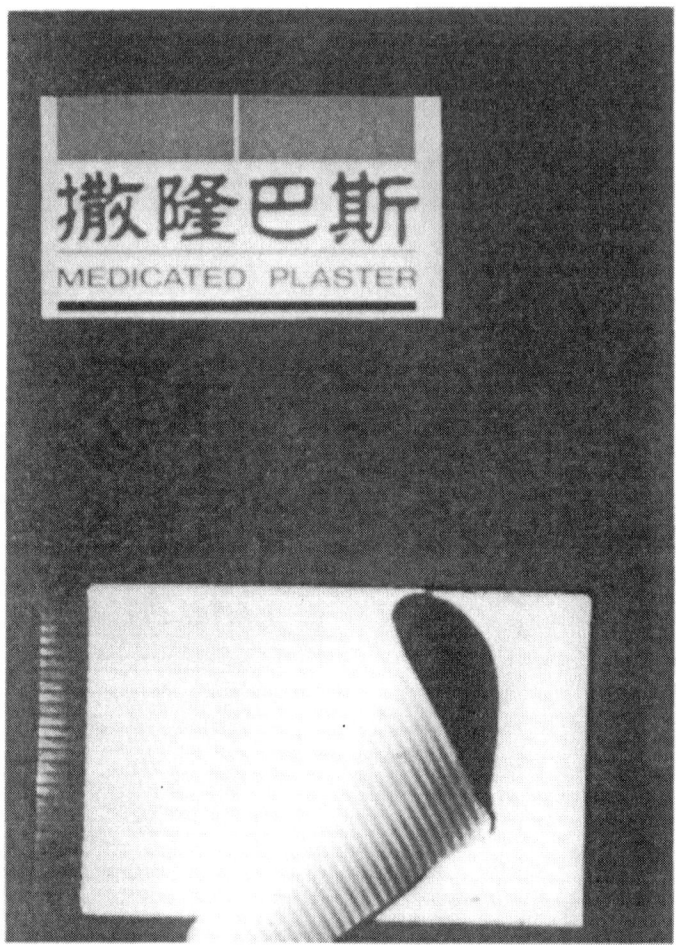

Figure 8 The Salonpas medicated plaster, manufactured by Hisamitsu Pharmaceutical Co., Inc., Saga, Japan, used for muscle ache.

Table 3   Salonpas Medicated Plaster

Active ingredients per 250 cm^2	Content (mg)
Methyl salicylate	330
l-Menthol	300
dl-Camphor	65
Glycol salicylate	50
Thymol	42
Tocopherol acetate	6

Directions: Clean and dry affected area. Remove
Salonpas plaster from the cellophane film and apply
to affected area. Change plaster once or twice a
day. Salonpas plaster is more effective if used
after a hot bath. Keep unused portions in a cool
place.

contains only purified drugs, not the herbal extracts as in Chinese
medicated plasters (Tables 1 and 2).
   Medicated plaster has also existed in Western medicine for several
decades. In the United States, for instance, three medicated plasters
have been documented in the official compendia as early as almost 40
years ago (14,15):

1. *Belladonna plaster*, which contains belladonna root extract
    (0.275%) and has been listed in the National Formulary (NF VIII,
    1946) as a local analgesic.
2. *Mustard plaster*, which contains black mustard powder and is
    capable of delivering allyl isothiocyanate after moistening with
    warm water. It has been listed in NF IX (1950) as an effective
    local irritant.
3. *Salicylic acid plaster*, which contains salicylic acid (10–40%) and
    has been listed in the U.S. Pharmacopoeia (USP XIV, 1950) as
    a keratolytic agent.

   It is interesting to note that these Western-type medicated plasters are rather simple in formulation and all contain a single active
ingredient, in great contrast to the Oriental-type medicated plasters

(Tables 1–3). However, like the Oriental plasters, the Western medicated plasters have been developed mainly for achieving a local therapeutic effect.

IV. RECENT DEVELOPMENTS IN TRANSDERMAL DRUG DELIVERY

The potential of using the intact skin as the port for continuous transdermal drug delivery beyond the boundary of topical medication has been recently recognized. The development of female syndromes in male operators working in the manufacturing areas of pharmaceutical dosage forms containing estrogenic steroids has challenged the old theory in biomedical sciences that skin is basically an impermeable barrier and also has triggered the research curiosity of biomedical scientists to investigate the feasibility of using the intact skin for transdermal delivery of systemically active drugs. The findings accumulated over the years have revolutionized the traditional belief in the impermeable skin barrier and also have motivated a number of pharmaceutical scientists to develop patch-type drug delivery systems for transdermal controlled administration of drugs for systemic medication (1,2,16).

Intensive R & D efforts over more than a decade have succeeded in the development and commercialization of several rate-controlled transdermal drug delivery systems (Fig. 9). They can be classified, according to the technological basis of their approach, into the following categories:

1. *Membrane permeation-controlled transdermal therapeutic systems*
   Transderm-Scop—delivers scopolamine for the prophylaxis of
      motion sickness
   Transderm-Nitro—delivers nitroglycerin for the medication of
      angina pectoris
   Clonidine–TTS—delivers clonidine for the treatment of hypertension
   Estraderm—delivers estradiol for the relief of postmenopausal
      syndromes
2. *Adhesive dispersion-type transdermal therapeutic systems*
   Deponit—delivers nitroglycerin for the treatment of angina
      pectoris
   Frandol—delivers isosorbide dinitrate for the medication of angina
      pectoris
3. *Matrix diffusion-controlled transdermal therapeutic systems*
   Nitro-Dur—delivers nitroglycerin for the medication of angina
      pectoris
   NTS—delivers nitroglycerin for the treatment of angina
      pectoris

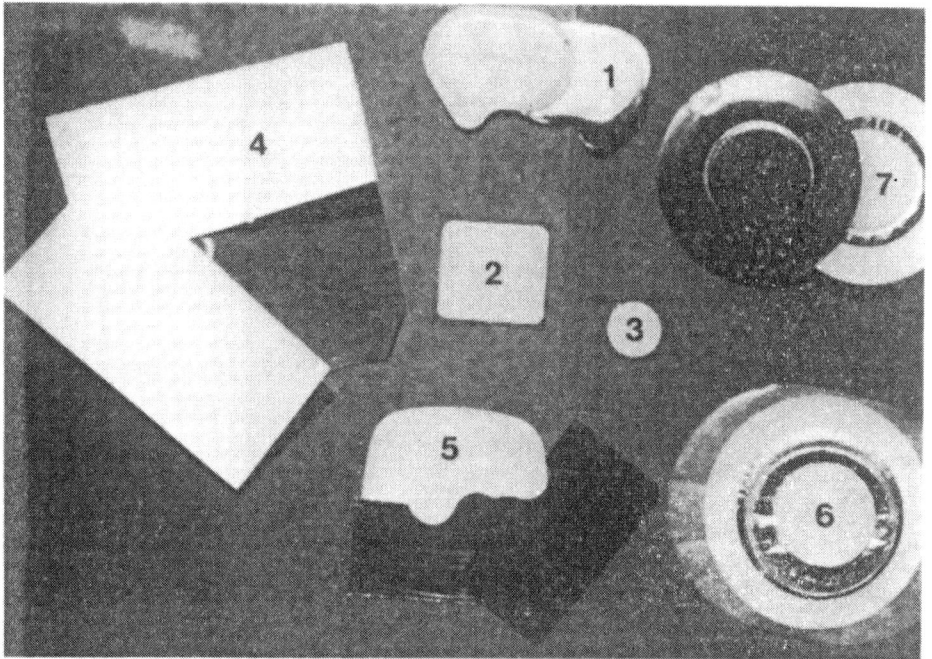

Figure 9   Examples of newly developed transdermal therapeutic systems. Membrane permeation-controlled transdermal therapeutic systems: (1), Transderm-Nitro; (2), Clonidine-TTS; (3), Transderm-Scop. Adhesive dispersion-type transdermal therapeutic systems: (4), Frandol tape; (5), Deponit system. Matrix diffusion-controlled transdermal therapeutic system: (6), Nitro-Dur. Microreservoir dissolution-controlled transdermal therapeutic system: (7), Nitrodisc.

4. *Microreservoir dissolution-controlled transdermal therapeutic system*
Nitrodisc—delivers nitroglycerin for the therapy of angina pectoris

So far, seven transdermal therapeutic systems have been launched on the worldwide prescription drug market: Transderm-Scop, Transderm-Nitro, and Clonidine-TTS (Fig. 10), Nitro-Dur (Fig. 11), and Nitrodisc (Fig. 12) in the United States, Deponit (Fig. 13) in Europe, and Frandol tape (Fig. 9) in Japan. The sciences and engineering involved in their development will be discussed in detail in Chapter 2.

The structural components of the newly developed transdermal patches and the old-fashioned medicated plasters are compared side by side in Table 4.

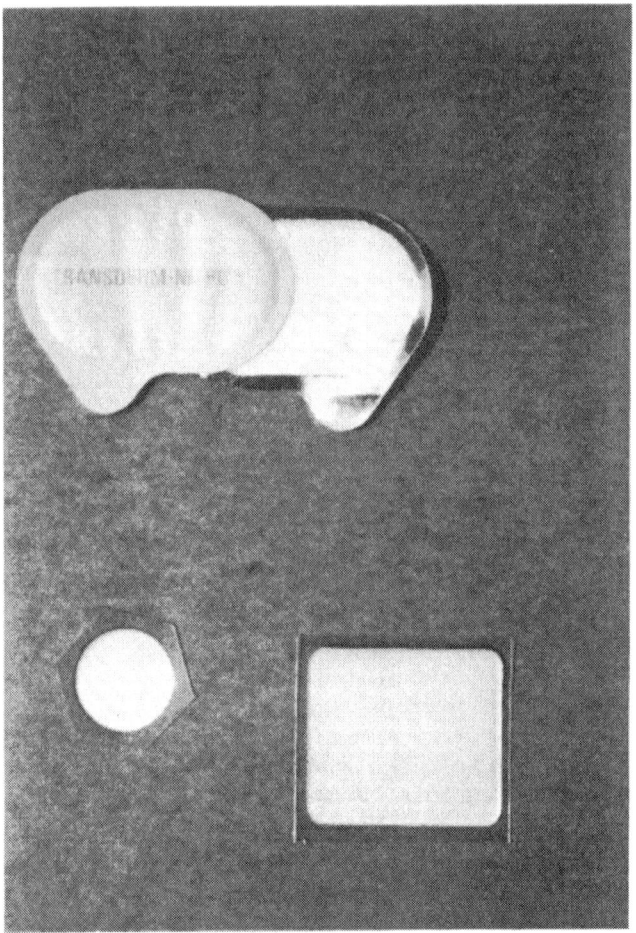

Figure 10   Three transdermal therapeutic devices developed from the membrane permeation-controlled drug delivery system. *Top*: Transderm-Nitro system (developed by Alza Corporation, Palo Alto, CA, and marketed by Ciba-Geigy Corporation, Summit, NJ). *Bottom, left*: Transderm-Scop system (developed by Alza Corporation and marketed by Ciba-Geigy Corporation). *Bottom, right*: Catapres-TTS system (developed by Alza Corporation and marketed by Boehringer Ingelheim Ltd., Ridgefield, CT).

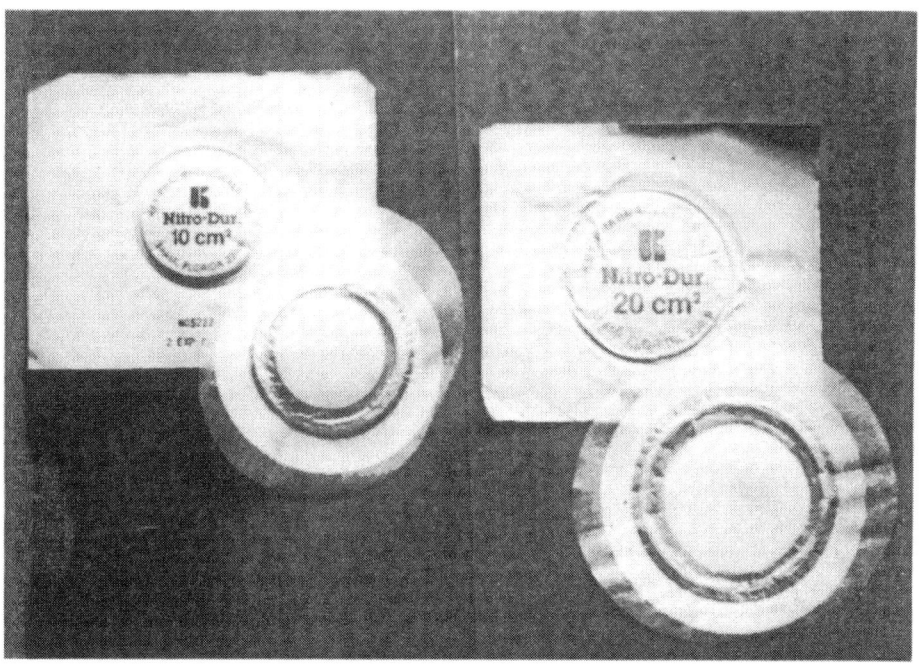

Figure 11   Two sizes of the Nitro-Dur system (developed by
A. Keith of Pennsylvania State University and marketed by Key
Pharmaceuticals, Inc., Miami, FL).

Transdermal rate-controlled drug delivery offers the following
potential advantages:

1. Avoidance of the risks and inconveniences of intravenous therapy,
   and of the varied conditions of absorption and metabolism associated with oral therapy
2. Continuity of drug administration, permitting the use of a drug
   with short biological half-life
3. Achievement of efficacy with lower total daily dosage of drug by
   continuous drug input and by bypassing hepatic first-pass
   elimination.
4. Less chance of over- or underdosing as the result of prolonged,
   preprogrammed delivery of drug at the required therapeutic
   rate
5. Provision of a simplified therapeutic regimen, leading to better
   patient compliance

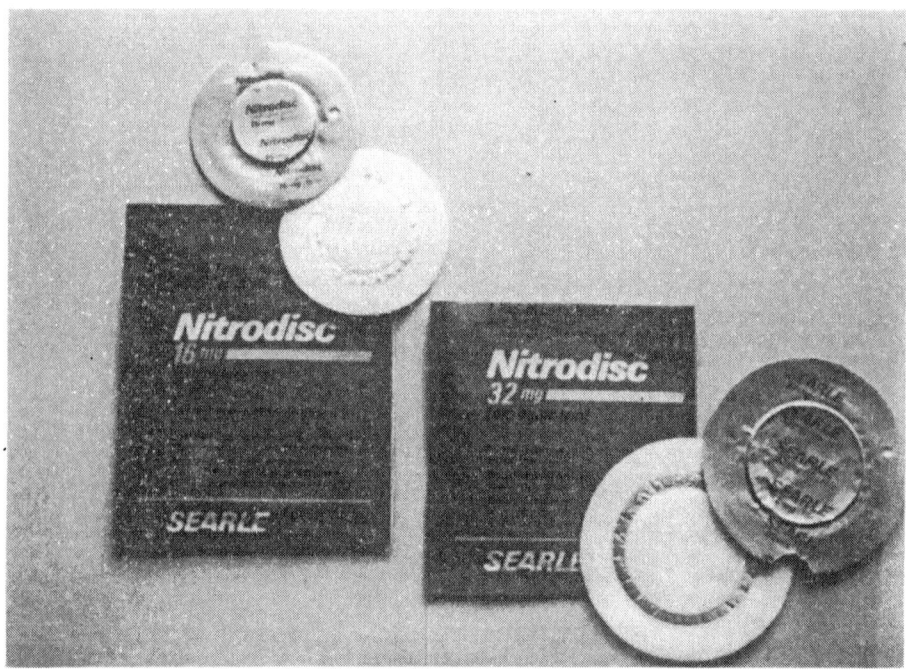

Figure 12 Two sizes of the Nitrodisc system (developed and marketed by Searle Pharmaceuticals, Inc., Chicago).

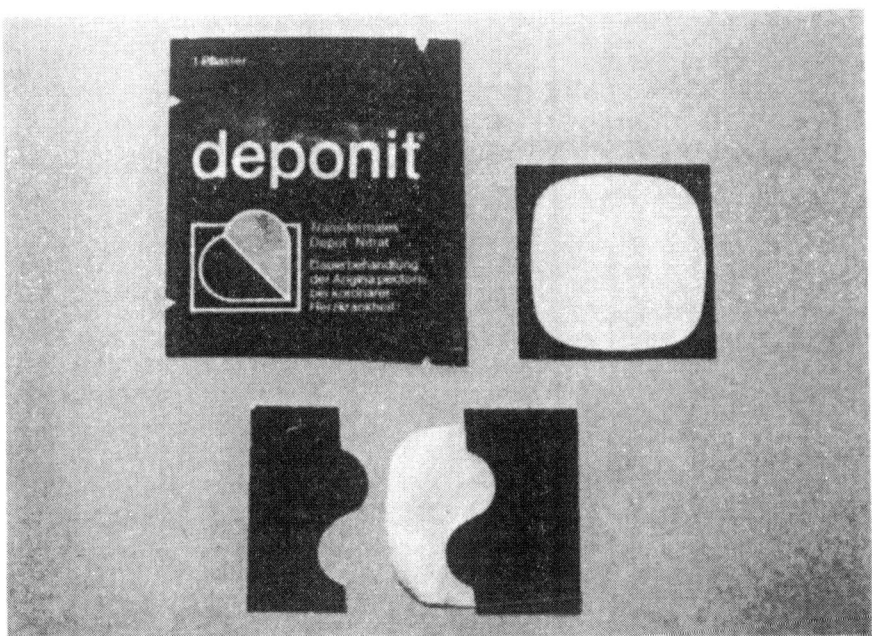

Figure 13   One size of the Deponit system (developed jointly by Pharma-Schwartz and Lohmann and marketed by Pharma-Schwartz GmbH, Monheim, West Germany).

Table 4 Transdermal Patches Versus Medicated Plasters

Structural component	Composition and functionality	
	Medicated plaster	Transdermal patch
Backing support	Nonocclusive (fabric, paper, etc.)	Occlusive (drug-impermeable plastic film, metallic plastic laminate)
Drug reservoir	Dispersion of multiple drugs in adhesive natural gum rubber base	Dispersion of single drug in liquid- or solid-state synthetic polymer base
Drug release mechanism	Matrix diffusion	Membrane permeation, microreservoir dissolution, or matrix diffusion
Adhesive film	No (adhesiveness derived from gum rubber base)	Yes (surface coating with pressure-sensitive adhesive polymer
Release liner	Cellophane, gauze	Occlusive (drug-impermeable plastic film, metallic plastic laminate with releasing surface)

6. Ability to easily terminate the medication as needed by simply removing the drug delivery device from the skin surface

This book consists of 18 chapters, which address five important areas of transdermal drug delivery:

1. Fundamentals of skin permeation (Chapters 2 and 3)
2. Development and manufacturing of transdermal therapeutic systems (Chapters 2 and 4)
3. Preclinical assessments of transdermal-controlled drug administration (Chapters 5-8)
4. Clinical assessments of transdermal pharmacodynamics and pharmacokinetics (Chapters 9-12)
5. Manufacturing of transdermal therapeutic systems (Chapters 13-15)
6. Regulatory requirements among international health authorities (Chapters 16-18)

REFERENCES

1. J. E. Shaw, S. K. Chandrasekaran, and P. Campbell, Percutaneous absorption: Controlled drug delivery for topical or systemic therapy, *J. Invest. Dermatol.*, *67*: 677 (1976).
2. J. E. Shaw and S. K. Chandrasekaran, Controlled topical delivery of drugs for systemic action, *Drug Metab. Rev.*, *8*: 223 (1978).
3. 1982 Industrial Pharmaceutical R & D Symposium on Transdermal Controlled Release Medication, Rutgers College of Pharmacy, Piscataway, NJ, January 14-15, 1982. Proceedings published in *Drug Dev. Ind. Pharm.*, *9* (4): 497-744 (1983).
4. World Congress of Clinical Pharmacology Symposium on Transdermal Delivery of Cardiovascular Drugs, Washington, DC, August 5, 1983. Proceedings published in *Am. Heart J.*, *108* (1): 195-236 (1984).
5. S. W. Jacob and C. A. Francone, *Structure and Function of Man*, 2nd ed., Saunders, Philadelphia, 1970, pp. 55-60.
6. P. Zanowiak and M. R. Jacobs, Topical anti-infective products, in *Handbook of Nonprescription Drugs*, 7th ed. (S. C. Laitin, ed.), American Pharmaceutical Association, Washington, DC, 1982, pp. 525-529.
7. Y. W. Chien, Logic of transdermal controlled drug administration, *Drug Dev. & Ind. Pharm.*, *9*: 497 (1983).
8. E. K. Kastrup and J. R. Boyd, *Drug: Facts and Comparisons*, 1983 ed., Lippincott, Philadelphia, 1983, pp. 1634-1708.
9. J. E. Shaw, W. Bayne, and L. Schmidt, Clinical pharmacology of scopolamine, *Clin. Pharmacol. Ther.*, *19*: 115 (1976).

10. P. W. Armstrong, J. A. Armstrong, and G. S. Marks, Pharmacokinetic-hemodynamic studies of nitroglycerin ointment in congestive heart failure, *Am. J. Cardiol.*, *46*: 670 (1980).

11. R. Sitruk-Ware, B. deLignieres, A. Basdevant, and P. Mauvais-Jarvis, Absorption of percutaneous oestradiol in postmenopausal women, *Maturitas*, *2*: 207 (1980).

12. A. Osol, *Remington's Pharmaceutical Sciences*, 16th ed., Mack, Easton, PA, 1980, pp. 1534.

13. First Transdermal Therapeutic System Symposium on Evaluation of External Adhesive Systems, Tokyo, Japan, July 26, 1985.

14. National Formulary (NF), 8th ed., 1946.

15. United States Pharmacopeia (USP), 14th ed., 1950.

16. A. S. Michaels, S. K. Chandrasekaran, and J. E. Shaw, *AIChE J.*, *21*: 985 (1975).

DEVELOPMENT AND PRECLINICAL ASSESSMENTS OF TRANSDERMAL THERAPEUTIC SYSTEMS

2

Developmental Concepts and Practice in Transdermal Therapeutic Systems

YIE W. CHIEN / Rutgers—The State University of New Jersey, Piscataway, New Jersey

I. INTRODUCTION

As discussed in Chapter 1, the potential of using the intact skin as the port of administration of systemically active drugs has been increasingly recognized, and several transdermal therapeutic systems have successfully been developed and recently commercialized to accomplish the goals of systemic medication. Typical examples of these transdermal therapeutic systems are scopolamine-releasing transdermal patches (Transderm-Scop system by Ciba) (1), nitroglycerin-releasing transdermal patches (Deponit system by Pharma-Schwartz/ Lohmann, Nitrodisc system by Searle, Nitro-Dur System by Key, and Transderm-Nitro system by Ciba) (2,3), isosorbide dinitrate-releasing transdermal patches (Frandol tape by Toaeiyo, Yamanouchi), and clonidine-releasing transdermal patches (Catapres-TTS by Boehringer Ingelheim) (3).

The intensity of interest in the potential biomedical applications of rate-controlled transdermal drug administration is also demonstrated by the tremendous increase in research and development activities in many health care institutions, private and public, aiming to develop novel and/or patentable transdermal therapeutic systems for the prolonged, continuous administration of systemically effective drugs (2-8). The candidates evaluated range from antihypertensive, antianginal, antihistamine, anti-inflammatory, and analgesic agents to antiarthritic, steroidal, and contraceptive drugs.

Using the transdermal patches recently marketed as the practical examples, this chapter analyzes the science and engineering underlying the successful development of various rate-controlled transdermal drug delivery systems. It aims to uncover the developmental concepts and to demonstrate how the fundamentals of transdermal controlled drug administration can be put into practical use in the development of rate-controlled transdermal therapeutic systems.

The primary structural components of various viable transdermal therapeutic systems will be outlined and the scientific rationales behind their uses will be discussed. The formulation design and optimization of transdermal drug delivery systems will be exemplified.

The relationship between rate-controlled drug release from a transdermal therapeutic system and the uptake, binding, and metabolism of drug by the cutaneous enzymes during the course of skin permeation will be illustrated and established. Enhancement of the transdermal permeation rate of the less-skin-permeable drugs by applying the prodrug approach in combination with the cutaneous bioconversion concept will also be explored and illustrated.

In addition, the chapter will discuss the feasibility of developing a new generation of transdermal therapeutic systems, capable of releasing one or more skin permeation enhancers prior to or simultaneously with the delivery of drugs. Development of such a system, which aims to modify the skin permeability and to enhance the transdermal bioavailability of drugs, will expand the spectrum of transdermal controlled drug administration to cover more classes of drugs.

On the basis of years of R & D experience, a generic program for the development and practice of transdermal patches is developed to include all the critical development activities in a logical sequence.

II. FUNDAMENTALS OF RATE-CONTROLLED TRANSDERMAL DRUG DELIVERY

A systemically active drug that will reach a target tissue far from the site of drug administration on the skin surface must possess some physicochemical properties that are capable of facilitating the sorption of drug by the stratum corneum, the penetration of drug through viable epidermis, and also the uptake of the drug by the capillary network in the dermal papillary layer (Fig. 1). The rate of permeation, dQ/dt, across the skin tissues can be expressed mathematically by the following relationship (9):

$$\frac{dQ}{dt} = P_s \, (C_d - C_r) \tag{1}$$

where C_d and C_r are, respectively, the concentrations of a skin penetrant in the donor compartment (e.g., the drug concentration on

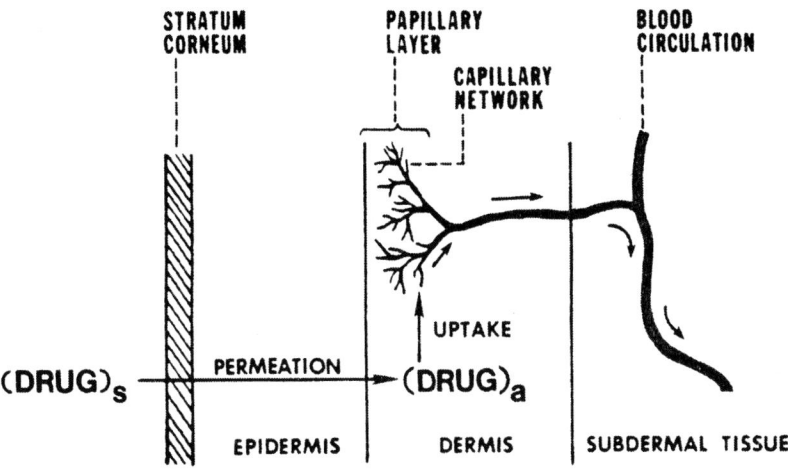

Figure 1   A multilayer skin model showing the sequence of transdermal permeation of drug: sorption by stratum corneum, permeation
across viable epidermis, and uptake by the capillary network in the
dermal papillary layer for systemic distribution.

the surface of stratum corneum) and in the receptor compartment
(e.g., body), and P_s is the overall permeability coefficient of the
skin tissues to the penetrant as defined by:

$$P_s = \frac{K_s D_{ss}}{h_s} \qquad (2)$$

where K_s is the partition coefficient for the interfacial partitioning
of the penetrant molecule from a solution medium or a transdermal
therapeutic system onto the stratum corneum, D_{ss} is the apparent
diffusivity for the steady-state diffusion of the penetrant molecule
through a thickness of skin tissues, and h_s is the overall thickness
of the skin tissues.   The permeability coefficient (P_s) for a skin
penetrant can be considered as a constant, since K_s, D_{ss}, and h_s
in Eq. (2) are essentially constant under given conditions.
    Analysis of Eq. (1) suggests that to achieve a constant rate of
drug permeation, one needs to maintain the drug concentration on
the surface of stratum corneum (C_d) consistently and substantially
greater than the drug concentration in the body (C_r), i.e., $C_d \gg$
C_r; under such a condition, Eq. (1) can be reduced to:

$$\frac{dQ}{dt} = P_s C_d \tag{3}$$

and the rate of skin permeation (dQ/dt) becomes a constant, if the magnitude of C_d remains fairly constant throughout the course of skin permeation. To maintain C_d at a constant value, it is necessary to make the drug release at a rate (R_r) that is either constant or always greater than the rate of skin uptake (R_a), i.e., $R_r \gg R_a$ (Fig. 2). By making R_r greater than R_a, the drug concentration on the skin surface (C_d) is maintained at a level equal to or greater than the equilibrium (or saturation) solubility of the drug in the stratum corneum (C_s^e), i.e., $C_d \geq C_s^e$; and a maximum rate of skin permeation $(dQ/dt)_m$, as expressed by Eq. (4), is thus achieved:

$$\left(\frac{dQ}{dt}\right)_m = P_s C_s^e \tag{4}$$

Apparently, the magnitude of $(dQ/dt)_m$ is determined by the skin permeability coefficient (P_s) of the drug and its equilibrium solubility in the stratum corneum (C_s^e). This concept of stratum-corneum-limited skin permeation was investigated by depositing various doses of pure, radiolabeled nitroglycerin, in a volatile organic solvent, onto a controlled skin surface area of rhesus monkeys (10). Analysis

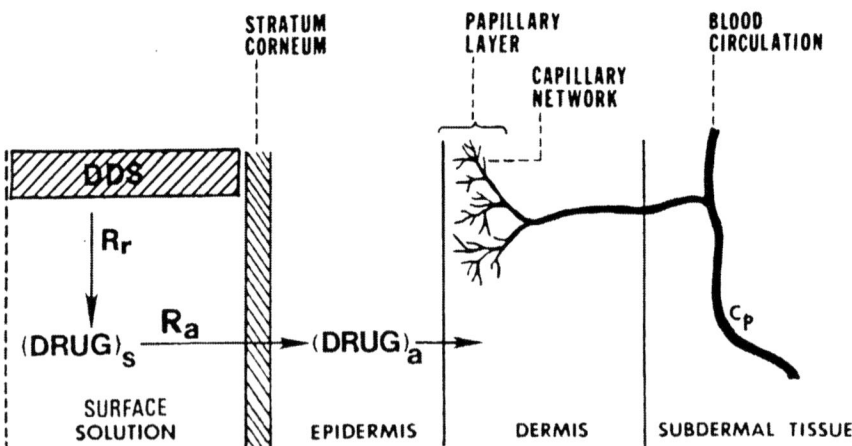

Figure 2   Schematic illustration of the relationship between the rate of drug release (R_r) from a transdermal drug delivery system (DDS) and the rate of drug absorption (R_a) by the skin.

of the urinary recovery data indicated that the rate of skin permeation (dQ/dt) increases with the increase in nitroglycerin dose (C_d) applied on a unity surface area of the skin (Fig. 3). It appears that a maximum rate of skin permeation (1.585 mg/cm^2/day) is achieved when the applied dose of nitroglycerin reaches the level of 4.786 mg/cm^2 or greater.

The kinetics of skin permeation can be more precisely analyzed by studying the time course for the permeation of drug across freshly excised skin mounted on a diffusion cell, such as the Franz diffusion cell (Fig. 4). A typical skin permeation kinetic profile is shown in Figure 5 for nitroglycerin. Results indicated that nitroglycerin penetrates through the freshly excised abdominal skin of

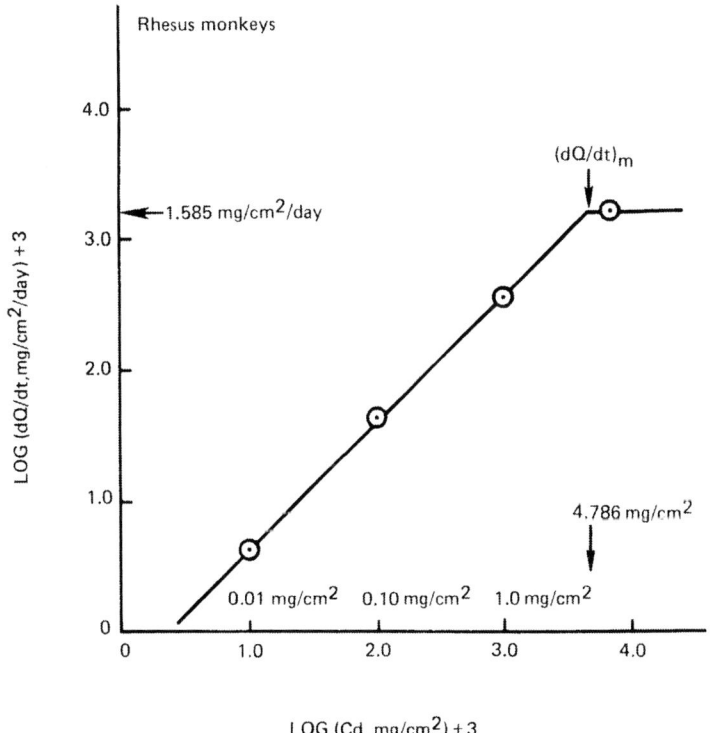

Figure 3 Linear relationship between the transdermal permeation rate of nitroglycerin (dQ/dt), determined from daily urinary recovery data, and the nitroglycerin dose applied to the rhesus monkey skin (C_d). (Plotted from data in Ref. 10.)

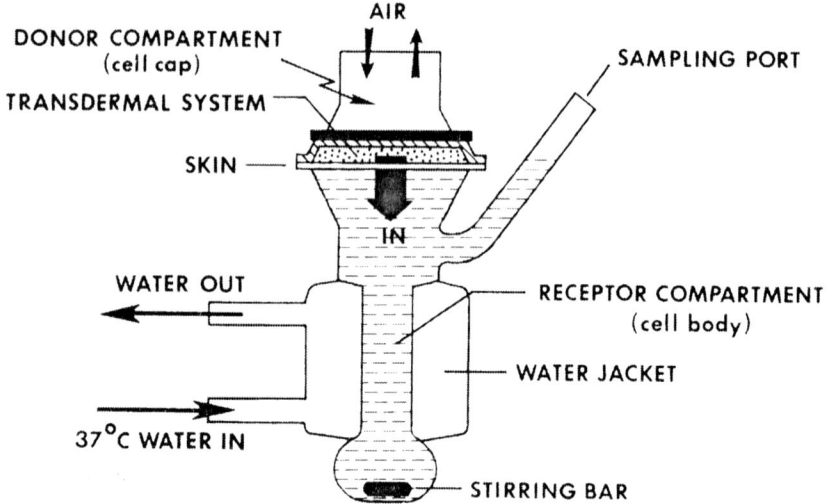

Figure 4   Diagrammatic illustration of the in vitro skin permeation system; this unit of the commercially available eight-cell Franz diffusion apparatus is shown with transdermal therapeutic system in intimate contact with the stratum corneum surface. (From Ref. 31.)

hairless mouse at a zero-order rate of 19.85 (±1.71) $\mu g/cm^2/hr$, as expected from Eq. (4), when pure nitroglycerin (oily liquid form) is directly deposited on the surface of the stratum corneum (in this case the skin permeation of drug is under *no* influence from an organic solvent or a drug delivery system) (11). Using a well-calibrated horizontal skin permeation cell, the same observations were also made in a series of long-term skin permeation kinetic studies for estradiol (12), which provides a critical analysis of the relationships among skin permeation rate, permeability coefficient, partition coefficient, diffusivity, and solubility. The effects of skin uptake, binding, and metabolism kinetics on skin permeation profiles were also evaluated and demonstrated (13).

To gain a fundamental understanding of skin permeation kinetics and to assist in the formulation and development of transdermal therapeutic systems, in vitro studies using a freshly excised skin sample mounted in a well-calibrated skin permeation cell are essential before any in vivo evaluations can be conducted in human volunteers. For detailed discussion of the design and calibration of skin permeation cells and in vitro evaluations of transdermal drug delivery, see Chapters 6 and 7.

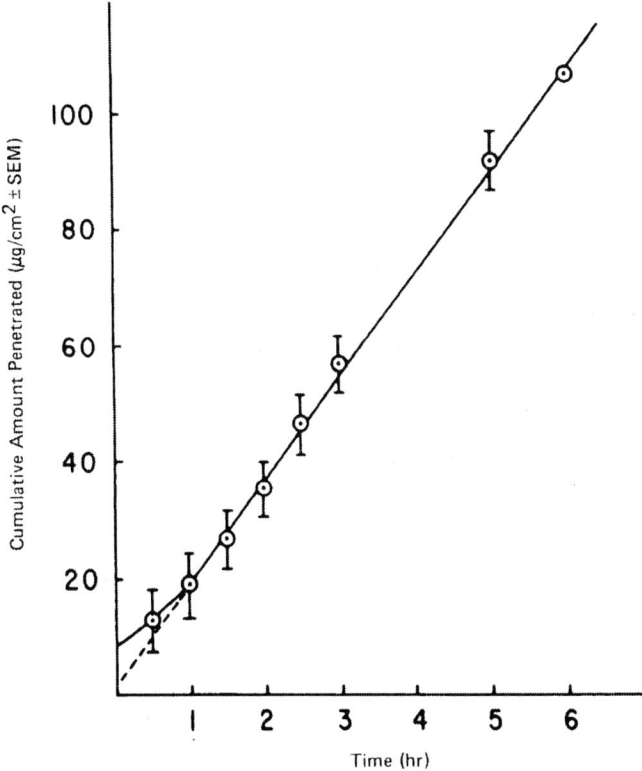

Figure 5   Permeation profile of pure nitroglycerin across the abdominal skin of hairless mouse mounted on the Franz diffusion apparatus at 37°C. A constant skin permeation profile was obtained with a permeation rate of 19.85 (±1.71) $\mu g/cm^2/hr$. (From Ref. 11.)

III. APPROACHES TO THE DEVELOPMENT OF TRANSDERMAL THERAPEUTIC SYSTEMS

Several technologies have been successfully developed to provide a mechanism of rate control over the release and the transdermal permeation of drugs. These technologies can be classified into four approaches, which are outlined as follows.

A. Membrane-Moderated Transdermal Drug Delivery Systems

In membrane-moderated systems, the drug reservoir is totally encapsulated in a shallow compartment molded from a drug-impermeable

metallic plastic laminate and a rate-controlling polymeric membrane
(Fig. 6). The drug molecules can be released only through the rate-
controlling polymeric membrane. In the drug reservoir compartment,
the drug solids are either dispersed homogeneously in a solid polymer matrix (e.g., polyisobutylene adhesive) or suspended in an un-
bleachable, viscous liquid medium (e.g., silicone fluid) to form a
pastelike suspension. The rate-controlling membrane can be either
a microporous or a nonporous polymeric membrane (e.g., ethylene-
vinyl acetate copolymer), with a defined drug permeability. On the
external surface of the polymeric membrane, a thin layer of drug-
compatible, hypoallergenic, pressure-sensitive adhesive polymer
(e.g., silicone or polyisobutylene adhesive) may be applied to provide intimate contact of the transdermal therapeutic system with the
skin surface.

The rate of drug release from this type of transdermal drug
delivery system can be tailored by varying the polymer composition,
the permeability coefficient, and/or the thickness of the rate-
controlling membrane and adhesive. Several transdermal therapeutic
systems have been successfully developed from this technology and
are best exemplified by the development and marketing of a nitroglycerin-releasing transdermal therapeutic system (Transderm-Nitro
by Ciba), which has been approved by the U.S. Food and Drug Administration (FDA) for once-a-day medication of angina pectoris
(14,15), a scopolamine-releasing transdermal therapeutic system
(Transderm-Scop by Ciba) for 3-day protection from motion sickness
(1), and a clonidine-releasing transdermal therapeutic system

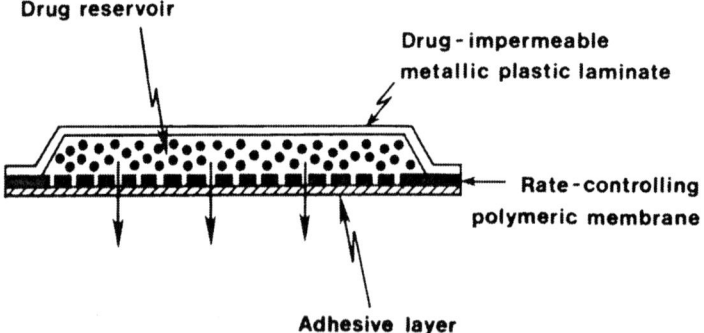

Figure 6 Cross-sectional view of a membrane-moderated transdermal
drug delivery system, showing major structural components. (From
Ref. 50.)

(Catapres-TTS by Boehringer Ingelheim) for weekly treatment of hypertension (16–18). The intrinsic rate of drug release from this type of drug delivery system is defined by:

$$\frac{dQ}{dt} = \frac{C_R}{1/P_m + 1/P_a} \tag{5}$$

where C_R is the drug concentration in the reservoir compartment, and P_a and P_m are the permeability coefficients of the adhesive layer and the rate-controlling membrane, respectively. For a microporous membrane, P_m is essentially the sum of permeability coefficients for simultaneous permeation across the pores and the polymeric material (19). The coefficients P_m and P_a are defined as follows:

$$P_m = \frac{K_{m/r} \cdot D_m}{h_m} \tag{6}$$

$$P_a = \frac{K_{a/m} \cdot D_a}{h_a} \tag{7}$$

where $K_{m/r}$ and $K_{a/m}$ are, respectively, the partition coefficients for the interfacial partitioning of drug from the reservoir to the membrane and from the membrane to the adhesive; D_m and D_a are the respective diffusion coefficients in the rate-controlling membrane and in the adhesive layer; and h_m and h_a are the thicknesses of the rate-controlling membrane and adhesive layer, respectively. In the case of microporous membrane, the porosity and tortuosity of the membrane should also be taken into consideration in the calculation of the D_m and h_m values.

Substituting the coefficients symbolized in Eqs. (6) and (7) for P_m and P_a in Eq. (5) gives:

$$\frac{dQ}{dt} = \frac{K_{m/r} K_{a/m} \cdot D_a \cdot D_m}{K_{m/r} D_m h_a + K_{a/m} D_a h_m} C_R \tag{8}$$

which defines the intrinsic rate of drug release from a membrane-moderated transdermal drug delivery system.

The membrane-permeation-controlled transdermal drug delivery technology has also been applied to the development of transdermal therapeutic systems for the rate-controlled percutaneous absorption of estradiol (20,21) and prostaglandin derivative (22).

The generalized scheme of manufacturing process and equipment for the production of Transderm-Nitro systems is outlined in Figure 7. A detailed discussion of the manufacturing and engineering aspects can be found in Chapter 13.

B. Adhesive Dispersion-Type Transdermal Drug Delivery Systems

In a simplified version of the membrane-moderated drug delivery system discussed above, instead of completely encapsulating the drug reservoir in a compartment fabricated from a drug-impermeable metallic plastic backing, the drug reservoir is formulated by directly dispersing the drug in an adhesive polymer (e.g., polyisobutylene or polyacrylate). Then the medicated adhesive is spread, by solvent casting or hot melt, onto a flat sheet of drug-impermeable backing support to form one or more layers of drug reservoir (Fig. 8). On the top of the drug reservoir layer, thin layers of nonmedicated, rate-controlling adhesive polymer of a specific permeability may be applied to produce a transdermal drug delivery system. The rate of drug release is defined by:

$$\frac{dQ}{dt} = \left(\frac{K_{a/r} \cdot D_a}{h_a} \right) C_R \tag{9}$$

where $K_{a/r}$ is the partition coefficient for the interfacial partitioning of drug from the reservoir layer to the rate-controlling adhesive layer.

This type of transdermal drug delivery system is best illustrated by the development and marketing of an isosorbide dinitrate-releasing transdermal therapeutic system (Frandol tape by Toaeiyo, Yamanouchi) in Japan, for once-a-day medication of angina pectoris.

The generalized scheme of the manufacturing process and the equipment for the fabrication of the multilaminate adhesive dispersion-type transdermal therapeutic system is outlined in Figure 9.

Alternatively, this type of transdermal therapeutic system can be modified to have the drug loading level varied at increments to form a gradient of drug reservoir along the multilaminate adhesive layers (Fig. 10). The rate of drug release from this drug reservoir gradient-controlled transdermal drug delivery system is defined by:

$$\frac{dQ}{dt} = \left(\frac{K_{a/r} D_a}{h_a(t)} \right) A (h_a) \tag{10}$$

In Eq. (10), the thickness of the adhesive layer for drug molecules to diffuse through increases with time $[h_a(t)]$. To compensate

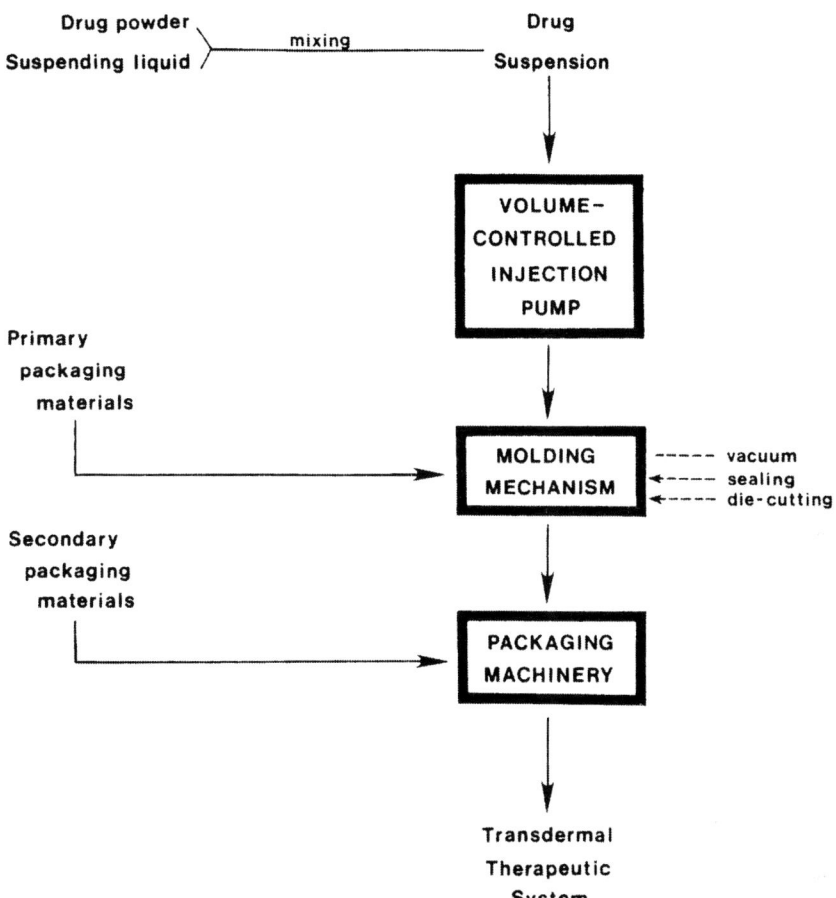

Figure 7   Schematic illustration of the process and equipment involved in the manufacture of the Transderm-Nitro system, a membrane-moderated transdermal therapeutic system.

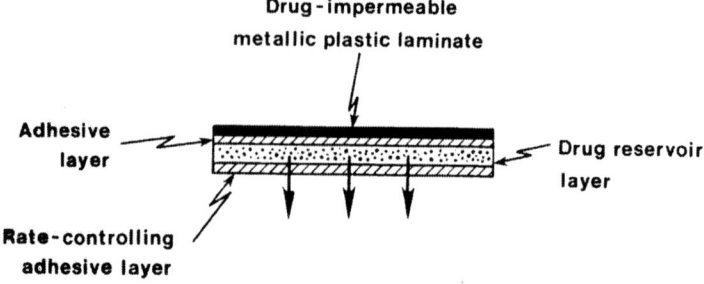

Drug-impermeable
metallic plastic laminate

Adhesive
layer

Drug reservoir
layer

Rate-controlling
adhesive layer

Figure 8   Cross-sectional view of an adhesive dispersion-type transdermal drug delivery system, showing major structural components.

for this time-dependent increase in diffusional path due to the depletion of drug dose by release, the drug loading level is also increased with the thickness of diffusional path [A (h_a)]. A constant drug release profile thus results. This type of transdermal drug delivery system is best illustrated by the development and marketing of a nitroglycerin-releasing transdermal therapeutic system (Deponit by PharmaSchwartz/Lohmann) in Europe. The New Drug Application (NDA) has recently been approved by the FDA for marketing approval in the United States.

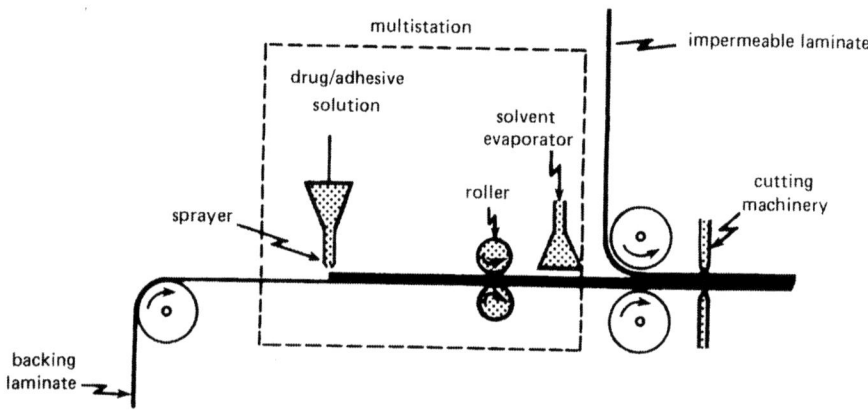

multistation

impermeable laminate

drug/adhesive
solution

solvent
evaporator

roller

cutting
machinery

sprayer

backing
laminate

Figure 9   Schematic illustration of the process and equipment involved in the manufacture of an adhesive dispersion-type transdermal therapeutic system.

Drug—impermeable

Metallic plastic laminate

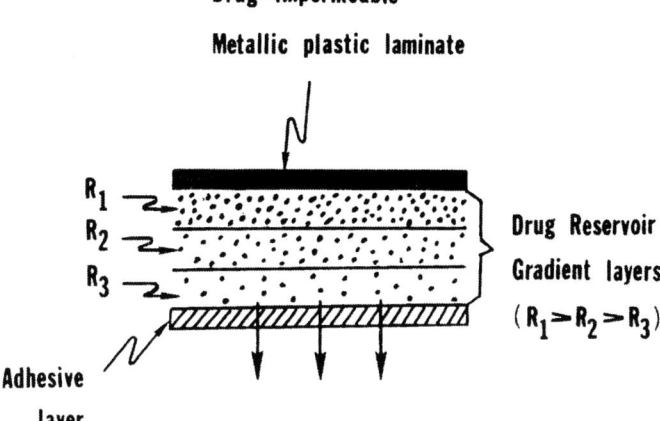

Figure 10   Cross-sectional view of a drug reservoir gradient-controlled transdermal drug delivery system, showing major structural components.

The science and technology involved in the biomedical application of pressure-sensitive adhesive polymers are discussed in great length in Chapter 4.

C. Matrix Diffusion-Controlled Transdermal Drug Delivery Systems

In the third approach, the drug reservoir is formed by homogeneously dispersing the drug solids in a hydrophilic or lipophilic polymer matrix; the medicated polymer is then molded into a medicated disc with a defined surface area and controlled thickness. This drug-reservoir-containing polymer disc is mounted onto an occlusive baseplate in a compartment fabricated from a drug-impermeable plastic backing (Fig. 11). Instead of applying the adhesive polymer directly on the surface of the medicated disc as discussed earlier in the first two types of transdermal drug delivery system, the polymer is spread along the circumference of the patch to form an adhesive rim around the medicated disc. The rate of drug release from this matrix diffusion-controlled transdermal drug delivery system is defined as follows:

$$\frac{dQ}{dt} = \left(\frac{ACpDp}{2t}\right)^{1/2} \tag{11}$$

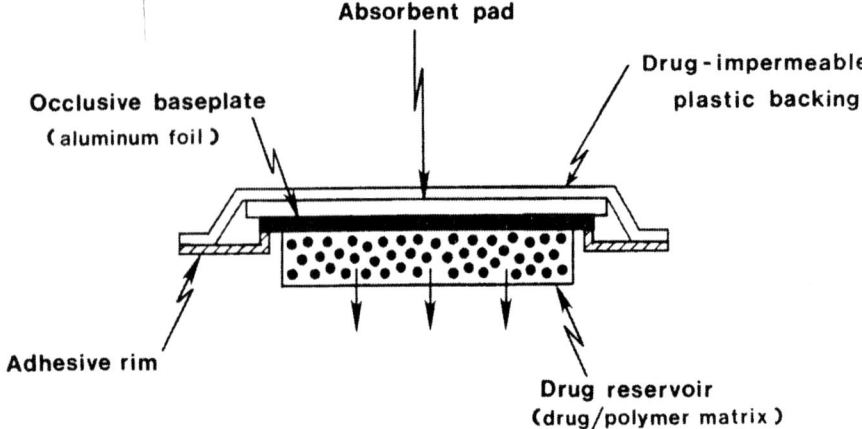

Absorbent pad

Occlusive baseplate
(aluminum foil)

Drug-impermeable plastic backing

Adhesive rim

Drug reservoir
(drug/polymer matrix)

Figure 11   Cross-sectional view of a matrix-diffusion-controlled transdermal drug delivery system, showing major structural components. (From Ref. 50.)

where A is the initial drug loading dose dispersed in the polymer matrix, and Cp and Dp are the solubility and diffusivity of the drug in the polymer, respectively. Since only the drug species dissolved in the polymer can release, Cp is essentially equal to C_R.

At steady state, a Q versus $\sqrt{t}$ drug release profile is obtained (23) as defined by:

$$\frac{Q}{\sqrt{t}} = [(2A - Cp)CpDp]^{1/2} \tag{12}$$

This type of transdermal drug delivery system is exemplified by the development and marketing of nitroglycerin-releasing transdermal therapeutic system (Nitro-Dur by Key), which has been approved by the FDA for once-a-day medication of angina pectoris (24). Patent application has also been filed for applying this drug delivery system in the transdermal controlled administration of estradiol diacetate and verapamil.

The generalized scheme of manufacturing process and equipment for the production of Nitro-Dur systems is outlined in Figure 12. For more detailed discussion, see Chapter 10.

D. Microreservoir Dissolution-Controlled Transdermal Drug Delivery Systems

The microreservoir-type drug delivery system can be considered a hybrid of the reservoir and matrix dispersion-type drug delivery systems. In this approach, the drug reservoir is formed by first suspending the drug solids in the aqueous solution of a water-soluble polymer (e.g., polyethylene glycol) and then dispersing the drug suspension homogeneously in a lipophilic polymer, by high-shear mechanical force, to form thousands of unleachable, microscopic spheres of drug reservoirs (Fig. 13). This thrrmodynamically unstable dispersion is quickly stabilized by immediately cross-linking the polymer chains in situ, which produces a medicated polymer disc with a constant surface area and a fixed thickness. A transdermal therapeutic system is then produced by positioning the medicated disc at the center of an adhesive pad (Fig. 14). This technology has been successfully utilized in the development and marketing of a nitroglycerin-releasing transdermal therapeutic system (Nitrodisc by Searle) that has been approved by the FDA for once-a-day treatment of angina pectoris (10,25-29).

Figure 15 outlines a generalized scheme of the manufacturing process and equipment for the production of Nitrodisc systems. For detailed discussion, see Chapter 13.

The rate of drug release from the microreservoir dissolution-controlled drug delivery system is defined (23,29) by:

$$\frac{dQ}{dt} = \frac{D_p D_s \alpha'K_p}{D_p \delta_d + D_s \delta_p \alpha'K_p} \left[\beta S_p - \frac{D_1 S_1 (1 - \beta)}{\delta_1} \left(\frac{1}{K_1} + \frac{1}{K_m} \right) \right] \quad (13)$$

where $\alpha' = \delta'/\beta'$; δ' is the ratio of drug concentration in the bulk of the elution solution to drug solubility in the same medium, and β' is the ratio of drug concentration at the outer edge of the polymer coating membrane to drug solubility in the same polymer composition; K_1, K_m, and K_p are the partition coefficients for the interfacial partitioning of drug from the liquid compartment to the polymer matrix, from the polymer matrix to the polymer coating membrane, and from the polymer coating membrane to the elution solution (or skin), respectively; D_1, D_p, and D_s are the drug diffusivities in the liquid compartment, polymer coating membrane, and elution solution (or skin), respectively; S_1 and S_p are the solubilities of the drug in the liquid compartment and in the polymer matrix, respectively; δ_1, δ_p, and δ_d are the thicknesses of the liquid layer surrounding the drug particles, the polymer coating membrane around the polymer matrix, and the hydrodynamic diffusion layer surrounding the polymer coating membrane, respectively; β is the ratio of

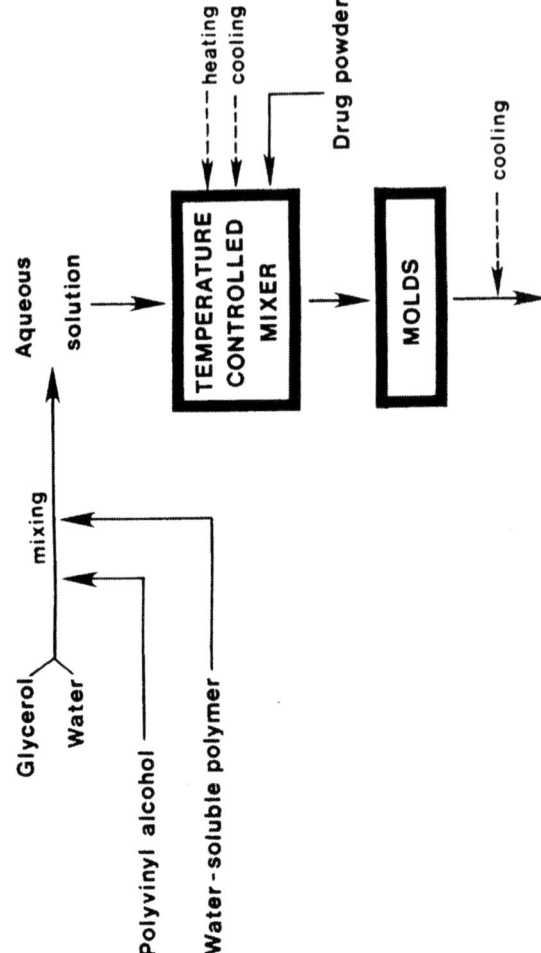

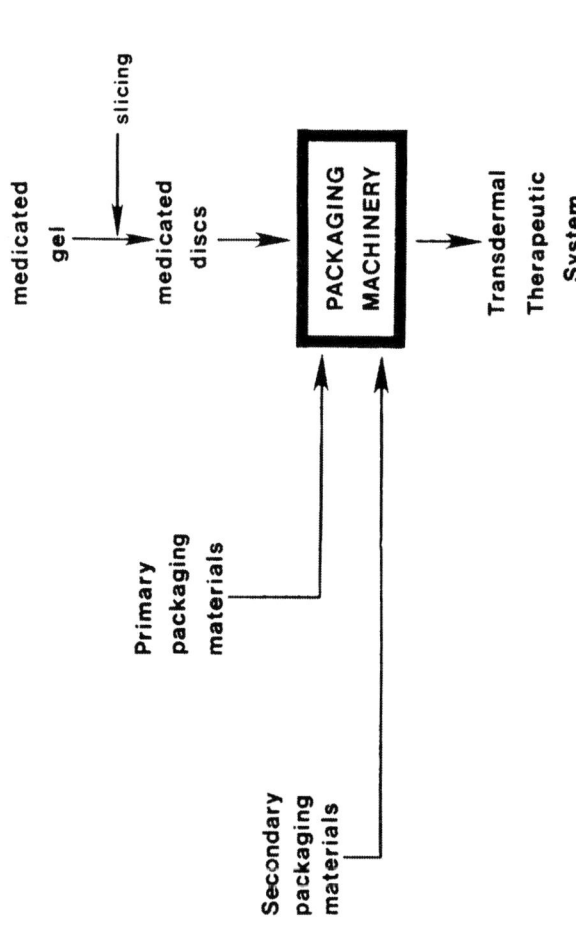

Figure 12   Schematic illustration of the process and equipment involved in the manufacturing of the Nitro-Dur system, a matrix-diffusion-controlled type transdermal therapeutic system.

polymer matrix
(cross-linked, solid)
drug reservoir
(microscopic liquid
compartments)
polymer/solution
interface

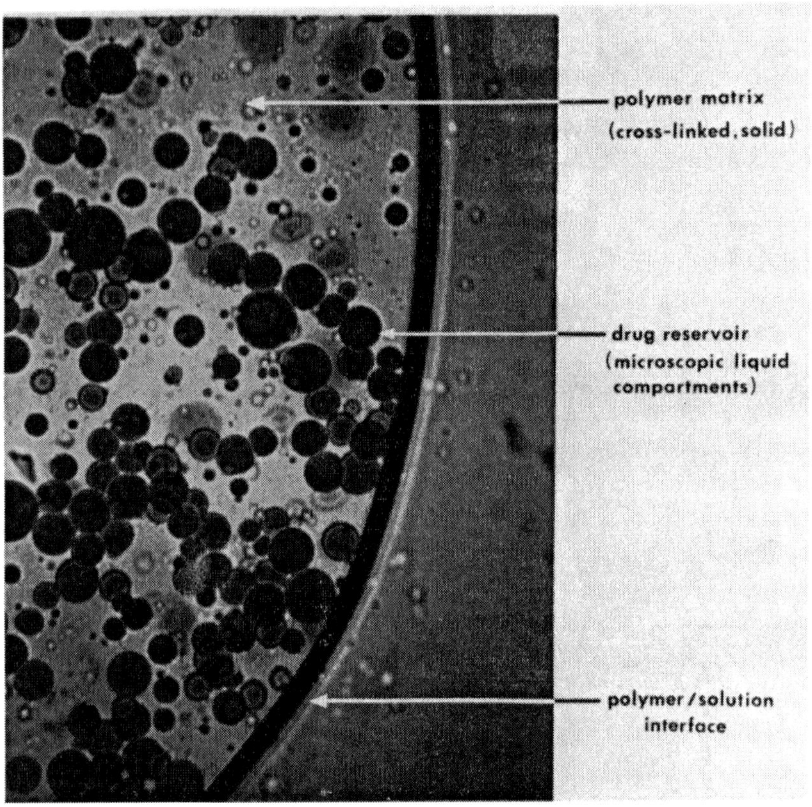

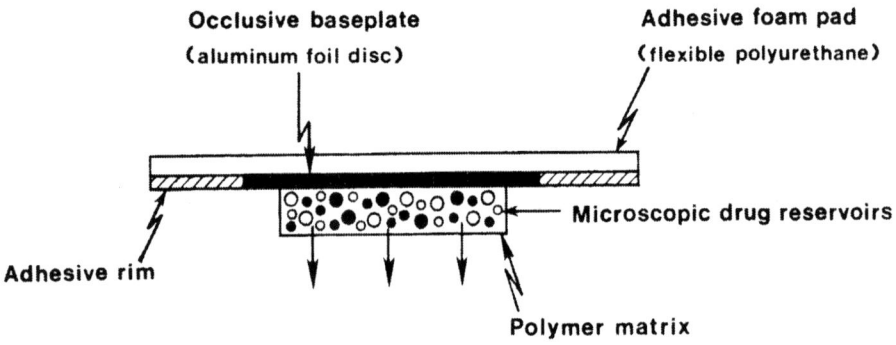

Figure 13 Photomicrograph of a microreservoir dissolution-controlled drug delivery system, showing its microscopic structure.

Occlusive baseplate
(aluminum foil disc)
Adhesive foam pad
(flexible polyurethane)
Microscopic drug reservoirs
Adhesive rim
Polymer matrix

Figure 14 Cross-sectional view of a microreservoir dissolution-controlled transdermal drug delivery system, showing major structural components. (From Ref. 50.)

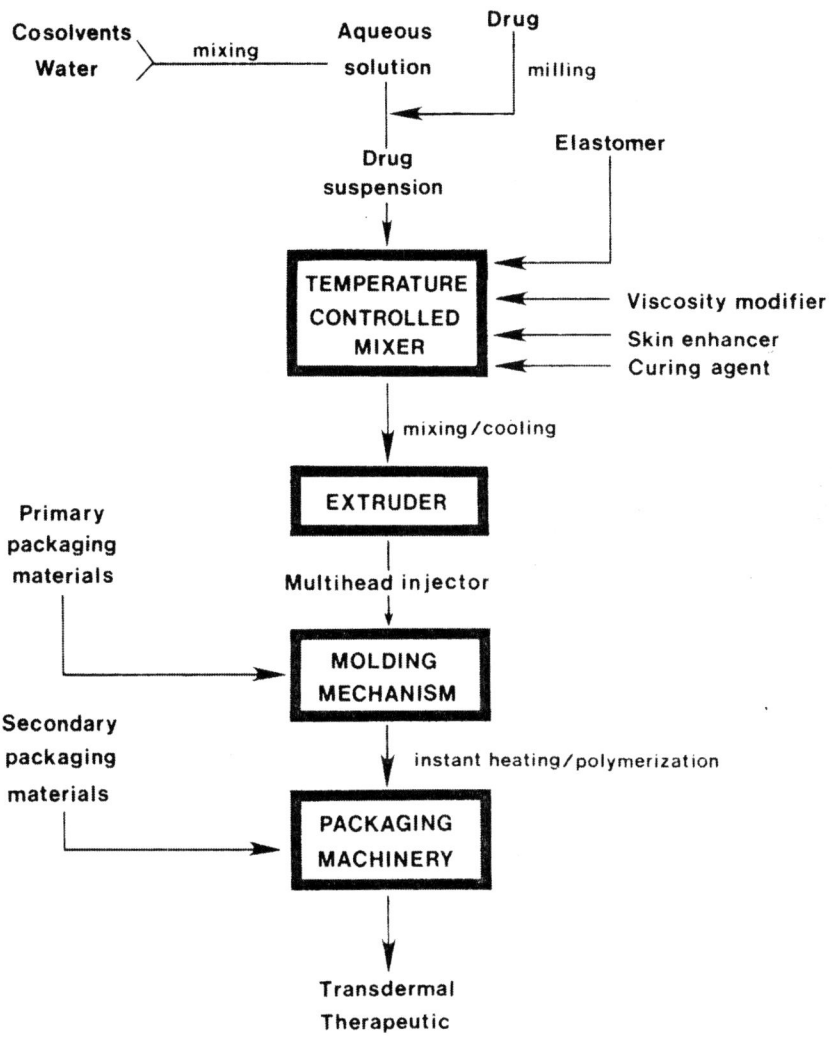

Figure 15   Schematic illustration of the process and equipment involved in the manufacture of the Nitrodisc system, a microreservoir dissolution-controlled transdermal therapeutic system.

drug concentration at the inner edge of the interfacial barrier to solubility in the polymer matrix.

Release of drugs from the microreservoir-type drug delivery system can follow either a partition-control or a matrix diffusion-control process, depending on the relative magnitude of S_l and S_p (29). Thus a Q versus t or a Q versus $\sqrt{t}$ release profile results (11,30,31).

Other types of potential drug delivery system are also undergoing development for possible applications in the transdermal controlled infusion of drugs. This area of research is exemplified by the disposition of drugs in poroplastic membranes (32) and the formation of hydrophilic polymeric reservoirs (33), both of which may be viewed as drug solution-saturated porous polymer matrices.

IV. KINETIC EVALUATIONS OF TRANSDERMAL THERAPEUTIC SYSTEMS

The release and skin permeation kinetics of drugs from these technologically different transdermal therapeutic systems can be evaluated using a two-compartment diffusion cell assembly, under identical conditions. Samples of full-thickness abdominal skin, which has been freshly excised from human cadaver or hairless mouse (34), are mounted individually on an eight-cell Franz diffusion assembly (Fig. 4). The drug delivery systems are then applied, with the drug-releasing surface in intimate contact with the stratum corneum surface of the skin (31). The skin permeation profile of the drug is obtained by sampling the receptor solution at predetermined intervals for 30 hr and assaying drug concentrations in the samples by a sensitive analytical method, such as high-performance liquid chromatography (HPLC) (11,31). The drug release profiles from these transdermal therapeutic systems can also be investigated using the same experimental setup without the skin (11).

In actual drug release and skin permeation kinetics studies, the rate profiles obtained could well be below the intrinsic rates calculated from Eqs. (8), (10), (12), and (13) due to the effect of mass transfer across the hydrodynamic diffusion layer on the surface of the drug delivery system or dermis. The magnitude of reduction is related to the thickness of the hydrodynamic diffusion layer and the physicochemical properties of the drugs (35). It is rather important to take these effects into consideration in the determination of drug release and skin permeation rate profiles. (For more detailed discussion, see Chapter 6.)

A. In Vitro Drug Release Kinetics

Using a Franz diffusion cell assembly, the mechanisms and release profiles of drugs from these technologically different transdermal therapeutic systems can be evaluated and compared (11). The results indicate that nitroglycerin release yields a constant rate profile (Q versus t) from transdermal therapeutic systems like Transderm-Nitro (a membrane-moderated transdermal drug delivery system) and Deponit (a drug reservoir gradient-controlled transdermal drug delivery system) (Fig. 16). The release rate of nitroglycerin from the Transderm-Nitro system (0.843 ± 0.035 mg/cm^2/day) is almost 3 times greater than that from Deponit (0.324 ± 0.011 mg/cm^2/day). This suggests that diffusion through the rate-controlling adhesive layers in the Deponit system plays a greater rate-limiting role in the release of nitroglycerin than does permeation across the rate-controlling membrane in the Transderm-Nitro system.

On the other hand, the release profiles of nitroglycerin from Nitrodisc and Nitro-Dur systems are not constant, but are observed to follow a linear Q versus $\sqrt{t}$ pattern as expected from matrix-diffusion-controlled drug release kinetics (23). The release flux of

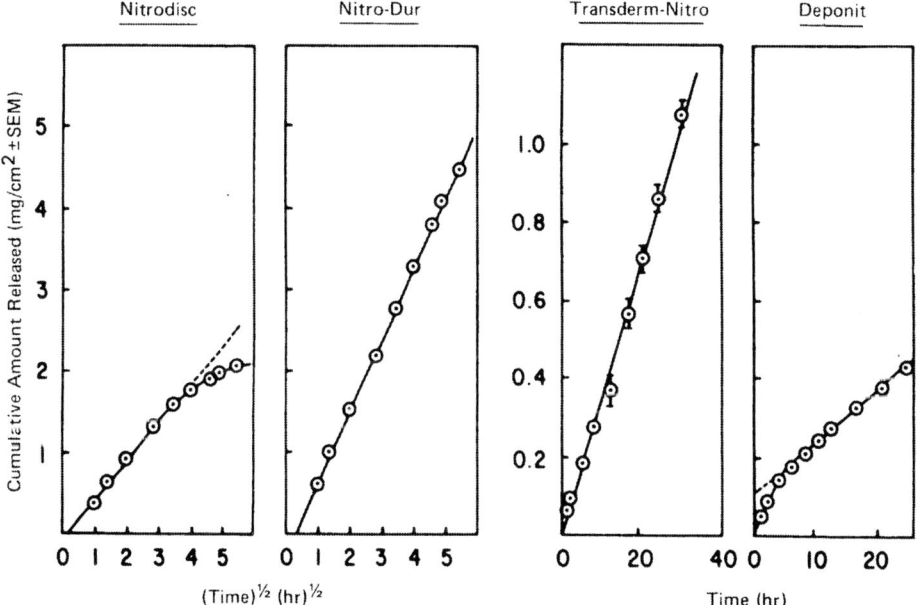

Figure 16   Comparative release profiles of nitroglycerin from various transdermal therapeutic systems into saline solution containing 20% polyethylene glycol 400 at 37°C. The release flux of nitroglycerin in each case is: Nitrodisc, 2.443 ($\pm$0.136) mg/cm^2/day$^{1/2}$; Nitro-Dur, 4.124 ($\pm$0.047) mg/cm^2/day$^{1/2}$; Transderm-Nitro, 0.843 (0.035) mg/cm^2/day; and Deponit 0.324 ($\pm$0.011) mg/cm^2/day. (From Ref. 11.)

nitroglycerin from the Nitro-Dur system (a matrix diffusion-controlled transdermal therapeutic system) is almost twice as great as that from the Nitrodisc system (a microreservoir-type transdermal therapeutic system) (4.124 ± 0.047 versus 2.443 ± 0.136 mg/cm^2/day$^{1/2}$). Apparently, the mechanisms and/or rates of nitroglycerin release from these four transdermal therapeutic systems are quite different from one another, as expected from Eqs. (8), (10), (12), and (13).

B. In Vitro Skin Permeation Kinetics: Animal Model

Skin permeation studies suggested that all four transdermal therapeutic systems provide a constant rate of skin permeation as expected from Eq. (3) (Fig. 17). The highest rate of skin permeation was observed with the Nitrodisc system (0.426 ± 0.024 mg/cm^2/day),

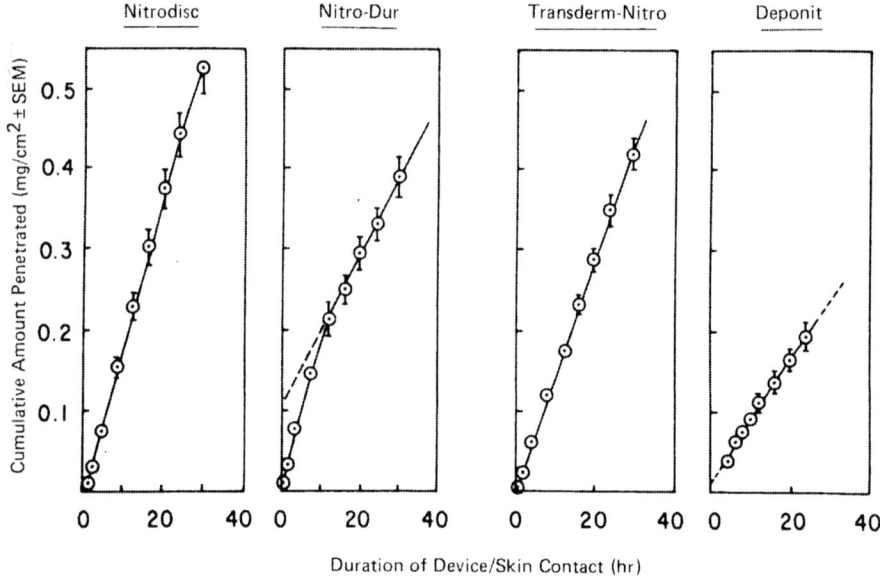

Duration of Device/Skin Contact (hr)

Figure 17   Comparative permeation profiles of nitroglycerin from various transdermal therapeutic systems through the abdominal skin of hairless mouse at 37°C. The rate of skin permeation in each case is: Nitrodisc, 0.426 (± 0.024) mg/cm^2/day; Nitro-Dur, 0.408 (± 0.024) mg/cm^2/day (< 12 hr), 0.248 (± 0.018) mg/cm^2/day (> 12 hr); Transderm-Nitro, 0.338 (± 0.017) mg/cm^2/day; and Deponit, 0.175 (± 0.016) mg/cm^2/day. (From Ref. 11.)

which is, however, statistically no different from the rate of skin permeation for pure nitroglycerin, which is freed from any mediation of a drug delivery system (0.476 ± 0.041 mg/cm^2/day, Fig. 5). For Nitro-Dur, practically the same rate of skin permeation (0.408 ± 0.024 mg/cm^2/day) was obtained initially; 12 hr later, however, the rate slowed to 0.248 (±0.018) mg/cm^2/day. On the other hand, the rate of skin permeation of nitroglycerin delivered by Transderm-Nitro (0.338 ± 0.017 mg/cm^2/day) was found to be 30% lower than the rate achieved by pure nitroglycerin (0.476 mg/cm^2/day) or 21% slower than that by Nitrodisc system (0.426 mg/cm^2/day). The lowest rate of skin permeation was observed with Deponit (0.175 ± 0.016 mg/cm^2/day), which achieved only one-third of the skin permeation rate for pure nitroglycerin.

Comparing the rate of skin permeation with the rate of release suggested that under sink conditions, all transdermal therapeutic systems release nitroglycerin at a rate greater than the rate of permeation across the skin (Fig. 2). For example, nitroglycerin was released from Transderm-Nitro, which is a membrane permeation-controlled drug delivery system, at a rate (0.843 mg/cm^2/day) that is 2.5 times greater than the rate of permeation across the skin (0.338 mg/cm^2/day). Likewise, the rate of release from the Deponit system, which is a multilaminate adhesive dispersion-type drug reservoir gradient-controlled drug delivery system and releases nitroglycerin at the slowest rate (Fig. 16), was also almost twofold faster than the rate of skin permeation (0.324 versus 0.175 mg/cm^2/ day). The same observations were true for Nitrodisc and Nitro-Dur. This phenomenon is indicative of the rate-limiting role of the stratum corneum in the skin permeation of drugs as a result of its low drug permeability.

C. In Vitro Skin Permeation Kinetics: Human Cadaver

The permeation of nitroglycerin across the skin of human cadaver was also investigated for Transderm-Nitro, the membrane-permeation-controlled transdermal therapeutic system, and for Nitro-Dur, the matrix-diffusion-controlled transdermal therapeutic system (36). The results (Fig. 18) indicated that the skin permeation of nitroglycerin through the human cadaver abdominal epidermis follows the same zero-order kinetic profile as observed with hairless mouse abdominal skin (Fig. 17). It is interesting to note that the rates of skin permeation generated from the freshly excised skin specimen of hairless mouse agree fairly well with the data obtained from human cadaver skin (Table 1), suggesting that hairless mouse skin could be an acceptable animal model for human skin in skin permeation kinetics studies of nitroglycerin (for more detailed discussion, see Chapter 7).

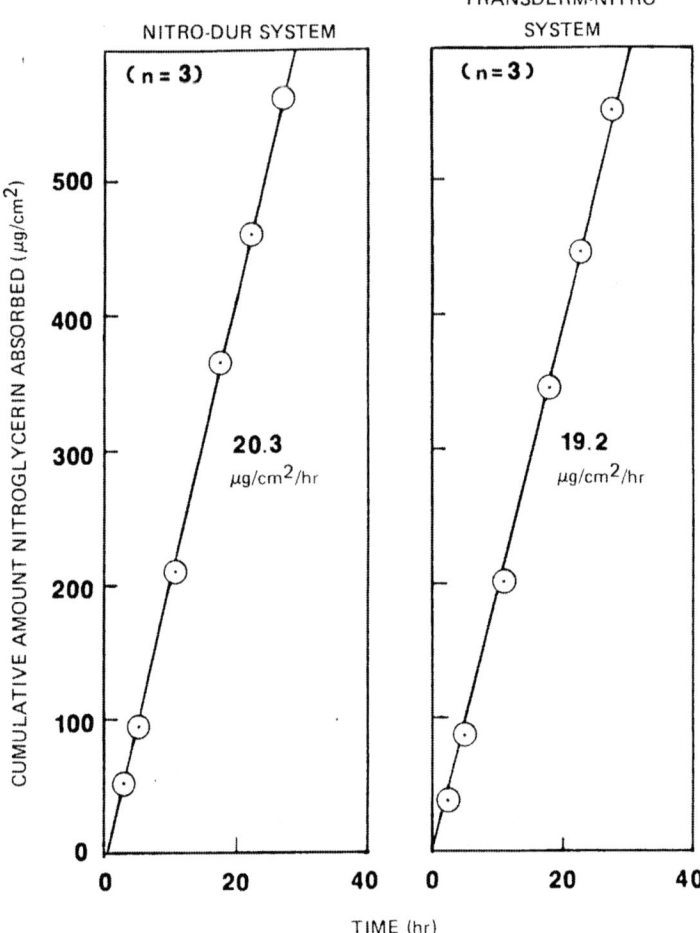

Figure 18   Comparative permeation profiles of nitroglycerin from the Nitro-Dur and Transderm-Nitro systems across the abdominal epidermis of human cadaver.   The rate of skin permeation is: Nitro-Dur (20.3 $\mu g/cm^2/hr$) and Transderm-Nitro (19.2 $\mu g/cm^2/hr$). (Plotted from data in Ref. 36.)

Table 1   In Vitro-In Vivo Comparison of Skin Permeation Rates
of Nitroglycerin

| | Skin permeation rates ($mg/cm^2/day$) | | | |
| | In vitro | | In vivo | |
Delivery system	Hairless mouse	Human cadaver[a]	A[b]	B[c]
Nitrodisc	0.426	—	0.714	0.67
Nitro-Dur	0.408	0.487	0.410	—
Transderm-Nitro	0.338	0.461	0.427	0.62
Deponit	0.175	—	0.318	0.45

[a]Determined from skin permeation studies at 37°C using the epidermis isolated from human cadaver abdominal skin (Ref. 36).
[b]Calculated from steady-state plasma profiles using Eq. (14), in which $k_e = 0.1575$ min^{-1} and $V_d = 179.6$ L (Ref. 39).
[c]Estimated from the residual drug content assay after 24-hr application on human volunteers (Refs. 28 and 41).

D. In Vivo Transdermal Bioavailability in Humans

The transdermal bioavailability of nitroglycerin resulting from 24–32 hr topical applications of various transdermal therapeutic systems in human volunteers, as indicated by the plasma levels of nitroglycerin, is shown in Figures 19–22. Results suggested that a prolonged, steady-state plasma level of nitroglycerin is achieved within 1–2 hr and maintained for at least 24 hr as a result of continuous transdermal infusion of drug at a controlled rate from the transdermal therapeutic system.

A comparative systemic bioavailability study was initiated (16), and the results demonstrated that there is no statistically significant difference among the plasma profiles of nitroglycerin delivered by the Transderm-Nitro, Nitrodisc, and Nitro-Dur systems (Fig. 23).

Plasma level was found to be linearly proportional to drug-releasing surface area of the transdermal therapeutic systems in contact with the skin (Fig. 24). For every unit area (cm^2) of the drug-releasing surface that is in intimate contact with the skin, a plasma nitroglycerin level of 14 pg/ml was achieved.

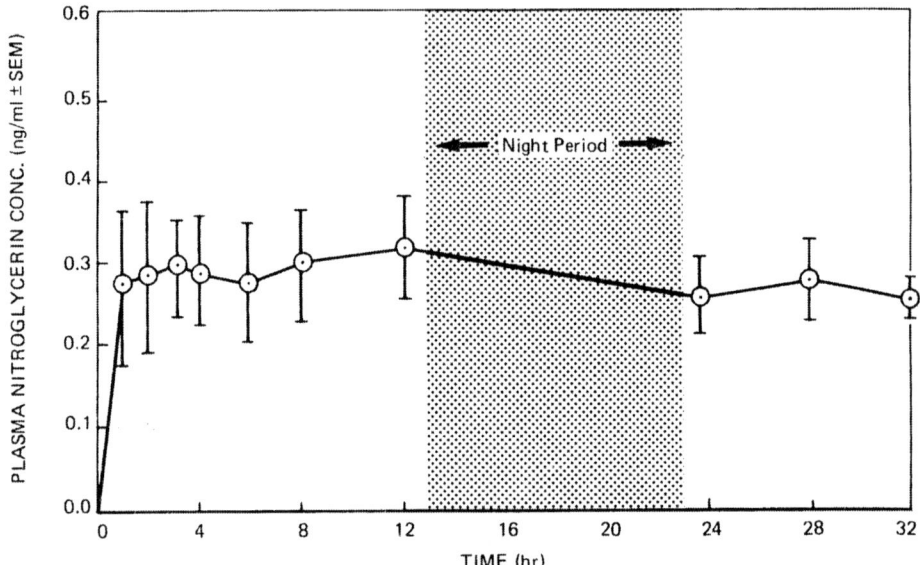

NITRODISC SYSTEM (16 cm^2, n=12)

Figure 19   Plasma profiles of nitroglycerin in 12 health male volunteers; each received one unit of the Nitrodisc system (16 cm^2) on the chest for 32 h. A steady-state plasma level, $(Cp)_{ss}$, of 280.6 ($\pm$18.7) pg/ml was achieved. (Plotted from data in Ref. 28.)

E.   In Vitro—In Vivo Correlations

To further examine the feasibility of using freshly excised hairless mouse skin as the animal model for studying the transdermal controlled permeation kinetics of drugs across the human skin, the in vivo rate of skin permeation $(Q/t)_{i.v.}$ should also be determined for comparison. It can be calculated from the steady-state plasma level $(C_p)_{ss}$ data (Figs. 19-22), using the following relationship (37):

$$\left(\frac{Q}{t}\right)_{i.v.} = \frac{(C_p)_{ss} \cdot K_e \cdot V_d}{A_s} \tag{14}$$

where K_e is the first-order rate constant for the elimination of drug, V_d is the apparent volume of distribution for the drug, and A_s is the surface area of drug-releasing surface in contact with the skin.

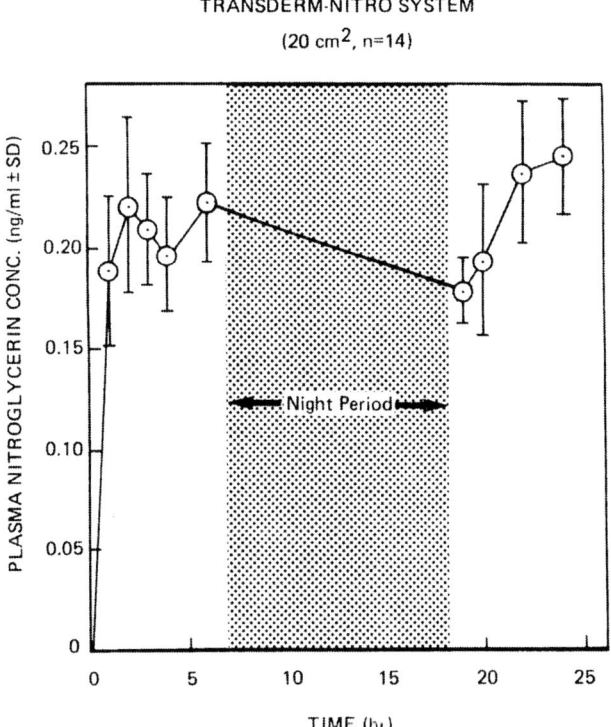

Figure 20   Plasma profiles of nitroglycerin in 14 healthy human subjects; each received one unit of the Transderm-Nitro system (20 cm²)
for 24 hr.   A $(Cp)_{ss}$ value of 209.8 (±22.8) pg/ml was obtained.
(Plotted from data in Ref. 15.)

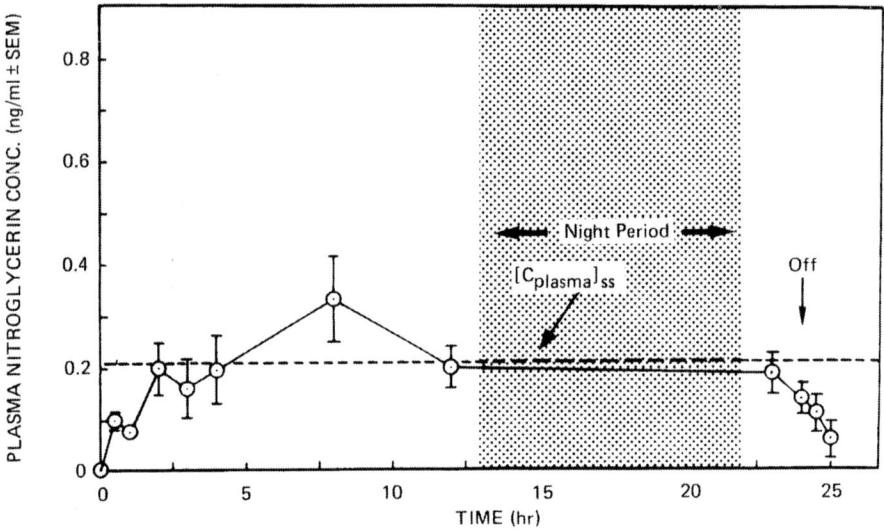

Figure 21   Plasma profiles of nitroglycerin in 6 normal male volunteers; each received one unit of the Nitro-Dur system (20 cm^2) over the chest for 24 hr.   A $(Cp)_{ss}$ value of 201.4 ($\pm$60.7) pg/ml resulted.   (Plotted from data in Ref. 40.)

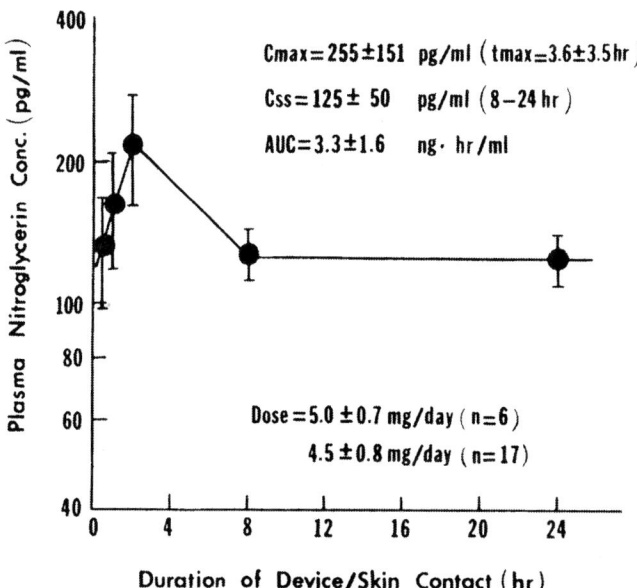

Figure 22   Plasma profiles of nitroglycerin in 6 healthy male volunteers; each received one unit of the Deponit system (16 cm^2) over the chest for 24 hr.   A (Cp)$_{ss}$ value of 125 ± 50 pg/ml resulted. (Plotted from data in Ref. 41.)

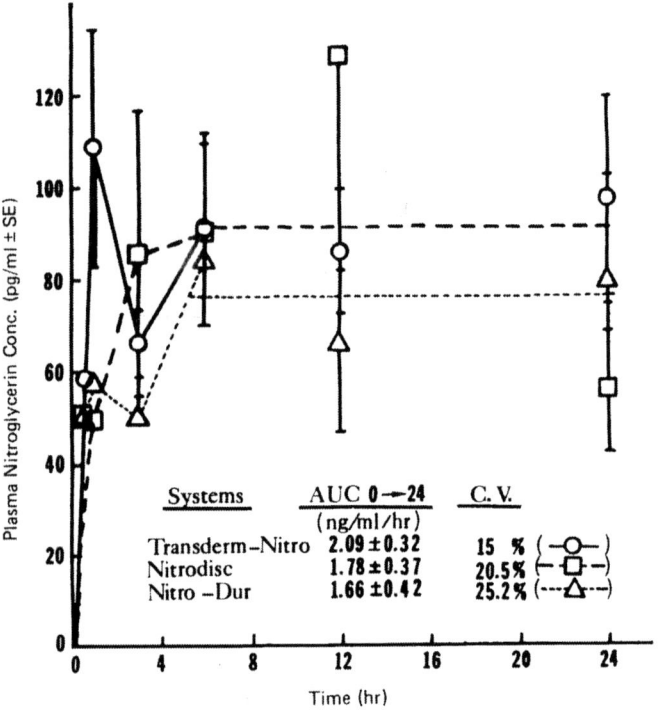

Figure 23 Comparative transdermal bioavailability of nitroglycerin delivered by the Transderm-Nitro, Nitrodisc, and Nitro-Dur systems in 6 normal volunteers in a three-way crossover study. AUC = area under the plasma concentration curve, CV = coefficient of variance. (Plotted from data in Ref. 16.)

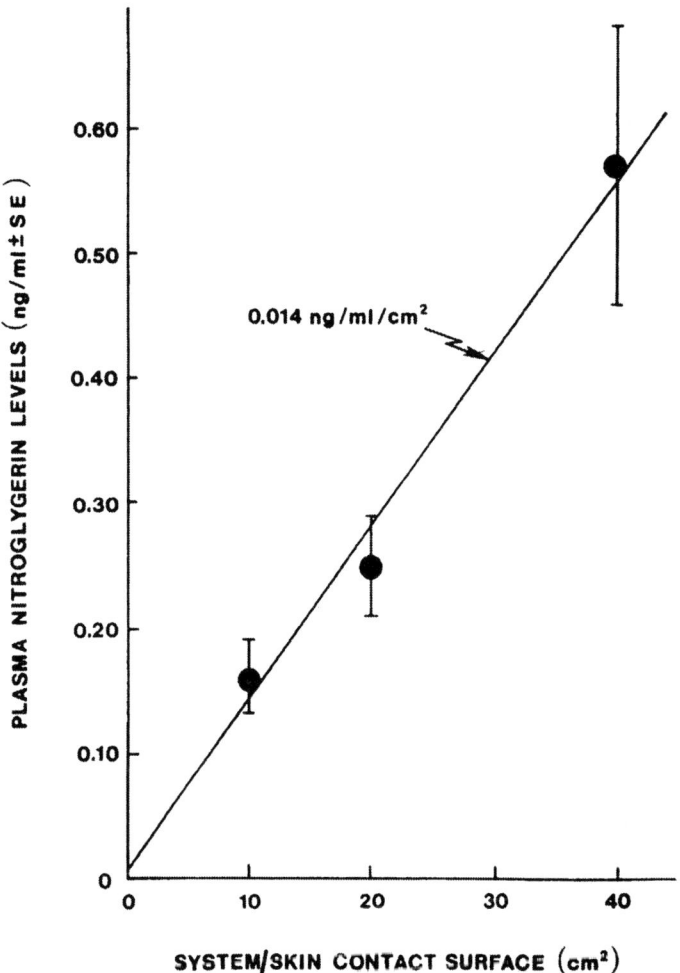

Figure 24 The linear relationship between the steady-state plasma nitroglycerin levels in humans and the drug-releasing surface of the Transderm-Nitro system in contact with the skin. A plasma nitroglycerin level of 14 pg/ml was achieved for every square centimeter of drug-releasing surface applied. (Plotted from data in Ref. 14.)

Results indicated that the in vivo skin permeation rates calculated on the basis of Eq. (14) show a reasonably good agreement with the in vitro data determined from either human cadaver epidermis or hairless mouse whole-thickness skin (Table 1). This in vivo—in vitro agreement provides additional evidence that hairless mouse skin could be an acceptable animal model for studying the skin permeation kinetics in humans of systemically effective drugs like nitroglycerin.

V. FORMULATION DESIGN AND OPTIMIZATION

To formulate a transdermal therapeutic system, one should take into consideration the relationship between the rate of drug delivery to the skin surface and the maximum achievable rate of drug absorption by the skin tissue. This is particularly important because the stratum corneum is known to be highly impermeable to many drugs. A properly designed transdermal therapeutic system should have a skin permeation rate that is determined by the actual rate of drug delivery to the skin surface, not by the skin permeability; in such a case, the transdermal bioavailability of a drug becomes independent of any possible intra- and/or interpatient variabilities in skin permeability.

The rate of skin permeation of a drug at steady state $(Q/t)_{ss}$ is mathematically related to the actual rate of drug delivery from a transdermal therapeutic system $(Q/t)_{tts}$ to the skin surface and the maximum achievable rate of skin absorption $(Q/t)_{m,s}$ by the following relationship (38):

$$\frac{1}{(Q/t)_{ss}} = \frac{1}{(Q/t)_{tts}} + \frac{1}{(Q/t)_{m,s}} \tag{15}$$

And, the actual rate of drug delivery from a transdermal therapeutic system to the skin surface (which acts as the receptor medium in clinical applications) can thus be determined from:

$$\frac{1}{(Q/t)_{tts}} = \frac{1}{(Q/t)_{ss}} - \frac{1}{(Q/t)_{m,s}} \tag{16}$$

If we consider the rate of skin permeation from the pure nitroglycerin, which is freed from any effect by the formulation or vehicle, as the value for $(Q/t)_{m,s}$, the actual delivery rate of nitroglycerin from various transdermal therapeutic systems can be calculated. Results in Table 2 indicated that the rates of delivery for Nitrodisc, Nitro-Dur, and Transderm-Nitro are three- to nine-fold greater than the maximum achievable rate of skin permeation (0.476 mg/cm^2/day)

Table 2   Delivery Rate of Nitroglycerin from
Various Transdermal Therapeutic Systems

Systems	Delivery rate $(mg/cm^2/day)^a$
Nitrodisc	4.058
Nitro-Dur	2.857
Transderm-Nitro	1.166
Deponit	0.277

[a]Calculated from the hairless mouse data in
Table 1 using Eq. (16) and $(Q/t)_{m,s}$ =
0.476 mg/cm^2/day.

for nitroglycerin. On the other hand, the rate of delivery from
Deponit is only 58% of the maximum rate of skin permeation. These
data suggest that the delivery rate of nitroglycerin from all four
transdermal therapeutic systems has not been optimized.

Using a matrix-diffusion-controlled transdermal therapeutic system, the relationship between the rate of drug delivery from the
transdermal therapeutic system and the rate of skin permeation can
be established. The skin permeation rate of a drug at steady state,
$(Q/t)_{ss}$, is related to the drug delivery rate from the matrix-type
transdermal therapeutic system, $(Q/\sqrt{t})$, as follows (42):

$$(Q/t)_{ss} = \frac{m(Q/\sqrt{t})^2}{1 + n(Q/\sqrt{t})^2} \qquad (17)$$

in which m and n are composite constants and defined as follows:

$$m = \frac{1}{2k} \qquad (18)$$

$$n = \frac{R_{sc}}{2K_1 kC_p} \left(1 + \frac{R_{vs}K_3 + R_{aq}}{K_2 K_3 R_{sc}} \right) \qquad (19)$$

where k is a constant; K_1, K_2, and K_3 are the partition coefficients
for the interfacial partitioning between the stratum corneum and the

polymer matrix, between viable skin and stratum corneum, and between aqueous layer and viable skin, respectively; C_p is the drug
solubility in the polymer matrix; R_{sc}, R_{vs}, and R_{aq} are the diffusional resistances for stratum corneum, viable skin, and aqueous
layer on the dermal surface, respectively.

As predicted by Eq. (17), a hyperbolic relationship was observed to exist between $(Q/t)_{ss}$ and $(Q/\sqrt{t})^2$. When the rate of
drug delivery from the transdermal therapeutic system is low, skin
permeation is controlled by the delivery system (Fig. 25). As the
rate of drug delivery increases, the rate of skin permeation increases, in a hyperbolic pattern, finally reaching a plateau at which

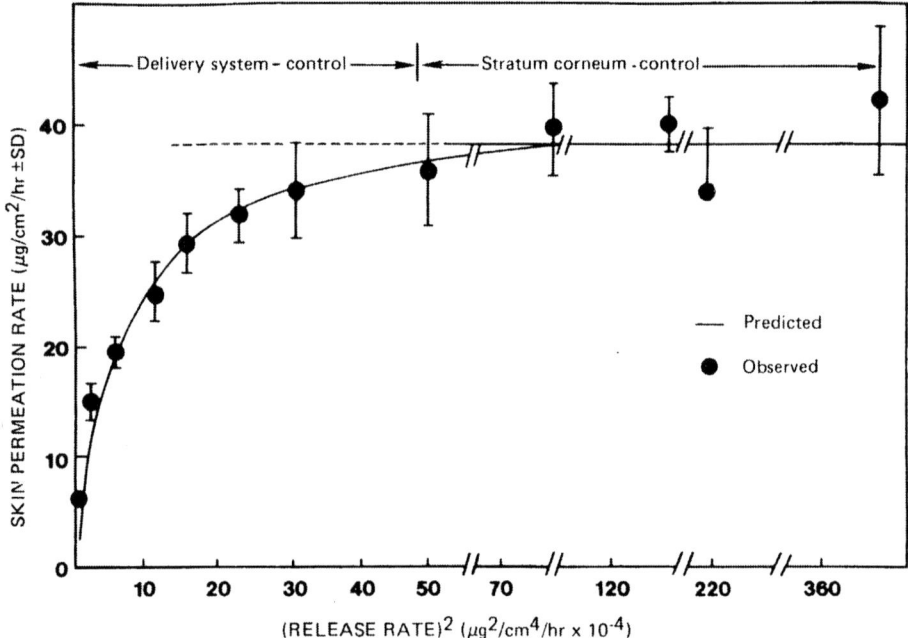

Figure 25   The hyperbolic relationship between skin permeation rate
and the square of the release flux of nitroglycerin delivered by the
matrix-diffusion-controlled transdermal therapeutic system, as predicted from Eq. (17). It was observed that when $(Q/\sqrt{t})^2$ is equal
to or less than 48 $\mu g^2/cm^4/hr$, the skin permeation rate of nitroglycerin is controlled by the delivery system; when $(Q/\sqrt{t})^2$ is
greater than 48 $\mu g^2/cm^4/hr$, the skin permeation rate becomes limited
by the stratum corneum. (From Ref. 42.)

the rate of skin permeation becomes rate-limited by the inherent permeability of stratum corneum to the drug species delivered. Using Eq. (17), one can optimize the formulation design of a transdermal therapeutic system with the rate of skin permeation controlled by the rate of drug delivery from the delivery system.

VI. ENHANCEMENT OF TRANSDERMAL CONTROLLED DRUG DELIVERY

It has become increasingly recognized that not every drug can be administered transdermally at a rate high enough to achieve a blood level that is therapeutically beneficial for systemic medication. An increasing number of biomedical researchers working in the field of transdermal controlled drug delivery have cautioned the scientific community about the potential limitations of transdermal systemic medications (2,6).

For instance, the smallest size of nitroglycerin-releasing transdermal therapeutic systems (8 cm^2 for Nitrodisc, 10 cm^2 for Transderm-Nitro and Nitro-Dur, and 16 cm^2 for Deponit) has been found to be capable of establishing a mean steady-state plasma level of less than 0.18 ng/ml (37), which is substantially lower than the plasma level (0.29–0.41 ng/ml) achieved by giving intravenous infusion of nitroglycerin at a rate of 3.4 µg/min (or 4.9 mg/day) (Fig. 26). To achieve the same plasma level as the intravenous infusion, it is estimated that a transdermal patch with a nitroglycerin-releasing surface of 20–30 cm^2 would be needed, depending on which type of transdermal therapeutic system is used. The same requirement is also applied to the ointment formulation containing 2% nitroglycerin, since the stratum corneum has the rate-limiting barrier properties in the transdermal delivery of a drug for systemic medication.

To achieve and maintain a plasma drug concentration above the minimum therapeutic level, the barrier properties of the skin must be overcome before the transdermal controlled delivery of drugs can be accomplished. Two approaches have shown potentially in accomplishing the goals of reducing skin's barrier properties and, hence, of enhancing the transdermal permeation of drugs (43–47). These approaches are discussed in the following sections.

A. Skin Permeability Enhancement by Bioconvertible Prodrugs

Prodrugs can be viewed as the therapeutically inactive derivatives of a therapeutically active drug that undergo bioconversion, either by chemical or enzymatic transformation, in a biological environment,

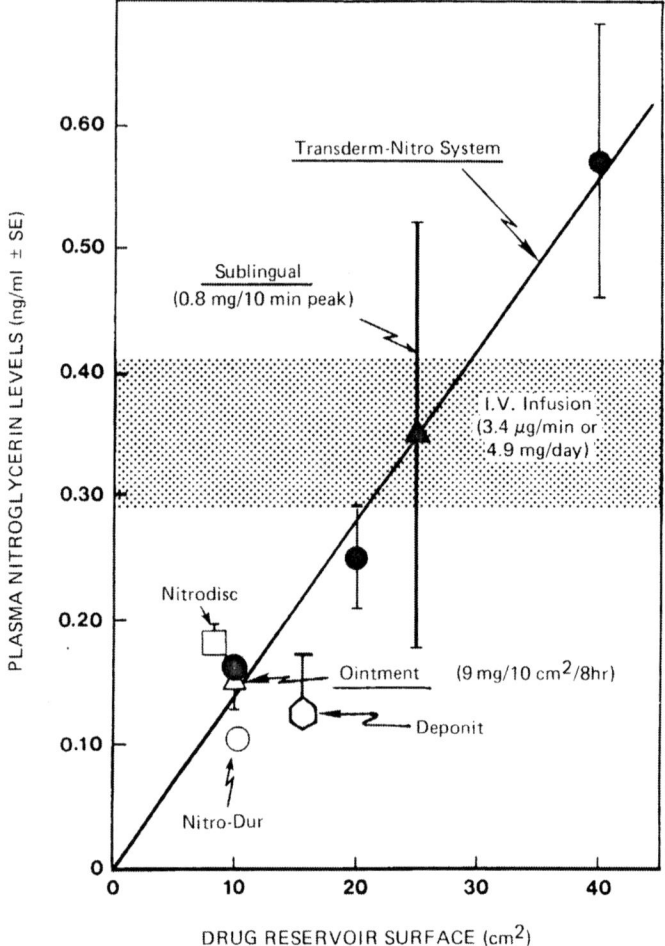

Figure 26 Comparison of the steady-state plasma levels of nitroglycerin achieved by various transdermal drug delivery systems in relation to those by sublingual admihistration and intravenous infusion. (Plotted from data in Refs. 14–16, 28, 39–41, 51.)

to regenerate the therapeutically active parent drug prior to exhibiting their pharmacological activities (48).

The prodrug concept can be applied in transdermal controlled drug delivery by altering skin permeability via modification of the physicochemical properties of the drug molecule to enhance its rate of transdermal permeation (44).

Prodrugs of a poorly skin-permeable drug may be synthesized to improve percutaneous absorption characteristics. During the course of transdermal permeation, the prodrugs can be transformed, by the metabolic processes within the skin tissue, back to the active parent drug (Fig. 27). In other words, if an active drug has a rather low affinity toward the skin, it will not easily partition into it to any great extent. The partition behavior of such a drug can be improved by simple chemical modification to form a lipophilic prodrug, thus substantially enhancing the transport of the drug into the skin. Upon absorption and penetration through the skin, the prodrug is rapidly metabolized to regenerate the active parent drug. One typical example of this approach is the esterification of less skin-permeable estradiol to form lipophilic estradiol esters (Table 3).

In vitro skin permeation studies (44) indicated that during the course of skin permeation, the five prodrug-type esters of estradiol are extensively metabolized by esterase in the skin tissue to regenerate estradiol (Fig. 28); the rate of regeneration of estradiol

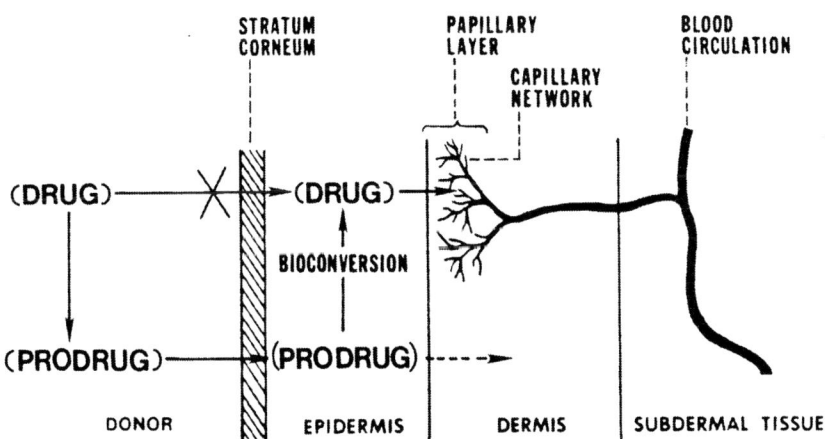

Figure 27 Multilayer skin model showing the enhanced skin permeation of drug by forming a more permeable prodrug. In the viable epidermis layers, the prodrug is metabolized to regenerate the parent drug.

Table 3   Chemical Structure of Estradiol and Its Esters

	R_1	R_2
Estradiol-17-β	—H	—H
Estradiol-17-acetate	$-\overset{\parallel}{\underset{O}{C}}-CH_3$	—H
Estradiol-3,17-diacetate	$-\overset{\parallel}{\underset{O}{C}}-CH_3$	$-\overset{\parallel}{\underset{O}{C}}-CH_3$
Estradiol-17-valerate	$-\overset{\parallel}{\underset{O}{C}}-(CH_2)_3-CH_3$	—H
Estradiol-17-heptanoate	$-\overset{\parallel}{\underset{O}{C}}-(CH_2)_5-CH_3$	—H
Estradiol-17-cypionate	$-\overset{\parallel}{\underset{O}{C}}-CH_2-CH_2-\langle\bigcirc\rangle$	—H

from esters by bioconversion was observed to follow the order of: diacetate > valerate > heptanoate > cypionate > acetate. The metabolism of estradiol esters was found to follow a first-order kinetics, and the rate constant for the enzymatic hydrolysis of the ester group at the third position was observed to be substantially greater than that at the seventeenth position (44,49).

Based on the results of simultaneous skin permeation and bioconversion profiles, a transdermal bioactivated hormone delivery (TBHD) device was developed, using the microreservoir dissolution-controlled drug delivery system (Figs. 13 and 14), for the transdermal controlled delivery of estradiol and its esters (43). Using a

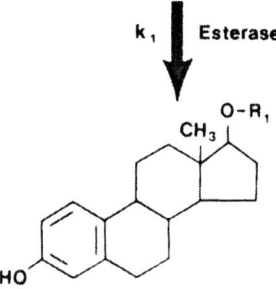

Estradiol-3,17-Diester

k_1 | Esterase

Estradiol-17-Ester

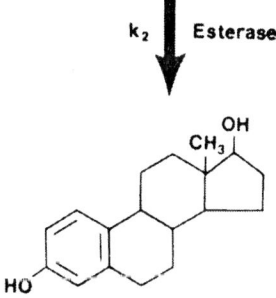

k_2 | Esterase

Estradiol

Figure 28 Schematic illustration of the bioconversion of estradiol-3,17-diester, by esterase in the cutaneous tissue, to estradiol-17-ester, as the intermediate, and then to the biologically active estradiol. (From Ref. 44.)

hydrodynamically well-calibrated horizontal-type skin permeation cell (Fig. 29), the in vitro drug release and skin permeation profiles of estradiol and its esters were investigated simultaneously (Fig. 30). Results indicated that estradiol and its esters are released from the TBHD device at a zero-order rate profile, and the rate of release increases as the hydrophilic OH groups at the 3- and 17-positions are esterified to form the lipophilic esters (Fig. 31). The release rate of estradiol from the lipophilic TBHD device was found to depend on the alkyl chain length of the ester at the seventeenth position (Table 4).

The skin permeation studies demonstrated that all the prodrugs of estradiol, except estradiol-3-acetate and 3,17-diacetate, are totally metabolized by the esterase to regenerate the biologically active estradiol during the course of skin permeation (Fig. 32). The rate of regeneration of estradiol from the prodrug-type esters was also

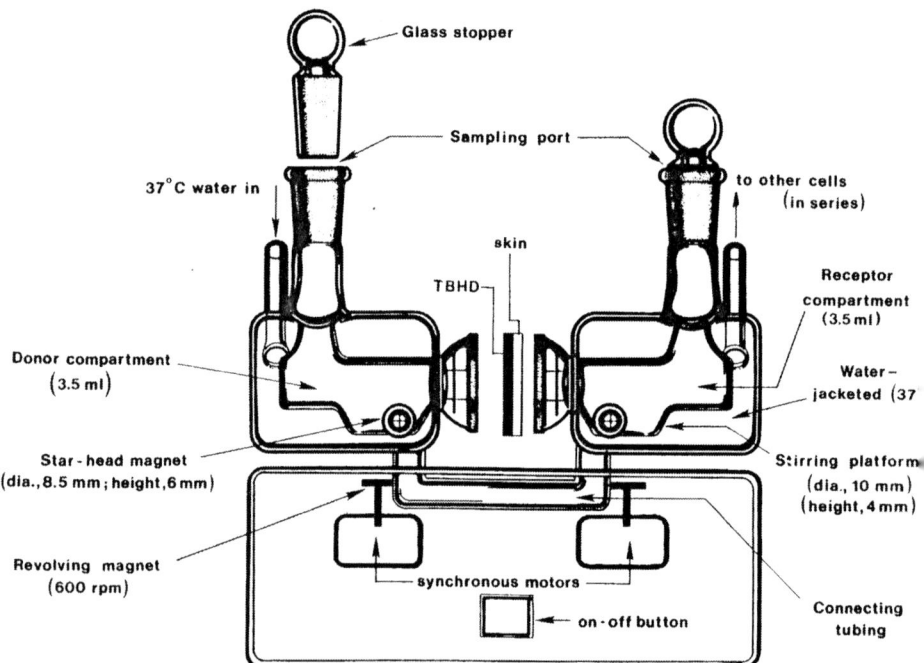

Figure 29   The experimental setup for the simultaneous study of the controlled release and the skin permeation of estradiol and esters from the transdermal bioactivated hormone delivery (TBHD) system. (From Ref. 43.)

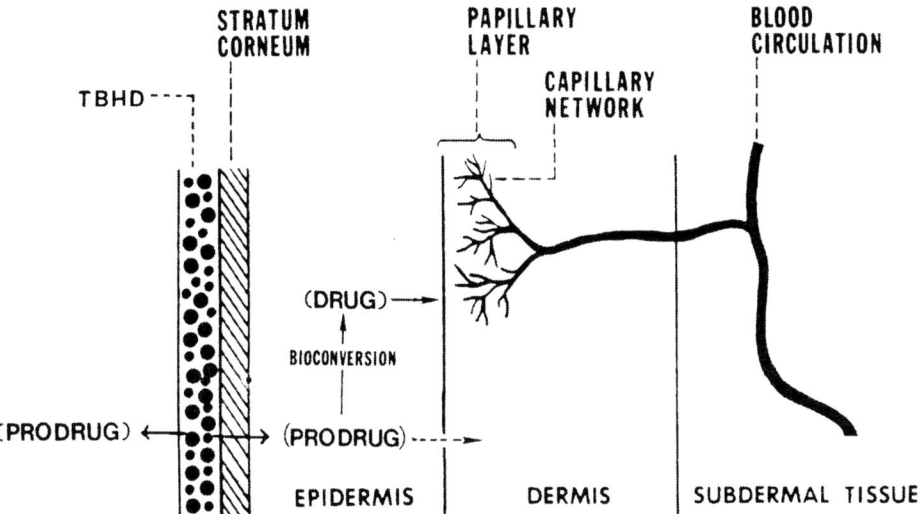

Figure 30   Expanded diagram of the TBHD system/skin tissue combination, illustrating the simultaneous kinetic processes of release and skin permeation of prodrugs from the TBHD system and of regeneration of drug by enzymatic metabolism of prodrugs.   (From Ref. 43.)

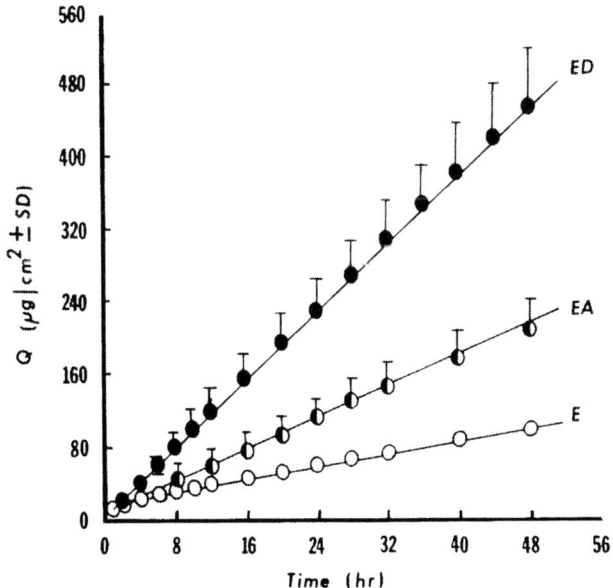

Figure 31   The time course for the cumulative release of estradiol and esters from TBHD system.   E = estradiol, EA = estradiol-17-acetate, ED = estradiol-3,17-diacetate.   (From Ref. 43.)

Table 4   Release Rate Profiles of Estradiol
and Estradiol Esters from Transdermal
Bioactivated Hormone Delivery System

Species	Release rate ($\mu g/cm^2/hr$ ±SD)
Estradiol	1.826 ± 0.074
Estradiol esters	
Diacetate	9.388 ± 1.160
Acetate	4.133 ± 0.525
Valerate	3.732 ± 0.662
Heptanoate	2.082 ± 0.768
Cypionate	0.567 ± 0.189

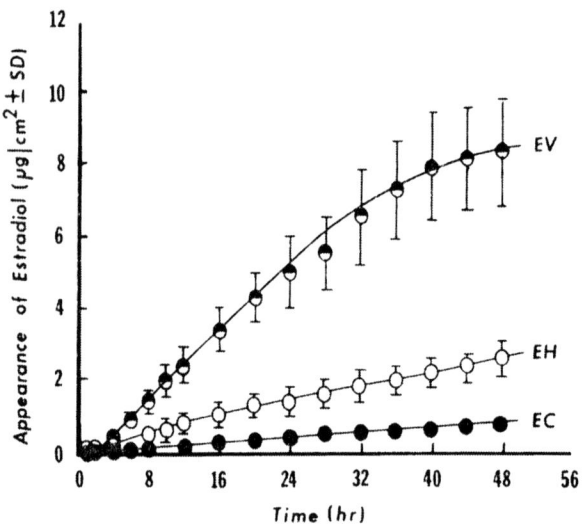

Figure 32   The time course for the regeneration of estradiol during
the skin permeation of various estradiol-17-esters by metabolism
following transdermal controlled administration from various ester-
releasing TBHD systems.   EV = estradiol-17-valerate, EH = estradiol-
17-heptanoate, EC = estradiol-17-cypionate.   No intact ester was
detected.   (From Ref. 43.)

Table 5   Appearance Rate Profiles of Estradiol
Following Transdermal Controlled Administration
of Estradiol and Esters from Transdermal
Bioactivated Hormone Delivery System

Species	Rate of appearance ($\mu g/cm^2/hr$ ±SD)
Estradiol	0.117 (±0.027)
Estradiol esters	
Diacetate	0.490 (±0.250)
Acetate	0.057 (±0.013)
Valerate	0.227 (±0.042)
Heptanoate	0.061 (±0.013)
Cypionate	0.016 (±0.002)

found to depend on the alkyl chain length (Table 5).   Diacetate and
valerate achieved rates that were, respectively, four- and twofold
greater than estradiol itself.

B. Skin Permeability Enhancement by Enhancers

The skin permeability of drugs can also be greatly improved by
treating the stratum corneum surface with an appropriate skin permeation enhancer.   Some representative classes of potential skin permeation enhancers are listed in Table 6.
   The concept of promoting the skin permeability of drugs by
enhancers has been incorporated into transdermal controlled drug
delivery in the development of a skin-permeation-enhancing (SPE)
transdermal therapeutic system (45).   This new type of transdermal
drug delivery system is capable of releasing one or more skin permeation enhancers to the surface of the stratum corneum to modify
the skin's barrier properties before the controlled delivery of the
active drug, and to render the skin more permeable to the drug
(Fig. 33).   In vitro skin permeation studies in a hydrodynamically
well-calibrated skin permeation cell (Fig. 34) demonstrated that
simple pharmaceutical excipients like propyl esters of myristic acid
and oleic acid can enhance the transdermal permeation rate of progesterone by approximately five times and also significantly reduce

Table 6 Some Representative Classes of Potential Skin Permeation Enhancers

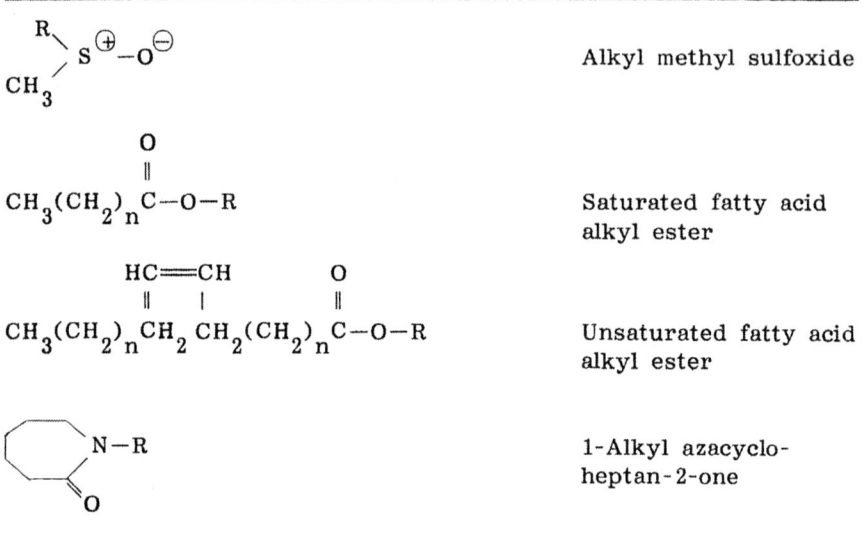

$\underset{CH_3}{\overset{R}{\diagdown}} S^{\oplus} - O^{\ominus}$	Alkyl methyl sulfoxide
$CH_3(CH_2)_n \overset{O}{\overset{\|}{C}} - O - R$	Saturated fatty acid alkyl ester
$CH_3(CH_2)_n CH_2 \overset{HC=CH}{\overset{\|}{CH_2}} (CH_2)_n \overset{O}{\overset{\|}{C}} - O - R$	Unsaturated fatty acid alkyl ester
azacycloheptanone ring with $N-R$ and $=O$	1-Alkyl azacyclo-heptan-2-one

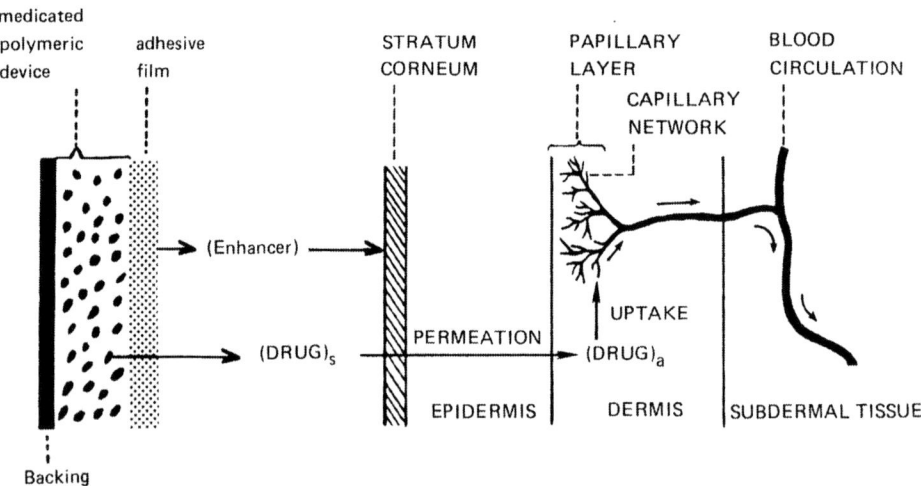

Figure 33 Expanded diagram to illustrate the concept of enhancing the skin permeation of drugs by releasing one or more enhancers to the skin surface to modify the permeability characteristics of stratum corneum prior to the controlled delivery of therapeutically active drug.

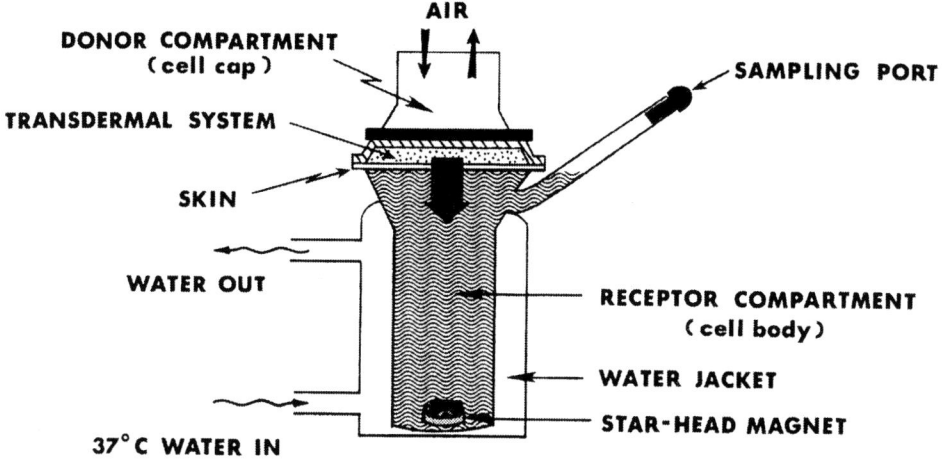

Figure 34 A hydrodynamically well-calibrated skin permeation cell consisting of two compartments arranged vertically: a donor compartment, which is exposed to an ambient condition, and a receptor compartment, which is maintained at 37°C by circulating thermostated water through the water jacket. The solution hydrodynamics in the receptor compartment is kept constant by a Teflon-coated star-head magnet rotated at 600 rpm by a synchronous motor mounted directly underneath the cell mounting block. One unit of the skin-permeation enhancing (SPE) transdermal therapeutic system is mounted between the donor and receptor compartments with its SPE-releasing adhesive layer in intimate contact with the stratum corneum surface. (From Ref. 42.)

the duration of time lag, while the zero-order skin permeation rate profile is still maintained (Fig. 35).

In addition to progesterone, which is relatively skin permeable, the propyl esters of myristic acid, a long-chain saturated fatty acid, and of oleic acid, a long-chain unsaturated fatty acid (Table 6), are also capable of promoting the rate of skin permeation for the less permeable steroidal anti-inflammatory agents (e.g., hydrocortisone), the nonsteroidal anti-inflammatory drugs (e.g., indomethacin), and the estrogenic steroids (e.g., estradiol) (Table 7).

The esters of saturated and unsaturated fatty acids, azone, and decylmethyl sulfoxide are very effective in enhancing the skin permeability of drugs (Table 7). In addition, however, results appear to suggest the existence of a relationship between the skin permeability enhancement of a drug and its molecular structure as well as the type of enhancer used. For more effective promotion of transdermal

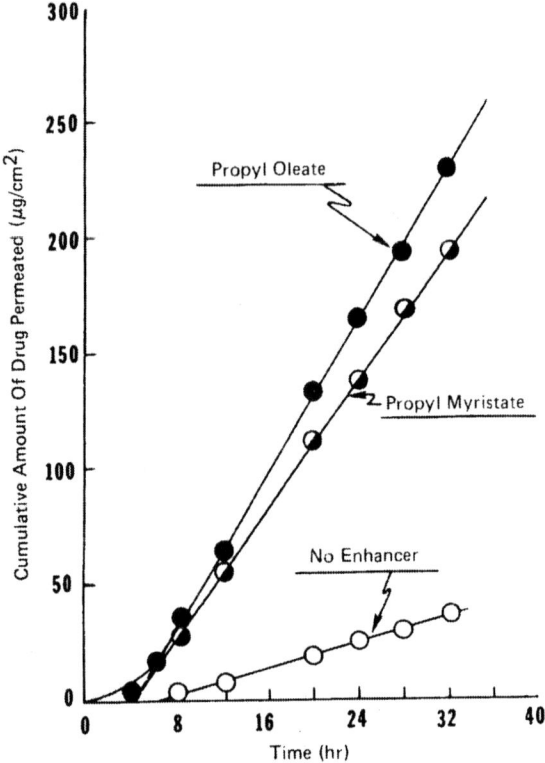

Figure 35 Enhancement in the skin permeation profiles of progesterone by the propyl esters of myristic acid, a long-chain saturated fatty acid, and of oleic acid, a long-chain unsaturated fatty
acid.

drug administration, the enhancing agent should be incorporated into
the adhesive layer, which will be in intimate contact with the stratum
corneum surface when applied (Table 8).

The extent of skin permeability enhancement seemed to depend
on the alkyl chain length of fatty acid (Fig. 36). A maximum enhancement was achieved with the fatty acid containing six units of
CH_2 groups. Free fatty acid was found to be more effective than
its propyl ester in promoting the skin permeation rate of progesterone.
The efficiency of skin permeation enhancement was noted to be a
function of the type and the concentration of enhancer released from

Table 7 Enhancement of Skin Permeability of Various Drugs by Different Types of Enhancer

Drugs	Skin permeation rate[a] (μg/cm^2/day)	Enhancement factor[b]			
		Propyl myristate[c]	Propyl oleate[c]	Azone[c]	Decylmethyl sulfoxide[c]
Progesterone	36.72 (±10.32)	4.56	5.36	5.96	11.04
Estradiol	29.29 (±24.48)	9.33	14.62	20.17	12.59
Hydrocortisone	1.10 (±0.12)	4.57	5.01	61.30	25.23
Indomethacin	9.36 (±0.08)	3.77	4.67	14.49	15.67

[a] The skin permeation rate of drugs from delivery systems containing no enhancer.

[b] Enhancement factor = $\dfrac{\text{(Normalized skin permeation rate) with enhancer}}{\text{(Normalized skin permeation rate) without enhancer}}$

[c] Enhancer concentration in the adhesive layer = 3.2 mg/cm^2.

Table 8 Effect of the Location of Skin Permeation Enhancer on the Enhancement of Progesterone Permeability

Location	Skin permeation rate ($\mu g/cm^2/day$)	Enhancement factor			
		Propyl myristate	Propyl oleate	Azone	Decylmethyl sulfoxide
Polymer matrix	34.6 (± 0.5)	2.67	4.05	2.56	3.81
Adhesive film	36.7 (± 10.3)	4.56	5.36	5.96	11.04

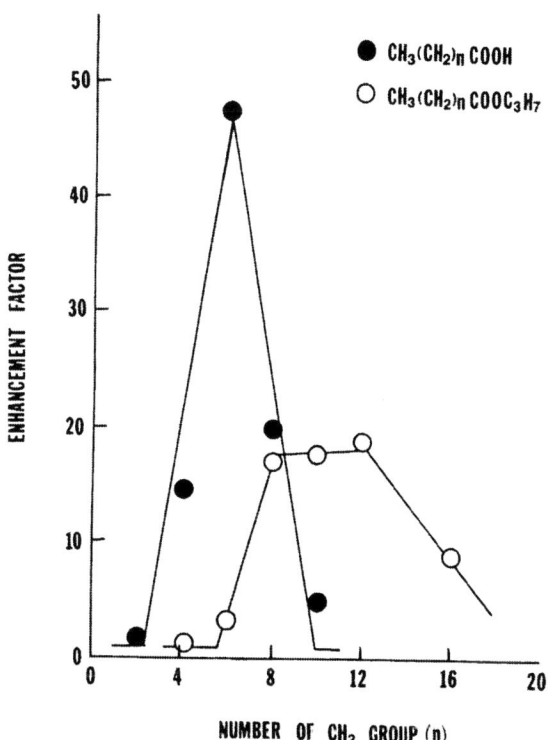

Figure 36   Dependence of the enhancement factor for the skin permeation of progesterone on the alkyl chain length of saturated fatty acid and the effect of esterification.

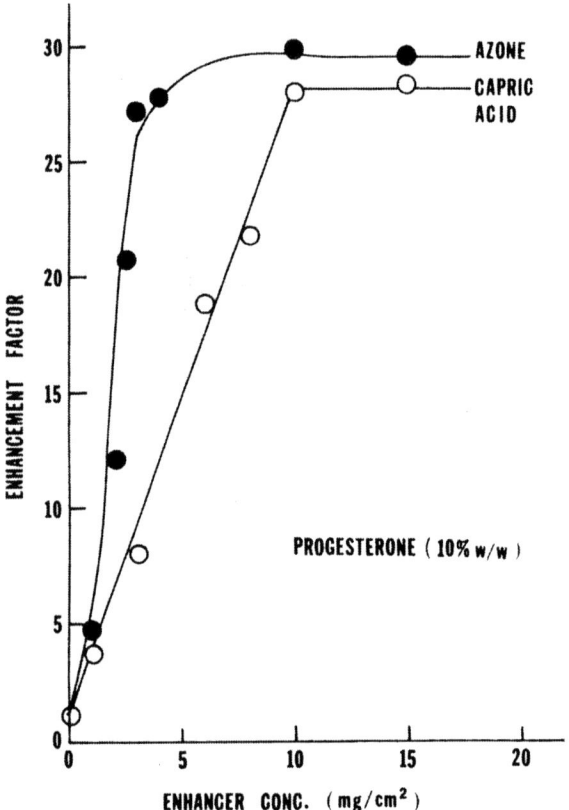

Figure 37   Relationship of the enhancement factor for the skin permeation of progesterone with the concentration of skin permeation enhancers.

Table 9   Skin Permeability Enhancement of Indomethacin by
Combination of Enhancers

Enhancers		
1: ($1.6 \ mg/cm^2$)	2: ($1.6 \ mg/cm^2$)	Enhancement factor
Azone	Azone	14.49
Azone	—	7.48
Azone	Propyl oleate	8.44
Azone	Oleic acid	13.47
Azone	Oleyl alcohol	15.25
Azone	Oleyl acetate	18.96
Azone	Mono-olein	7.19
Azone	Propyl myristate	8.98
Azone	Myristyl alcohol	5.10
Azone	Myristyl N,N- dimethylamide	12.02

the adhesive layer (Fig. 37). A synergistic effect in skin permeability enhancement could be achieved by incorporating two or more
enhancers in the adhesive layer (Table 9).

For more detailed discussions of the mechanisms and actions of
skin permeation enhancers, see Chapter 3.

VII.   GENERIC PROGRAM FOR TRANSDERMAL DRUG
DELIVERY SYSTEM DEVELOPMENT

To successfully develop a transdermal therapeutic system, a program
should be established to carry out the preclinical and clinical investigations of transdermal controlled drug administration in a scientific and logical manner. It is believed that the development program for transdermal drug delivery research should consist of the
three major phases of research and development outlined as follows.

Phase I: *Feasibility studies*

1. Compilation of a technical database on the drug candidate, including:
   (a) Daily effective dose by intravenous infusion
   (b) Minimum therapeutic plasma level
   (c) Dose-response relationship by intravenous administration
   (d) Biological half-life
   (e) Volume of distribution
   (f) Rate constant for plasma elimination
   (g) Skin permeability or (skin/vehicle) partition coefficient
   (h) Molecular structure and physicochemical properties
   (i) Stability-indicating analytical method
   (j) Physicochemical compatibility and stability profiles
2. Improvement and optimization of a sensitive analytical method for skin permeation kinetics studies of the drug candidate
3. In vitro evaluations of long-term skin permeation rate profiles of the drug candidate, including:
   (a) Determination of skin permeability
   (b) Determination of cutaneous metabolism profile
   (c) Determination of tissue-binding capacity
   (d) Effect of skin sources
   (e) Effect of vehicles
   (f) Effect of environmental conditions
   (g) Effect of skin permeation enhancers
   (h) Effect of drug analogues and derivatives

Phase II: *Formulation development*

1. Development of transdermal therapeutic systems; kinetic evaluations and system optimization, including the following:
   (a) Effect of system design
   (b) Effect of polymer composition
   (c) Effect of adhesive formulation
   (d) Preliminary stability testing
2. In vivo evaluations of transdermal therapeutic systems (6-8 healthy subjects or model animals), including:
   (a) Development of a stability-indicating bioassay
   (b) Monitoring of the onset, level, and duration of plasma concentration profiles of drug and metabolites versus reference dosage forms
   (c) Quantitation of steady-state plasma drug level and patch size relationship (using 3-4 patch sizes and one selected skin site)
   (d) Establishment of in vitro-in vivo correlation and formulation optimization

(e) Establishment of steady-state plasma drug level and skin site relationship (using one selected patch size and different skin sites)

(f) Evaluation of the skin sensitization–drug delivery rate relationship

Phase III: *Regulatory submission, clinical evaluations, and production*

1. Submission of Investigational New Drug Application (INDA) to the regulatory agency
2. Clinical trials in patient population, including:
   (a) Comparative pharmacokinetic profiles following single transdermal system application versus reference dosage forms (single and multiple doses)
   (b) Variability in steady-state pharmacokinetic profiles following single transdermal system application with respect to:
       (i) Effect of skin site
       (ii) Effect of age
       (iii) Effect of sex
   (c) Establishment of pharmacokinetics–pharmacodynamics relationship
   (d) Comparative pharmacodynamic profiles following single transdermal system application versus multiple-dosing reference dosage forms
   (e) Steady-state pharmacokinetic and pharmacodynamic profiles following multiple applications of transdermal therapeutic system on one selected skin site
3. Pharmaceutical engineering; development of manufacturing process and equipment, including:
   (a) Equipment—design, calibration, and validation
   (b) Process—scaling up, challenging, and qualification
   (c) Contract manufacturing—evaluation and qualification
   (d) Raw materials—establishment of quality control specifications
   (e) Total stability program
4. Submission of New Drug Application (NDA) to the regulatory agency
5. Regulatory approval and marketing

REFERENCES

1. J. E. Shaw and S. K. Chandrasekaran, Controlled topical delivery of drugs for systemic action, *Drug Metab. Rev.*, *8*: 223 (1978).

2. 1982 Industrial Pharmaceutical R & D Symposium on Transdermal Controlled Release Medication, Rutgers University College of Pharmacy, Piscataway, NJ, January 14-15, 1982. Proceedings published in *Drug Dev. Ind. Pharm.*, 9(4): 497-744 (1983).

3. World Congress of Clinical Pharmacology Symposium on Transdermal Delivery of Cardiovascular Drugs, Washington, DC, August 5, 1983. Proceedings published in *Am. Heart J.*, 108(1): 195-236 (1984).

4. Y. W. Chien, Logics of transdermal controlled drug administration, *Drug Dev. Ind. Pharm.*, 9: 497 (1983).

5. R. Sitruk-Ware, B. deLignieres, A. Basdevant, and P. Mauvais-Jarvis, Absorption of percutaneous oestradiol in postmenopausal women, *Maturitas*, 2: 207 (1980).

6. Symposium on Problems and Possibilities for Transdermal Drug Delivery, Schools of Medicine and Pharmacy, University of California, San Francisco, February 2-3, 1985.

7. 1985 International Pharmaceutical R & D Symposium on Advances in Transdermal Controlled Drug Administration for Systemic Medications, Rutgers Unviersity, College of Pharmacy, Piscataway, NJ, June 20-21, 1985.

8. APhA/APS 39th National Meeting, "Pharm. Sci. 85," Minneapolis, October 20-24, 1985.

9. Y. W. Chien, *Novel Drug Delivery Systems: Fundamentals, Developmental Concepts and Biomedical Assessments*, Dekker, New York, 1982, Chapter 5.

10. D. R. Sanvordeker, J. G. Cooney, and R. C. Wester, Transdermal nitroglycerin pad, U.S. Patent 4,336,243, June 22, 1982.

11. P. R. Keshary, Y. C. Huang, and Y. W. Chien, unpublished data, personal communication, (1984).

12. K. H. Valia and Y. W. Chien, Long-term skin permeation kinetics of estradiol. I. Effect of drug solubilizer—polyethylene glycol 400, *Drug. Dev. Ind. Pharm.*, 10: 951 (1984).

13. K. H. Valia and Y. W. Chien, Long-term skin permeation kinetics of estradiol. II. Kinetics of skin uptake, binding and metabolism, *Drug Dev. Ind. Pharm.*, 10: 991 (1984).

14. W. R. Good, Transderm-Nitro: Controlled delivery of nitroglycerin via the transdermal route, *Drug. Dev. Ind. Pharm.*, 9: 647 (1983).

15. A. Gerardin, J. Hirtz, P. Fankhauser, and J. Moppert, Achievement of sustained plasma concentrations of nitroglycerin (TNG) in man by a transdermal therapeutic system, in APhA/APS 31st National Meeting Abstracts, 11(2): 84 (1981).

16. J. E. Shaw, Pharmacokinetics of nitroglycerin and clonidine delivered by the transdermal route, *Am. Heart J.*, 108: 217 (1984).

17. M. A. Weber and J. I. M. Drayer, Clinical experience with rate-controlled delivery of antihypertensive therapy by a transdermal system, *Am. Heart J.*, *108*: 231 (1984).

18. D. Arndts and K. Arndts, Pharmacokinetics and pharmacodynamics of transdermally administered clonidine, *Eur. J. Clin. Pharmacol.*, *26*: 79 (1984).

19. S. Hwang, E. Owada, L. Suhardja, N. F. H. Ho, G. L. Flynn, and W. I. Higuchi, Systems approach to vaginal delivery of drugs. V. In situ vaginal absorption of 1-Alkanoic acids, *J. Pharm. Sci.*, *66*: 781 (1977).

20. L. Schenkel, J. Balestra, L. Schmitt, and J. Shaw, Transdermal oestrogen substitution in the menopause, in *Second International Conference on Drug Absorption—Rate Control in Drug Therapy*, University of Edinburgh, Edinburgh, Scotland, September 21–23, 1983, p. 41.

21. L. R. Laufer, J. L. De Fazio, J. K. H. Lu, D. R. Meldrum, P. Eggena, M. P. Sambhi, J. M. Hershman, and H. L. Judd, Estrogen replacement therapy by transdermal estradiol administration, *Am. J. Obstet, Gynecol.*, *146*: 533 (1983).

22. T. J. Roseman, R. M. Bennett, J. J. Biermacher, M. E. Tuttle, and C. H. Spilman, Design criteria for carbopost methyl controlled release devices, in *Proceedings of 11th International Symposium on Controlled Release Bioactive Materials* (W. E. Meyers and R. L. Dunn, eds.), Controlled Release Society, Inc., Lincolnshire, IL, 1984, p. 50.

23. Y. W. Chien, *Novel Drug Delivery Systems*, Dekker, New York, 1982, Chapter 9.

24. A. D. Keith, Polymer matrix considerations for transdermal devices, *Drug Dev. Ind. Pharm.*, *9*: 605 (1983).

25. Y. W. Chien and H. J. Lambert, Microsealed pharmaceutical delivery devices, U.S. Patent 3,946,106, March 23, 1976.

26. Y. W. Chien and H. J. Lambert, Method for making a microsealed delivery device, U.S. Patent 3,992,518, November 16, 1976.

27. Y. W. Chien and H. J. Lambert, Microsealed pharmaceutical delivery device, U.S. Patent 4,053,580, October 11, 1977.

28. A. Karim, Transdermal absorption: A unique opportunity for constant delivery of nitroglycerin, *Drug Dev. Ind. Pharm.*, *9*: 671 (1983).

29. Y. W. Chien, Microsealed drug delivery systems: Theoretical aspects and biomedical assessments, in *International Symposium, Recent Advances in Drug Delivery Systems* (J. M. Anderson and S. W. Kim, eds.) Plenum Press, New York, 1984, p. 367.

30. Y. W. Chien, Long-term controlled navel administration of testosterone, *J. Pharm. Sci.*, *73*: 1064 (1984).

31. Y. W. Chien, P. R. Keshary, Y. C. Huang, and P. P. Sarpotdar, Comparative controlled skin permeation of nitroglycerin from

marketed transdermal delivery systems, *J. Pharm. Sci.*, *72*: 968 (1983).

32. S. J. Davidson, L. D. Nichols, A. S. Obermayer, M. B. Allen, E. J. Murphy, and R. N. Hurd, Developing a controlled release dual-antibiotic wound dressing, in *Proceedings of 11th International Symposium on Controlled Release Bioactive Materials* (W. E. Meyers and R. L. Dunn, eds.), Controlled Release Society, Inc., Lincolnshire, IL, 1984, pp. 58 and 60.

33. A. C. Hymes, A hydrophilic polymeric reservoir for transdermal drug delivery, in APhA/APS Midwest Regional Meeting, April 2, 1984, Chicago.

34. H. Durrheim, G. L. Flynn, W. I. Higuchi, and C. R. Behl, Permeation of hairless mouse skin. I. Experimental methods and comparison with human epidermal permeation by alkanols, *J. Pharm. Sci.*, *69*: 781 (1980).

35. K. Tojo, M. Ghannam, Y. Sun, and Y. W. Chien, Intrinsic Rates of permeation and release through polymeric drug delivery systems, in APS/APhA 37th National Meeting Abstracts, *14(2)*: 193 (1984).

36. D. E. Magnuson, personal communication, 1983.

37. Y. W. Chien, Pharmaceutical considerations of transdermal nitroglycerin delivery: The various approaches, *Am. Heart J.*, *108*: 207 (1984).

38. J. E. Shaw, S. K. Chandrasekaran, A. S. Michaels, and L. Taskovich, Controlled transdermal delivery, in vitro and in vivo, in *Animal Models in Dermatology* (H. Maibach, ed.) Churchill-Livingston, Edinburgh, 1975, Chapter 14.

39. P. W. Armstrong, J. A. Armstrong, and G. S. Marks, Blood levels after sublingual nitroglycerin, *Circulation*, *59*: 585 (1979).

40. A. D. Keith, personal communication, (1983).

41. M. Wolff, G. Cordes, and V. Luckow, In vitro and in vivo release of nitroglycerin from a new transdermal therapeutic system, *Pharm. Res.*, *1*: 23–29 (1985).

42. P. R. Keshary, Y. C. Huang, and Y. W. Chien, Mechanism of transdermal controlled nitroglycerin administration. III. Control of skin permeation rate and optimization, *Drug. Dev. Ind. Pharm.*, *11*: 1213–1254 (1985).

43. Y. W. Chien, K. H. Valia, and U. B. Doshi, Long-term permeation kinetics of estradiol. V. Development and evaluation of transdermal bioactivated hormone delivery system, *Drug Dev. Ind. Pharm.*, *11*: 1195–1212 (1985).

44. K. H. Valia, K. Tojo, and Y. W. Chien, Long-term permeation kinetics of estradiol. III. Kinetic analyses of the simultaneous skin permeation and bioconversion of estradiol esters, *Drug Dev. Ind. Pharm.*, *11*: 1133–1173 (1985).

45. Y. W. Chien, Developmental concepts and practice in transdermal therapeutic systems, Abstracts of 1985 International Pharmaceutical R & D Symposium on Advances in Transdermal Controlled Drug Administration for Systemic Medications, Rutgers University, College of Pharmacy, Piscataway, NJ, June 20–21, 1985, pp. 8–11.

46. Y. W. Chien and C. S. Lee, Enhancement in transdermal controlled drug delivery. I. Development of a skin-permeation-enhancing transdermal therapeutic system, presented at the Academy of Pharmaceutical Sciences' 39th National Meeting and Exposition, Minneapolis, October 20–24, 1985. *Abstracts*, p. 109.

47. E. R. Cooper, Permeability enhancement in skin permeation, Abstracts of 1985 International Pharmaceutical R & D Symposium on Advances in Transdermal Controlled Drug Administration for Systemic Medications, Rutgers University, College of Pharmacy, Piscataway, NJ, June 20–21, 1985, p. 7.

48. T. Higuchi and V. Stella, Prodrugs as novel drug delivery systems, American Chemical Society, Washington, DC, (1975).

49. K. Tojo, K. H. Valia, G. Chotani, and Y. W. Chien, Long-term permeation kinetics of estradiol. IV. A theoretical approach to the simultaneous skin permeation and bioconversion of estradiol esters, *Drug Dev. Ind. Pharm.*, *11*: 1175–1193 (1985).

50. Y. W. Chien, The use of biocompatible polymers in rate-controlled drug delivery systems, *Pharm. Techn.*, *9*(5): 50–66 (1985).

51. P. W. Armstrong, J. A. Armstrong, and G. S. Marks, Pharmacokinetic–hemodynamic studies of nitroglycerin ointment in congestive heart failure, *Am. J. Cardiol.*, *46*: 670 (1980).

3

Alterations in Skin Permeability

EUGENE R. COOPER / Alcon Laboratories, Inc., Fort Worth, Texas

I. INTRODUCTION

This chapter discusses various methods for promoting skin permeation. Although there are enhancement methods specific for skin, there are general considerations that apply for the enhancement of permeation across any membrane (e.g., the cornea, the skin, etc.). By permeation, one really means flux, and one is thus concerned with the problem of increasing the flux across membranes. For any region within a membrane the flux, J, can be written as follows:

$$J = -D\frac{\partial C}{\partial x}$$ (1)

for flow in one dimension. Here D is the diffusion coefficient, C is the permeant concentration, and x is the spatial coordinate. Although the solution for J with various boundary conditions and membrane heterogeneities can be very complex (1), the basic concepts regarding flux enhancement can be found in Eq. (1). The concentration gradient is thermodynamic in origin, and the diffusion coefficient is related to the size and shape of the permeant and to the energy required to make a hole for diffusion. Thus enhancement of flux across membranes reduces to considerations of:

1. Thermodynamics (lattice energies, distribution coefficients)
2. Molecular size and shape
3. Reducing the energy required to make a molecular hole in the membrane

Although these basic concepts can be used to develop systems for enhanced transport, such practical considerations as vehicle evaporation and excipient interactions make useful systems somewhat evasive. Most of the discussion in this chapter deals with technology for altering membranes, but a brief look at thermodynamic factors is included as well.

II. ENHANCEMENT RECOGNITION

There are two basic kinds of enhancement measurement—the comparison of fluxes of the same molecule from two different vehicles and the comparison of the fluxes of two different molecules from the same vehicle. The latter case often results from an attempt to alter the structure to gain improved penetration. The amount of increase in penetration is simply the ratio, R, where

$$R = \frac{J_1}{J_2} \tag{2}$$

Here J_1 is the flux from vehicle 1 (or molecule 1) and J_2 is the flux from vehicle 2 (or molecule 2). Often these fluxes will not be at steady state, since the membrane barrier properties will be changing with time if enhancement is occurring.

For R to be a true measure of vehicle enhancement, the drug in each vehicle must be at the same thermodynamic activity. This result is most easily achieved by using saturated solutions or equal fractions of saturation. One demonstrates this fact by equating the activities, a, in each vehicle, where

$$a_1 = a_2 \tag{3}$$

The activity coefficient is $a = \gamma c$, where γ is the activity coefficient and C is the concentration. Thus Eq. (3) can be written as:

$$\frac{C_1}{C_2} = \frac{\gamma_2}{\gamma_1} = \frac{S_1}{S_2} \tag{4}$$

where S is the solubility. The concentration ratio must always be the same as the solubility ratio. A similar result follows for comparing

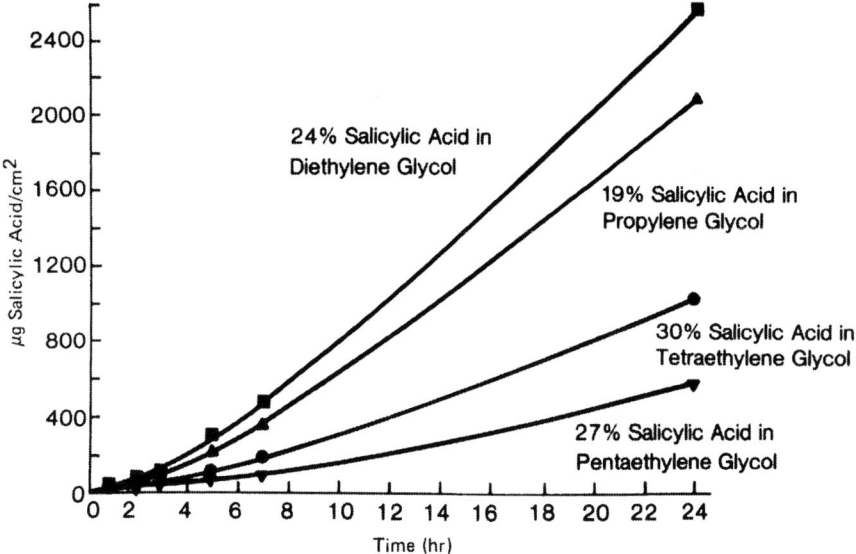

Figure 1   Effect of polar solvents on the transport of salicylic acid across human epidermis from saturated solutions.

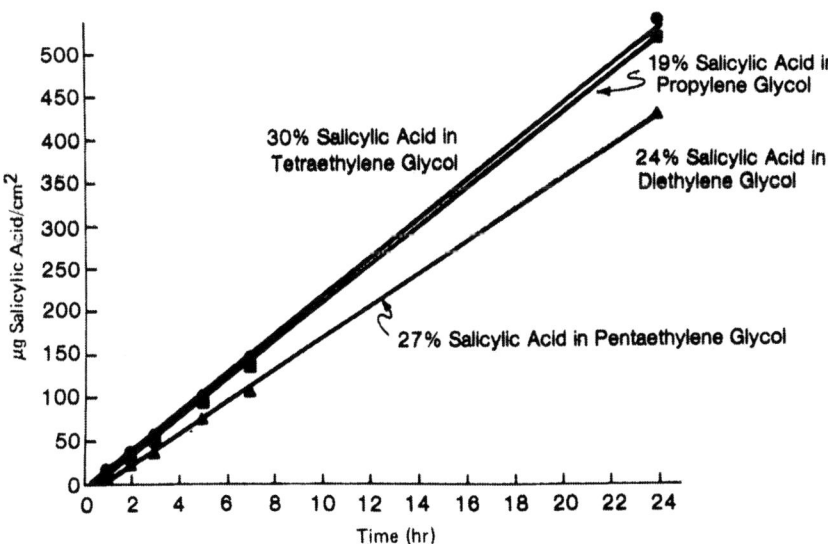

Figure 2   Effect of polar solvents on the transport of salicylic acid across silicone membrane from saturated solutions.

two different drugs from the same vehicle. Here one is interested in comparing the maximum fluxes, which occurs at saturation. The same comparison can also be made at equal fractions of saturation. An example of different solvent effects is shown in Figure 1, which plots the flux of salicylic acid across human epidermis from different polyols. The flux decreases with increasing number of ethoxylates for skin but is the same from all vehicles for transport across a Silastic membrane (Fig. 2).

III. MEMBRANE ALTERATIONS

A. Proteins

As noted previously, if vehicle-induced penetration enhancement is to occur, the energy for making diffusion holes must be altered. This process can take place if a solvent swells the barrier and is most obvious for water-swellable polymer films, where transport is very sensitive to hydration. For skin one must alter the protein and/or the lipids to make it "easier" for a molecule to diffuse through these media. It is well known that surfactants can alter the proteins of the stratum corneum (2-6), and thus increase penetration. This effect appears to be much larger for polar molecules than for non-polar molecules, as in Figures 3 and 4. In Figure 3 one sees that the flux of salicylic acid at pH 2.65 (nonpolar form) is only slightly affected by treatment with decylmethyl sulfoxide ($C_{10}MSO$). At pH 9.9 (polar form) the flux is greatly enhanced (Fig. 4). The stratum corneum proteins can be denatured by heat, and again one observes a pronounced effect on the polar molecules (Fig. 5). The interaction of the surfactant with the stratum corneum appears to be governed by the hydrophilicity (5) of the surfactant. The more hydrophilic surfactants (ionic and zwitterionic) interact strongly with the keratin and alter transport, and the less hydrophilic surfactants (long-chain alcohols) interact weakly and do not alter the transport of polar molecules.

Pursuit of this general approach would lead one to look for solvents and other agents that can interact strongly with keratin. Urea has been reported to enhance skin penetration (7), and at high concentrations it can also denature proteins. Many agents and solvents that interact strongly with proteins (e.g., disulfide reducing agents), however, can be extremely irritating, and thus one is left with the difficult task of searching for materials that can localize in the stratum corneum and not penetrate significantly into the viable tissue below the stratum corneum.

B. Lipids

To alter the fluid properties of the stratum corneum lipids, one must be able to "swell" the lipids or increase the volume per molecule.

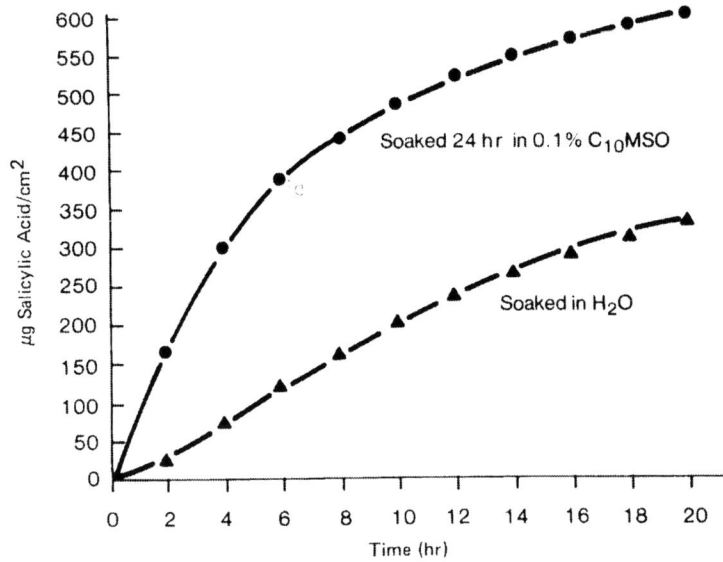

Figure 3   Effect of decylmethyl sulfoxide ($C_{10}MSO$) on the penetration of salicylic acid across human epidermis from 0.2% aqueous solution at pH 2.65.

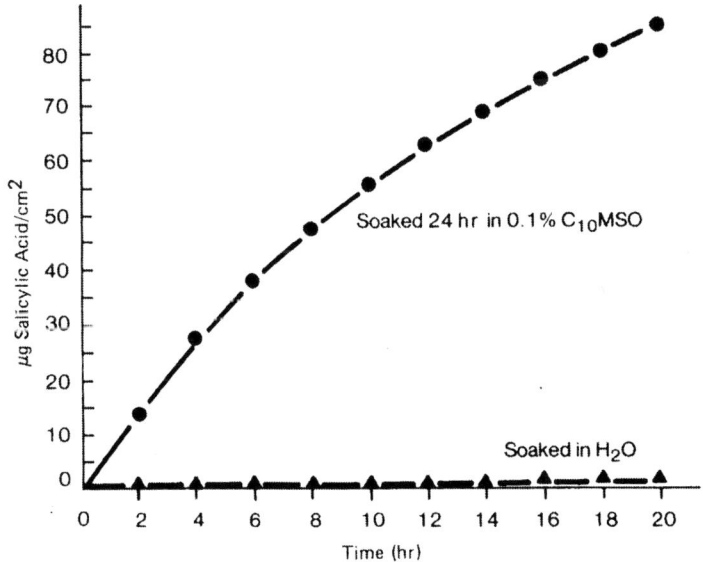

Figure 4   Effect of decylmethyl sufoxide ($C_{10}MSO$) on the penetration of salicylic acid across human epidermis from 0.2% aqueous solution at pH 9.9.

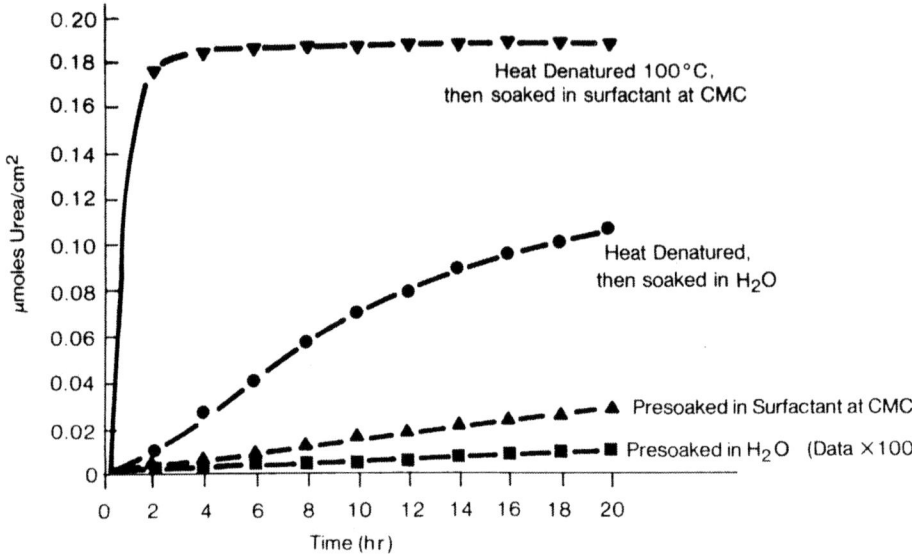

Figure 5 Effect of nonionic surfactants and heat denaturation on the penetration of urea across human epidermis.

The process is analogous to a solid-to-liquid phase change. This concept is quite obvious if one just considers how impermeable a solid, crystalline material is compared to a liquid or semisolid. The lowering of melting points in multicomponent systems is well known from phase diagram studies, and this process must somehow be utilized to fluidize the lipids.

An example of what is believed to be enhancement via the lipid fluidization mechanism is shown in Figure 6 (8), where oleic acid acts as an enhancer for salicylic acid. (Figure 7 illustrates how oleic acid may be altering the lipid packing.) Other fatty acids can also enhance penetration, and it seems quite probable that Azone acts by a similar mechanism. The polarity of the head group appears to play little role in the enhancement of lipophilic molecules (8). If a very hydrophilic head group is used, however, the penetration of both polar and nonpolar molecules can be accomplished.

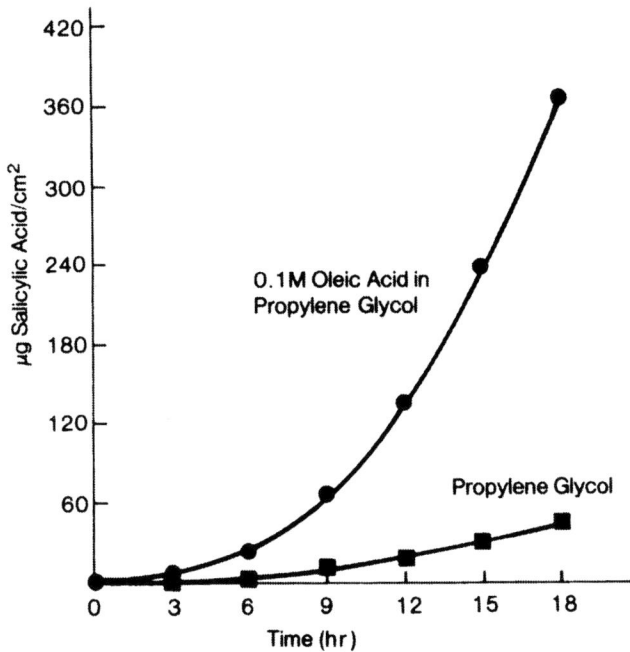

Figure 6   Effect of oleic acid on the penetration of salicylic acid across human epidermis.

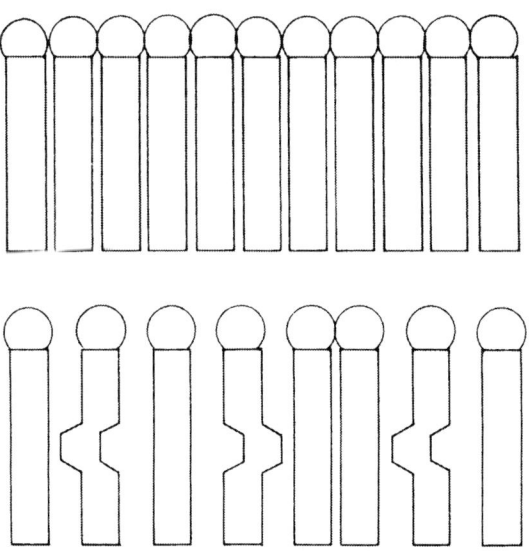

Figure 7   Model for oleic acid-induced lipid disruption.

IV. REDUCTION OF PENETRATION

In many cases one desires to enhance penetration, but in some instances reduced penetration is desired. This problem is really more challenging than the enhancement problem. Figure 1 may serve to point out some of the issues. Here one observes that the polyethylene glycols reduce penetration relative to propylene glycol. This result might be simply interpreted to indicate that propylene glycol enhances penetration and the other solvents do not. However, polyethylene glycols appear to have a "protective" effect on skin with respect to reducing the barrier damage of surfactants. Ethoxylated surfactants can have a similar effect (9). For example, the swelling effect of sodium dodecyl sulfate can be inhibited by treatment with polyethylene glycol. Thus there may be something to the concept that penetration can be reduced by means other than reduction in driving force via thermodynamic considerations.

Formulation excipients can render penetration enhancers ineffective. These effects are probably thermodynamic in origin but are very much a practical consideration. Thus, the identification of an enhancer is the first step, but reduction in penetration can occur as a multicomponent formulation is developed. For example if a surfactant is used as an enhancer, its effect can be greatly reduced by the addition of other surfactants.

V. SUMMARY

The enhancement of penetration across membranes is conceptually rather simple. The discovery of agents to alter the barrier energy to hole formation can be a somewhat empirical process, but the task can also be approached from a basic study of the thermodynamics and kinetics of expanding the structure of protein and lipids. For example, the effect of agents on the compressibility of monolayer films can easily be studied with a Langmuir trough. In addition, various spectroscopic techniques can be employed to investigate detailed molecular interactions. Once a more basic understanding of the interactions of chemical agents with proteins and lipids has been achieved, the shopping list for enhancers will be greatly expanded.

REFERENCES

1. R. M. Barrer, Diffusion and permeation in heterogeneous media, *Diffusion in Polymers* (J. Crank and G. S. Park, eds.), Academic Press, New York, 1968, p. 165.
2. F. R. Bettley and E. Donoghue, Effect of soap on the diffusion of water through isolated human epidermis, *Nature*, *17*: 185 (1960).

3. F. R. Bettley, The influence of detergents and surfactants on epidermal permeability, *Br. J. Dermatol.*, *77*: 98 (1965).
4. R. J. Scheuplein and L. Ross, Effects of surfactants and solvents on the permeability of epidermis, *J. Soc. Cosmet. Chem.*, *21*: 853 (1970).
5. E. R. Cooper, Effect of decylmethyl sulfoxide on skin penetration, in *Solution Behavior of Surfactants* (K. L. Mittal and E. J. Fendler, eds.), Plenum Press, New York, 1982, p. 1505.
6. R. J. Scheuplein and P. H. Dugard, Effects of ionic surfactants on the permeability of human epidermis: An electrometric study, *J. Invest. Dermatol.*, *60*: 263 (1973).
7. P. J. W. Ayres and G. Hooper, Assessment of the skin penetration properties of different vehicles for topically applied cortisol, *Br. J. Dermatol.*, *99*: 307 (1978).
8. E. R. Cooper, Increased skin permeability for lipophilic molecules, *J. Pharm. Sci.*, *73*: 1153 (1984).
9. Unpublished observations by the author.

4

Pressure-Sensitive Adhesives: Science and Engineering

MARTIN C. MUSOLF / *Dow Corning Corporation, Midland, Michigan*

I. INTRODUCTION

A. Historical Development of Pressure-Sensitive Adhesives

A pressure-sensitive adhesive is generally defined as a material that will adhere to a substrate when a light pressure is applied and will leave no residue when removed. Since the first patent issued more than 140 years ago (in 1845), pressure-sensitive adhesives have found widespread use in both industrial and consumer markets. It was not long before the potential of medical applications was recognized with the first application of a tackified, zinc oxide-filled natural rubber for hospital tape in 1899. During World War II, isobutylene-and butyl rubber-based pressure-sensitive adhesives were developed to replace the waning supply of natural rubber. Acrylic adhesives were developed in the postwar years. Since 1950, a great number of polymers have been developed and used as pressure-sensitive adhesives, including a relative newcomer, silicone adhesives.

Apart from the use in tapes and labels, other specific applications of pressure-sensitive adhesives have continued to be developed, and some of them have rigorous property requirements. One of the recent applications is in the area of transdermal drug delivery (TDD) systems, which requires the use of pressure-sensitive adhesives to maintain an intimate contact of TDD systems with the skin surface

(Chapter 2). In addition to the usual requirements of pressure-sensitive properties, a TDD system also requires that an adhesive be nonirritating to skin, physically and chemically compatible with the drugs, and moisture resistant. It must adhere to all skin types, leave no residue upon removal, and conform to skin contour and accommodate skin movement.

B. Important Application in Transdermal
   Drug Delivery Systems

There are three basic designs of TDD systems, and each requires the pressure-sensitive adhesive to perform under slightly different conditions. In one system, a drug-loaded matrix or reservoir is totally covered by a rate-controlling membrane and the drug-releasing surface is coated with an adhesive film, which is protected by a release liner (Fig. 1). To use this device, the release liner is stripped from the adhesive layer and the device is placed on the body at the desired location.

Since the adhesive layer is positioned across the drug-releasing surface of the device, the drug must be able to diffuse through the adhesive without adversely affecting the adhesive properties of the adhesive film, and the adhesive polymer used should not have any physicochemical incompatibility with the diffusing drug, nor should it affect the overall delivery rate of the drug.

Two commercial systems based on this design are Transderm-Nitro, which delivers nitroglycerin for the 24-hr alleviation of angina

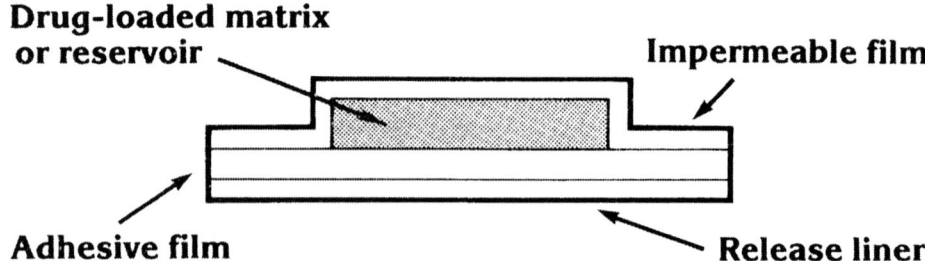

Adhesive Across the Face

Figure 1   Transdermal drug delivery systems with adhesive film coating over the drug-releasing surface.

Adhesive Around Edges

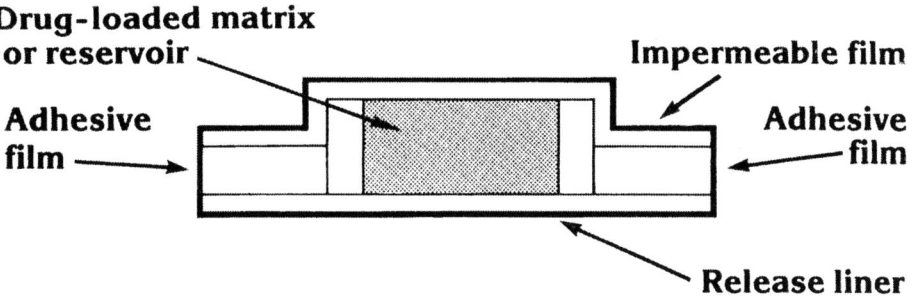

Figure 2   Transdermal drug delivery systems with adhesive film coating around the edge of the drug-releasing surface.

symptoms, and Transderm-Scop, which delivers scopolamine for the 72-hr prevention of motion sickness. Both these products are marketed by Ciba Pharmaceutical Corporation.

A second type of TDD system also uses a drug-loaded matrix or reservoir, but the adhesive film is located around the edge of the drug-releasing device (Fig. 2). Since the adhesive does not come in direct contact with the drug, only its adhesive properties and biocompatibility characteristics are of concern. Two commercial products are based on this design, both delivering nitroglycerin. One is Nitro-Dur by Key Pharmaceuticals, and the other is Nitro-disc by Searle Pharmaceuticals.

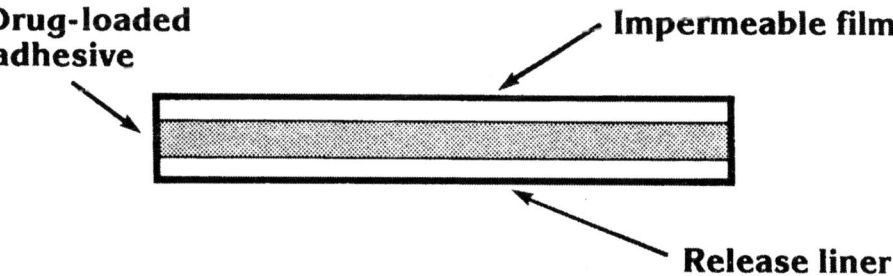

Figure 3   Transdermal drug delivery systems with drug dispersed in the adhesive film.

The third type is rather simple in system design in that the drug is directly loaded or dispersed into the pressure-sensitive adhesive polymer. The drug-dispersed adhesive is protected on one side by an impermeable film and on the other side by a removable release liner (Fig. 3). As in the first design, the adhesive must be inert to and permeable to the drug, and the adhesive properties must not be adversely affected by the drug. Deponit, manufactured by Pharma-Schwarz/Lohmann in West Germany, is representative of this type of TDD system. This device is also designed to deliver nitroglycerin.

The evaluation of pressure-sensitive adhesives for these systems is an exacting task, involving the evaluations of general adhesive properties as well as specific testing of dermal toxicity and human wear. Initial screening involves the use of standard pressure-sensitive adhesive test methods, but many more specific tests are still under development.

II. PRESSURE-SENSITIVE ADHESIVES

A. Preparation of Test Laminates

Typical adhesive evaluations are carried out by using adhesive laminates, which are the composites made of a backing sheet or membrane, an adhesive film, and a release liner. They can be prepared easily in the laboratory by a direct coating process in which the adhesive is applied onto the backing sheet and the adhesive film formed is then covered by a release liner. This process has a disadvantage, however: when one tries to coat a solvent-based adhesive, the backing sheet may be sensitive to the adhesive solvent, which could result in warped, nonuniform laminates.

Another technique of preparing adhesive laminates, involving a transfer coating process, is more commonly used and eliminates the potential solvent-backing sheet compatibility problems. In this process the adhesive is applied on the release liner, the solvent is allowed to evaporate, and then the backing sheet is applied to the adhesive film. Release liners are usually prepared from materials that have been made resistant to solvents.

The laboratory-scale transfer coating process outlined in Figure 4 can be easily carried out. A release liner (8.5 in. × 11 in.) is taped to a flat, smooth surface or held in place on a vacuum table. A sample of adhesive solution or emulsion is placed across the top edge of the release liner. The adhesive film is metered onto the liner by drawing a doctor blade or a Mayer rod from the top edge to the bottom. A Mayer rod is a metal rod, tightly wrapped with a wire. Large-diameter wires increase the spaces between the touching wires and the release liner, which produces a heavier coating. The correct

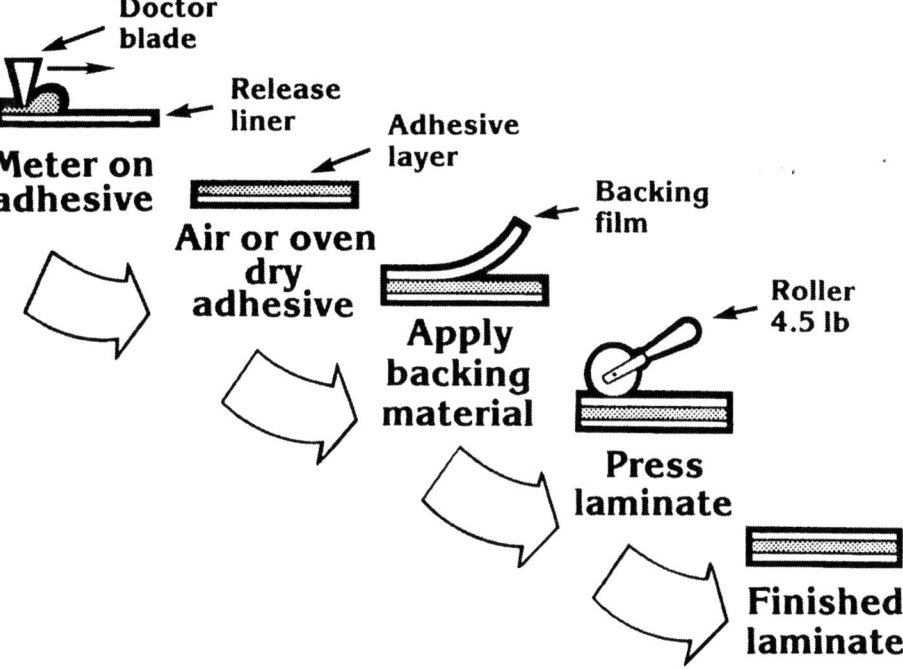

Figure 4   Transfer coating process used in the laboratory for making adhesive laminate (Dow Corning procedure).

Mayer rod is chosen to give a dry adhesive film with thickness ranging from 0.0015 to 0.002 in. (0.04−0.05 mm).

The wet adhesive film is then allowed to dry, either at room temperature or in an oven. Appropriate oven safety precautions must be exercised if a flammable solvent is being used. If oven drying is used, the oven temperature should be properly controlled to prevent the production of nonuniform and possibly foamed adhesive films caused by the rapid evaporation of solvent at high temperature.

A backing sheet is carefully placed on the dry adhesive. The laminate is smoothed by rolling a 4.5-pound roller, with no additional pressure, once from the top to the bottom and once from the bottom to the top. The finished laminate is usually aged for three days at standard conditions, such as 25°C and 50% relative humidity, before testing. The laminate is then cut into strips and is ready for testing.

B. Evaluations of Adhesive Properties

The evaluation of pressure-sensitive adhesives begins with the following three basic properties: peel adhesion, tack, and shear strength.
Every application requires a different combination of these properties. Although the possible combinations cf properties can be virtually endless, obtaining the correct one is often difficult. The improvement of one property must be carefully balanced against the possible destruction of another.

1. Peel Adhesion Properties

Peel adhesion is the force required to remove an adhesive coating from a test substrate. It is important in TDD system applications because the bond must provide adequate adhesion to the skin, yet allow nontraumatic removal. Some of the variables that can influence the peel adhesion properties include the molecular weight of adhesive polymer, the type and amount of additives (e.g., tackifiers), and polymer composition.

The most widely used test for peel adhesion is PSTC test no. 1: Peel Adhesion for Single-Coated Tapes, 180-Degree Angle (1). This test is one of many specified by the Pressure-Sensitive Tape Council (PSTC) and accepted as the industry standards. A single-coated tape is applied to a stainless steel plate or a backing of choice, and the tape is then pulled from the substrate at a 180° angle, typically using an Instron tester to measure the force (Fig. 5). The force is expressed in ounces (or grams) per inch width of tape, with higher values indicating greater bond strength. Test sample preparation and test conditions are specified in the method (1). If the pulled tape does not leave any residue on the plate, it indicates "adhesive failure," which is desirable for most applications, especially for TDD system. If some residue is left behind, it suggests "cohesive failure," which often signifies a lack of cohesive strength.

2. Tack Properties

Tack is the ability of a polymer to adhere to a substrate with little contact pressure. It is important in TDD systems, which are applied with finger pressure.

Tack is affected by the molecular weight and the composition of polymer, among other factors, but is particularly influenced by the use of tackifying resins. The polymer, such as polyisobutylene, has a low glass transition temperature and provides cohesive strength with some latent tack. Tack may be increased through the addition of a tackifying resin. There are a number of theories concerning the role of tackifying resins. Current thought suggests that the resin dissolves out the low-molecular-weight species (the tacky

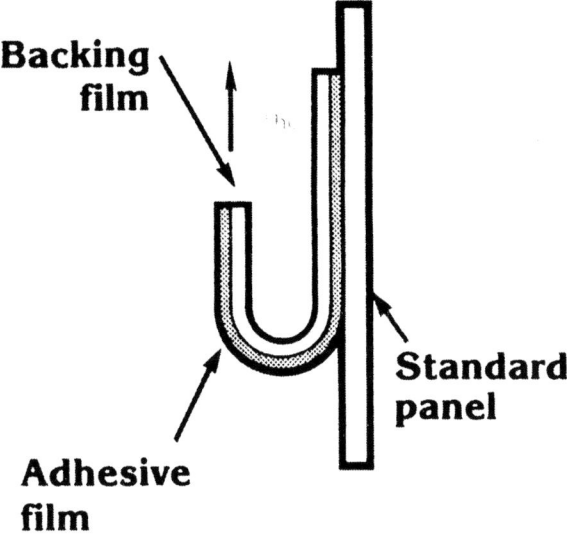

Backing film

Adhesive film

Standard panel

180° Peel test

Figure 5   Peel adhesion test (PSTC no. 1) for adhesive evaluation. (From Ref. 1.)

portion) in the polymer and brings them to the surface, where they are available to adhere to the substrate. Not all polymers require tackifiers to achieve tack.

There are four generally accepted tests for tack: the thumb, rolling ball, quick-stick (peel-tack), and probe tack tests. Each one assesses a different aspect of the property.

Thumb Tack Test: One simply presses the thumb briefly into the adhesive. The tack property can be detected. By experience, one can develop an "educated" thumb and differentiate between degrees of tack. However, the test is rather subjective and, at best, qualitative.

Rolling Ball Tack Test: This test measures the softness of a polymer and relates this to tack. In PSTC test no. 6 (Tack Rolling Ball Method) (1), a stainless steel ball of 7/16-in. diameter is released on an inclined track so as to roll down and come into contact with the horizontal, upward-facing adhesive (Fig. 6). The distance the ball travels along the adhesive provides the measurement of tack, which is usually expressed in inches. The less tacky the adhesive, the farther the ball will travel. Although this is currently

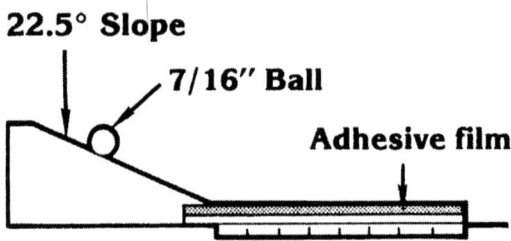

Figure 6   Rolling ball tack test (PSTC no. 6) for adhesive evaluation.   (From Ref. 1.)

the most widely used tack test, its usefulness is becoming limited as more types of adhesive are being evaluated.   Rolling ball tack is highly dependent on the glass transition temperature of an adhesive polymer.   Although it produces a good correlation for tackified natural rubbers, it is not as useful for polymers that exhibit low tack.

   Quick-Stick (or Peel-Tack) Test: This is an extension of the peel adhesion test (PSTC test no. 1).   The primary difference is that in the quick-stick test the coated tape is adhered to the substrate by its own weight.   In PSTC test no. 5 (Quick-Stick test) (1), the tape is pulled away from the substrate at 90° at a speed of 12 in./min (Fig. 7).   The peel force required to break the bond between adhesive and substrate is measured and recorded as the tack value, which is expressed in ounces (or grams) per inch width, with higher values indicating increasing tack.

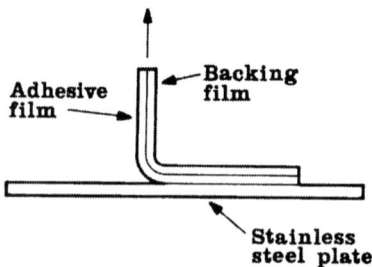

Figure 7   Quick-stick (peel-tack) test (PSTC no. 5) for adhesive evaluation.   (From Ref. 1.)

PSTC test no. 5 can offer a good method of comparing adhesive tapes if the end-use application conditions are similar to those in the test. However, the test is highly influenced by the backing on which the adhesive is coated. For example, different results may be obtained with plastic backing and with cloth backing. It is advisable to prepare test samples in such a way that they simulate the end-use application as closely as possible.

Probe Tack Test: A commonly used tester for this adhesive property is the Polyken Probe Tack Tester (The Kendall Company, Fig. 8). The tip of a cleaned probe with a defined surface roughness is brought into contact with an adhesive, and when a bond has formed between probe and adhesive, it is broken by removing the probe mechanically (2). Rate, pressure, temperature, and test duration must be specified in this ASTM test. The force required to pull the probe away from the adhesive at a fixed rate is recorded as tack (expressed in grams).

3. Shear Strength Properties

Shear strength is the measurement of the cohesive strength of an adhesive polymer. If a transdermal device has adequate cohesive strength, it will not slip after application and will leave no residue upon removal. It can be influenced by the molecular weight, the degree of cross-linking, and the composition of polymer, as well as by the type and the amount of tackifier added. The most widely used test for shear strength is PSTC test no. 7 (Shear Strength test) (1), which outlines the method of preparation for an adhesive-coated tape to be applied onto a stainless steel plate (Fig. 9). A specified weight is hung from the tape, with the pulling in a direction parallel to the plate. Shear strength, which is also called creep

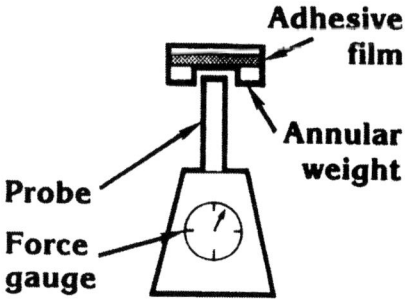

Figure 8 Schematic illustration of the Polyken Probe Tack Tester (ASTM D 2979-71) for adhesive evaluation.

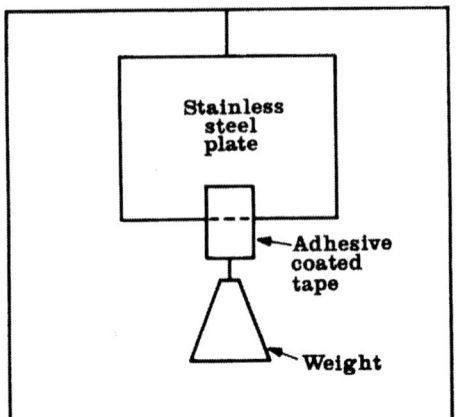

Figure 9   Shear strength test (PSTC no. 7) for adhesive evaluation. (From Ref. 1.)

resistance, is determined by measuring the time it takes to pull the tape off the plate. The longer the time, the greater the shear strength.

Although peel adhesion, tack, and shear strength are basic properties in the screening and characterization of pressure-sensitive adhesives, they are useful mainly for making comparison between products. Any correlation or extrapolation of these properties to practical applications on human skin should not be made without first completing the tests that are more specific to transdermal systems, including human wear testing.

C.   Requirements for Transdermally Applied Adhesive Polymers

1.   Biocompatibility

The pressure-sensitive adhesives used in a transdermal drug delivery (TDD) system must exhibit no skin irritation or systemic toxicity when applied to the skin. This requirement also applies to any materials or agents contained in the TDD system. Potential irritants that may be present include residual solvents, unreacted monomers, antioxidants, tackifiers, and other additives. Although the individual components of a system may have been evaluated for safety, the finished TDD system must be submitted for toxicological testing, which is the only way to predict the biocompatibility of the final product.

Toxicological testing tends to be product specific. That is, testing programs are geared toward specific products, with manufacturing processes and individual components taken into consideration. For such evaluations, the standard toxicological tests, like the irritancy test in albino rabbits and repeat-insult patch tests in humans, are considered to be the minimum testing required.

An example of the product-specific toxicological testing program for adhesive polymers is presented by the studies carried out on Dow Corning 355 medical adhesive (3). In this program, the following tests were performed: rabbit skin and eye irritation (dermal administration to rabbits at 200 mg/kg/day for 28 days) and a guinea pig maximization test for sensitization. Also included were the USP Class V tests for toxic extractables from plastics, rabbit pyrogen tests for saline extracts, and tissue cell cultures for cytopathology. Intramuscular and subcutaneous implantations were performed in rabbits for 90 days. Finally, a human repeat-insult test was performed in 50 patients at nine repetitions.

Another example for the product-specific toxicological testing program is illustrated by the studies conducted on Scothpak 1022 release liner (3M Company), in which two acute ocular and primary skin irritation tests were performed: Magnusson–Kligmann maximization-sensitization tests and a modified Draize–Schelanski–Jordan patch test using 200 subjects. Additional testing included the standard Ames *Salmonella* in vitro mutagenicity assay and recombinogenicity via *Saccharomyces cerevisiae* D_3 assay (3).

2. Skin Adhesion

While adhesion to standard substrates can be defined and is usually reproducible, actual adhesion to human skin is another story. Human skin can be oily, wet, wrinkled, and hairy, representing a wide range of substrates that must be considered. As a result, a proper combination of sufficient adhesion and good removability can be difficult to obtain. Although tests on substrates like pig skin have been done, there still is no substitute for controlled tests on human skin.

Human skin adhesion tests can consist of placing strips of tape on the backs of human subjects and removing them at several intervals over 96 hr, during which skin irritation as well as the adhesive properties are checked (3). To further establish a quantitative measurement on the TDD systems, new tests are under development (4).

3. Environmental Resistance

The adhesive must retain its physicochemical properties under typical environmental conditions. The adhesion properties must tolerate high humidity or water immersion, as well as cold and heat. The adhesive polymer and the total system must also tolerate the normal flexing that would be experienced on the human body.

4. Removability

The adhesive system must be removable without inducing trauma to the skin. The primary irritation test is generally considered as the minimum testing to evaluate an adhesive of its potential suitability for skin contact (5). Such a test, conducted on both abraded and nonabraded skin area of specially bred albino rabbits (Draize rabbit test), consists of observation after a single application of the test adhesive in the form of a patch. The site is rated, after removal, on a scale of 0.00 (nonirritating) to 8.00 (extremely irritating) based on the degree of erythema (reddening), eschar (scar formation), or edema (swelling from fluid accumulation). The test, however, does not take into consideration the possibility of induced sensitization after multiple contact. This would require a test panel of human subjects.

5. Porosity

It is generally accepted that most of the trauma to the skin upon use of adhesive systems is caused by occlusion. Covering the skin with an adhesive barrier, which causes moisture to build up in the outer layers (stratum corneum) of the skin, will induce hydration. When hydrated, these normally dry and strongly bound layers become weakened and are easily damaged, and they become separated from each other as the tape is removed. This can be avoided, in part, by the use of perforated tapes, which limit the trauma only to the space between perforations. More recently, nonwoven porous backings have been developed. These backings can be used along with porous or permeable adhesives. So, the porosity of both backings and adhesives should be taken into consideration.

III. PRESSURE-SENSITIVE ADHESIVES FOR TRANSDERMAL APPLICATIONS

The major pressure-sensitive adhesive polymers that have been evaluated for potential medical applications are polyisobutylenes, acrylics, and silicones. While these polymers are quite different from one another in both molecular structure and chemistry, they are rather similar with respect to their acceptability for use in medical applications where skin contact is required. Adhesive systems prepared from representative polymers have been shown not to possess primary skin sensitization or irritation properties.

A. Polyisobutylene-Type Pressure-Sensitive Adhesives

1. Chemistry and Performance

Polyisobutylenes are a group of inherently tacky polymers that are widely used as pressure-sensitive adhesives and as tackifiers and modifiers. They are homopolymers of isobutylene, polymerized using a Lewis acid type of catalyst, such as aluminum chloride (Fig. 10). The hydrocarbon backbone is relatively long and straight, with only terminal unsaturation (6). Because of the scarcity of double bonds and reactive sites, polyisobutylenes are very stable and resist the effects of weathering, aging, and heat. They have good resistance to vegetable and animal oils and to the attack by chemicals, which are the two factors in their favor for medical applications. The all-hydrocarbon, nonpolar nature of polyisobutylenes makes them soluble in typical hydrocarbon solvents. Since their water permeability is known to be rather low, permeation of the adhesive to moisture must be achieved through means other than the inherent permeability of the polymer.

Polyisobutylenes have little tendency to crystallize and show less dependency on molecular entanglement or cross-linking for their adhesive strength (6). Their amorphous character imparts an internal mobility that leads to their flexibility, permanent tack, and resistance to shock. Even though tack is high in these polymers, their lack of polarity results in a weak adhesion to substrates. This weakness can be overcome by the addition of resins and other tackifiers.

Polyisobutylenes have been produced over a wide range of molecular weights (6). The low-molecular-weight grades are permanently tacky semiliquids, which have a broad acceptability in FDA-regulated applications. While the low-molecular-weight polyisobutylenes are primarily utilized as tackifiers to provide tack, softness, and flexibility of other adhesive polymers, and to improve "wetting out" on various hard-to-adhere substrates, the high molecular-weight grades

$$CH_3\!-\!\underset{\substack{|\\Isobutylene}}{C}\!=\!CH_2 \longrightarrow \left[\underset{\substack{|\\CH_3}}{\overset{\substack{CH_3\\|}}{C}}\!-\!CH_2\right]_x$$

Polyisobutylene

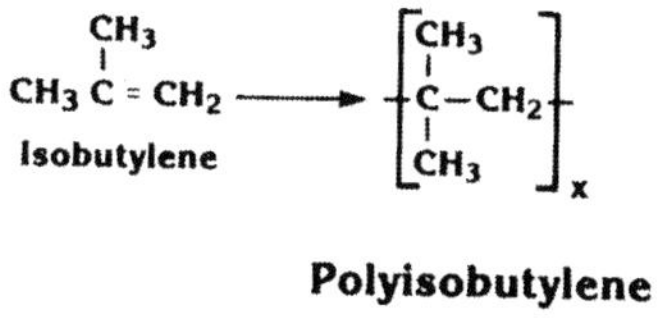

Figure 10 Schematic illustration of the synthetic process for polyisobutylene-type pressure-sensitive adhesives.

are used as high-strength backbone polymers in the pressure-
sensitive adhesives.

2. Formulation

Unlike many other pressure-sensitive adhesives, polyisobutylene-
type adhesives are routinely formulated in-house by device manufacturers or formulators, not by the polymer producers. Although a
wide range of properties can be obtained by varying the composition
using polymers of differing molecular weights, the addition of tackifiers, plasticizers, fillers, and stabilizers can also extend this range.

The low-molecular-weight polyisobutylene can be handled like
any other viscous, tacky material (6). They blend readily with oils,
waxes, solvents, and other polymers. High-molecular-weight grades
of polyisobutylene are normally shredded before formulation. Preparation of a concentrated solution of the polymer and the additives is
advisable prior to solvation. Polyisobutylenes are generally soluble
in nonpolar hydrocarbon solvents and insoluble in polar solvents.
Such solvents as aliphatic and aromatic hydrocarbons, carbon disulfide, and halogenated solvents are good solvents for polyisobutylenes

Tackifier resins are added to the high-molecular-weight polyisobutylenes to improve the balance between tack and internal strength
to tailor the properties desired. Hydrocarbon resins and hydrogen-
ated esters as well as low-molecular-weight grades of polyisobutylene
have been used as the tackifier for the high-molecular-weight
polyisobutylenes.

Other additives can also be added: plasticizers, which modify
the tack and cohesive strength of the adhesive; fillers, which reduce
cost and improve handling; and antioxidants, which improve the adhesive's resistance to oxidative degradation, particularly during
compounding.

A representative formulation for a surgical tape is shown in
Table 1. It should be recognized that any additive to the basic
polyisobutylene must also fulfill the biocompatibility requirements for
the final adhesive system.

3. Manufacturers

Major suppliers of polyisobutylene polymers include Exxon Chemical Company and BASF Wyandotte Corporation.

B. Acrylic-Type Pressure-Sensitive Adhesives

1. Chemistry and Performance

Acrylic-type pressure-sensitive adhesives are produced through
the copolymerization of acrylic esters with acrylic acid and other
functional monomers (Fig. 11). Polyacrylates can be synthesized

Table 1 Polyisobutylene Adhesive Formulation for Surgical Tape

Component	Content
Vistanex MM L-100	100 parts
Zinc oxide	50 parts
Hydrated alumnina	50 parts
White oil, USP	50 parts
Amberol ST 140F	70 parts
Hydrocarbon solvent	To coatable viscosity

Source: From Ref. 6.

through either emulsion or solution polymerization, using free-radical-initiated processes. This produces a polymer with a saturated-hydrocarbon backbone. The ester group of the monomer is attached in a pendant fashion from the polymer backbone and provides a unique method of tailoring the adhesive properties of the polymer.

Since the acrylics are saturated polymers, they are highly resistant to oxidation and do not require the addition of stabilizers, which potentially can cause biocompatibility problems. The polymers are moderately polar, due to their acrylate–ester structure, and, thus, have a degree of moisture permeability.

The copolymerization process is the key to synthesizing acrylic polymers with a wide range of adhesive properties. The copolymers produced have physical properties roughly equivalent to the corresponding combined properties of the homopolymers (7). Since

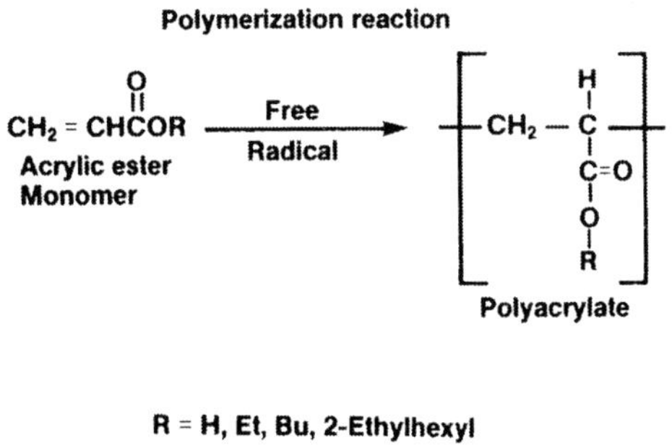

Polymerization reaction

$$CH_2 = CHCOR \xrightarrow[\text{Radical}]{\text{Free}} \left[-CH_2 - \underset{\substack{| \\ C=O \\ | \\ O \\ | \\ R}}{\overset{\substack{H \\ |}}{C}} - \right]$$

Acrylic ester Monomer   Polyacrylate

R = H, Et, Bu, 2-Ethylhexyl

Figure 11 Schematic illustration of the synthetic process for acrylic-type pressure-sensitive adhesives.

there are many types of monomer available for this vinyl-type polymerization, the possible combination of properties is extensive. The most commonly used monomers are ethyl-, butyl-, and 2-ethylhexylacrylate. Incorporation of the ester groups with longer chain lengths increases the randomness of the acrylate polymer, which reduces the crystallinity and lowers the glass transition temperature. The resulting polymers are softer and more flexible, and have increased tackiness. Addition of a small amount of acrylic acid and other functional monomers promotes the adhesion and increases the moisture permeability of the polymer. Increased permeability of moisture may be desirable from the standpoint of minimizing the effects of occlusion.

Advantages of this single-component adhesive system include its low level of low-molecular-weight species and impurities that may migrate to the surface of adhesive polymer and affect its adhesion. Modification of the system, apart from copolymerization, can also be achieved through cross-linking and molecular weight control.

2. Formulation

Both emulsion- and solvent-based acrylics are commercially available. Typical solvents for the solvent-based acrylics are toluene and ethanol. Since acrylics, as a rule, do not require tackifiers, variation in properties is achieved by the manufacturer through copolymerization, rather than by in-house formulation. However, it is also possible to modify acrylics to some extent using plasticizers and fillers. There are also a few tackifying resins that can be used with acrylics.

3. Manufacturers

Major suppliers of acrylic adhesives include Monsanto Polymer Products Company, Rohm & Haas Company, and National Starch and Chemical Company.

C. Silicone-Type Pressure-Sensitive Adhesives

1. Chemistry and Performance

Silicone-type pressure-sensitive adhesives are preformulated and available as solvent-based products that use the fluid/resin concept to develop adhesive properties. They are prepared by the reaction of a linear polydimethylsiloxane fluid with a solvent-soluble, low-molecular-weight silicate resin (Fig. 12). The linear polydimethylsiloxane fluid possesses a backbone of alternating silicon and oxygen
bonds ($-Si-O-$) and is terminated by silanol groups ($-Si-OH$).
Each silicon atom is also attached with two methyl groups. Although linear siloxane fluids possessing some phenyl substitution are formulated

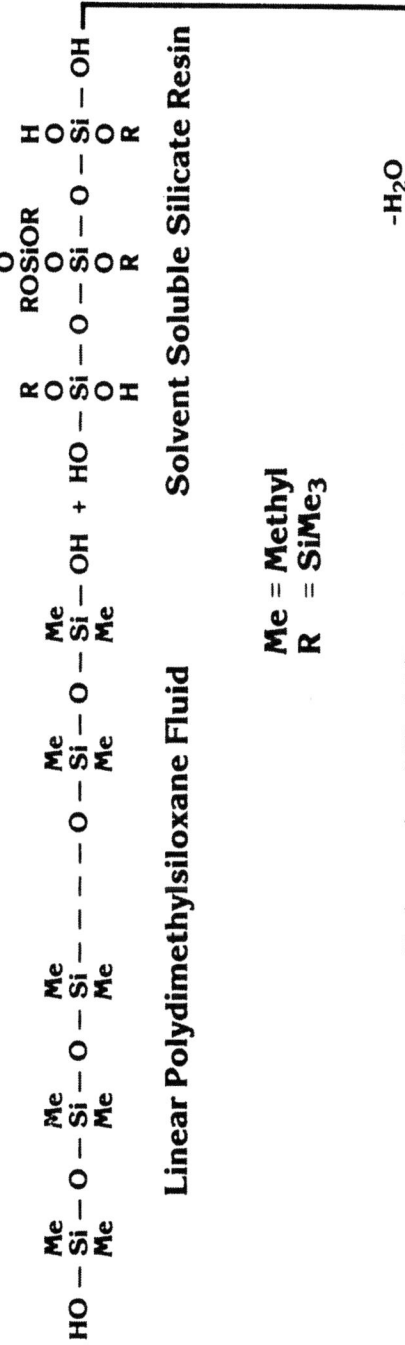

Figure 12   Schematic illustration of the synthetic process for silicone-type pressure-sensitive adhesives.

into certain industrial silicone pressure-sensitive adhesives, the adhesives are not used in medical applications.

The resin portion of the adhesive is a solvent-soluble silicate. The linear fluid and resin are combined and allowed to condense in solvent medium to make an adhesive network. During the reaction, the silanol groups in both polydimethylsiloxane and silicate resin

condense to form a stable siloxane bond ($-Si-O-Si-$). The silicate resin, unlike the resins in the organic pressure-sensitive adhesives, becomes chemically bonded to the polydimethylsiloxane. In this respect, the two-component system actually acts as a one-component system.

The molecular architecture of polydimethylsiloxane is responsible for some unique properties of silicone-type pressure-sensitive adhesives. The polymer chain has a very low glass transition temperature ($-127°C$), hence a great degree of flexibility (8,9). This structure is also responsible for the low surface energy of the polymer and is important in "wetting out" the surface of a substrate to which an adhesive is applied. The chain mobility also produces openings in the network to create free volume for molecular diffusion. Thus, silicone adhesives have high permeability to moisture and oxygen, which is important in reducing the degree of occlusion. This may also be indicative of high permeability to drugs, which is an important factor to be considered for TDD systems in which the drug-releasing surface is covered with adhesive.

Silicone-type pressure-sensitive adhesives are serviceable at both high and low temperatures and possess good moisture resistance and good electrical insulation properties. Other characteristics include good adhesion to both high- and low-energy surfaces, excellent chemical stability, and low toxicity. The excellent skin compatibility of the polydimethylsiloxane-based silicone adhesives is reflected in their extensive use in medical applications since 1965.

The adhesive properties of the silicone adhesives are a function of the fluid/resin ratio (Fig. 12). Increasing the fluid content gives a softer, more tacky adhesive, while high resin levels produce a drier adhesive with less tack but higher adhesion. At resin levels of 50-70% (w/w), a pressure-sensitive adhesive is produced with a useful range of pressure-sensitive adhesive properties.

2. Formulation

Silicone adhesives are commercially available in preformulated products.

3. Manufacturers

Medical-grade silicone adhesives are available from Dow Corning Corporation.

IV. SUMMARY

The adhesives used in a transdermal drug delivery (TDD) system must fulfill requirements beyond those delineated by typical property testing of a general-purpose, pressure-sensitive adhesive. For this reason, it is important that the adhesives be considered in the early stage of the development of a TDD device.

General-purpose, pressure-sensitive adhesives must be permanently tacky at room temperature; they must adhere spontaneously to the surfaces they contact with only light finger pressure; and they must possess sufficient cohesive strength that upon removal from a surface, they leave no adhesive residue. A pressure-sensitive adhesive intended for use in a TDD device must not cause any irritation to the skin, must be chemically compatible with drugs, and must function in the presence of moisture. It must also adhere to all skin types and conform to and accommodate skin movement. While the tests for general adhesive properties are well established, the tests specific to the adhesives for transdermal applications are still under development.

Representative polyisobutylene-, polyacrylate-, and silicone-type pressure-sensitive adhesives have been found to be nonirritating to the skin. Extensive toxicological testing is required, however, to confirm this in the final TDD product. Polyisobutylenes are inherently tacky and flexible. They have low moisture and gas permeability and a high resistance to chemicals. They are the only adhesives among those discussed that can be formulated in-house; and since they are easily blended by varying polymer composition, they can offer an extensive range of adhesive properties.

Acrylics exhibit good adhesive tack and generally require no addition of tackifying resins. They are single-component systems with low levels of low-molecular-weight species and impurities. Since the polymer is a saturated hydrocarbon, it is very stable and requires no stabilizers for protection against degradation. A wide range of adhesive properties is made possible through copolymerization.

Silicones are flexible and will adhere to high- and low-energy surfaces. They are moisture resistant, and yet are permeable to vapor, gases, and many drugs. They are resistant to oxidation and, therefore, require no stabilizing additives. They are preformulated products, and their biocompatibility has been established through many years of service in medical applications. Their chemical inertness is documented both in the scientific literature and in numerous and varied industrial applications.

The choice of an adhesive lies in the properties required for a specific TDD device. Also important are the facilities available for development and ultimate production. Whether the manufacturer of a transdermal device has selected a preformulated adhesive product or is intending to formulate it in-house, the numerous variables involved in the adhesive technology make it advisable for the device manufacturer to work closely with the adhesive producers (10).

REFERENCES

1. *Test Methods for Pressure-Sensitive Tapes*, 7th ed., Pressure-Sensitive Tape Council, Glenview, IL, 1976.
2. ASTM D 2979-71, Standard Test Method for Pressure-Sensitive Tack of Adhesives Using an Inverted Probe Machine, American Society for Testing and Materials, Philadelphia, 1971.
3. S. A. Huie, P. F. Schmidt, and J. S. Warren, Testing adhesive and liner for transdermal drug-delivery, *Adhesives Age, 32*: (June 1985).
4. H. M. Leeper and D. Enscore, Creep test developed for adhesive-backed skin patch used to deliver drugs, *Adhesive Age, 16*: (February 1982).
5. J. A. Fries and D. A. Nadler, Pressure-sensitive adhesives for medical applications, in *TAPPI Polymers, Laminations, and Coatings Conference*, Boston Proceedings (Book 2), September 24-26, 1984, pp. 479-483.
6. N. E. Stucker and J. J. Higgins, Butyl rubber and polyisobutylene, in *Handbook of Adhesives* (I. Skeist, ed.), Van Nostrand Reinhold, New York, 1977, p. 255.
7. D. Satas, Acrylic adhesives, in *Handbook of Pressure-Sensitive Adhesives Technology* (D. Satas, ed.), Van Nostrand Reinhold, New York, 1982, p. 298.
8. M. J. Owen, Why silicones behave funny, *Chemtech, 11*: 288 (1981).
9. E. L. Warrick, O. R. Pierce, K. E. Polmanteer, and J. C. Saam, Silicone elastomer developments, 1967-1977, *Rubber Chem. Technol., 52*: 437 (1979).
10. *Adhesives Age Directory*, Vol. 28, Communication Channels, Inc., Atlanta, GA, May 1985.

5

Polymeric Materials: Assessment of Skin Biocompatibility

KEVIN S. WEADOCK / UMDNJ—Robert Wood Johnson Medical School, Piscataway, New Jersey
JAMES M. PACHENCE / Pachence Associates, Lawrenceville, New Jersey
RICHARD A. BERG and FREDERICK H. SILVER / UMDNJ—Robert Wood Johnson Medical School, Piscataway, New Jersey

I. INTRODUCTION

The early development of synthetic materials used as skin replacements or transdermal drug delivery devices primarily focused on providing either a barrier to infection and protection against reinjury or a stable, controlled delivery surface. Consequently, the mechanical characteristics of the material were the most important to investigate. However, the rapid increase in the number and application of synthetic materials used in contact with skin has led to developments of more sophisticated testing procedures to establish the biocompatibility of the materials.

Guidelines for establishing biocompatibility exist only in very broad terms (1). In general, each new material, device, and device application should have its own unique protocol to establish biocompatibility. This chapter discusses the general issues of skin biocompatibility with respect to materials used in transdermal devices and gives specific examples of testing procedures.

To choose appropriate testing procedures to establish biocompatibility and to evaluate the risk/benefit ratio, it is useful to classify a medical device according to its application. Medical devices can be classified in terms of the duration of contact with living tissue, that is, whether the contact is permanent, long term (less than 5 years), or temporary (less than 1 year). Transdermal delivery devices would, for the most part, be considered to be temporary devices.

Transdermal devices also can be classified according to the drug to be delivered (e.g., as to whether the drug is used in chronic or acute applications) and according to the design of the device. It has been previously noted that a transdermal delivery system can be designed as either a monolithic system (usually a device in which the drug is dispersed within the polymer matrix) or a membrane system in which a core of drug is enveloped by a polymeric membrane (2). The design of the device will determine whether the skin contact material is a pressure-sensitive adhesive such as silicone, polyisobutylene, or polyalkylacrylate (3) or a barrier-type polymer such as silicone elastomers, polyethylene, polyvinyl alcohol, or hydrogels. The types of biocompatibility assay and the parameters of the testing protocol (animal models, duration, etc.) can then be determined.

II. BIOCOMPATIBILITY TESTING OF POLYMERS

The FDA requires that the safety of all materials used for medical or dental applications be established prior to clinical use. As mentioned above, the tests used to establish safety will depend on the type of transdermal device, the drug to be delivered, and its application. The in vitro and in vivo testing on transdermal devices would be designed to investigate the polymer–skin interface reactions, effects on subsurface tissue, and systemic effects.

In vivo procedures usually involve, at the minimum, a subcutaneous and/or intramuscular implant test and a surface patch test. If the material is a biopolymer such as collagen, bioabsorption and immunogenicity must also be investigated. Rodents are most often used in screening assays, for periods ranging from months to years. In critical applications, higher mammals are used, since they are considered to be more accurate models for the human response to materials.

For implant tests, the animals are sacrificed at predetermined time periods and the sample with the surrounding tissue is excised and fixed. Scoring systems have been used based on the number of specific cell types within a specific area of the implant (4). Such histological assessments tend to be subjective. Autian (5) proposed a series of in vitro and in vivo tests to screen for primary acute toxicity. Based on these methods, the severity of the response was given a score. A grading method for histological examination was used by Sewell et al. (6) to effectively compare the biocompatibility of polymers by implanting a powdered form of the polymer in gelatin capsules (7). More recently, a cage implant system has been proposed to provide quantitative data for evaluating biocompatibility of a material using an in vivo test (8).

In some instances, histological examination of lymph nodes has been necessary in addition to evaluation of the subcutaneous site. For example, polyvinylidene fluoride (PVDF) films used to immobilize urokinase were implanted subcutaneously in rats and examined after 3 months to evaluate the histology of the implant site (9). In this study, both the subcutaneous sites and the lymph nodes were examined. Although cytotoxicity at the site of the implant was minimal, a histological examination of the lymph nodes indicated that an immunologically modulated response was induced, as seen by the proliferation of lymphocytes. More highly sulfonated PVDF was accompanied by an increased plasma cell population near the implant, and therefore such a material would not be suited for long-term or permanent use (9).

Skin patch tests are common tests for preclinical and clinical device evaluations, and a number of procedures have been described, including the Draize test (10). Primary irritation is usually measured by a patch test on intact or abraded skin of an albino rabbit clipped free of hair. The material is applied to the skin, and an occlusive dressing is wrapped around the entire trunk of the animal. The patches are removed after 24 hr and the resulting reactions are evaluated using a standardized visual grading system. The Draize test has been useful in identifying strong to moderate irritants, but it has been less effective in detecting weak irritants on either rabbits or human skin (11). Several modifications were proposed and successfully tested, including the repeated application of weak irritants (11). A large number of cosmetic and topically applied materials have since been tested using the accumulative irritant method in both rabbits and humans (12).

The lack of knowledge of the basic mechanisms of irritation development makes it difficult to rate the relative merits of available assays for polymer-tissue interactions. However, it is now known that skin thickness, vascularity, and location of the patch are all important variables that affect patch tests (13). Primary differences in the percutaneous absorption of animal and human skin are also important in understanding the differences with respect to various responses (14,15).

Acute dermal (percutaneous) toxicity is generally measured by applying a test material to a shaved intact or abraded skin patch followed by occlusion. Various biological parameters such as body weight, mortality, and gross pathological evaluation are usually assessed. This method has been modified to include multiple doses over longer periods of time to recognize both acute and chronic toxicity of various chemicals (16). The testing of polymers in mammals to simulate human usage is expensive in both time and resources, and therefore some form of rapid prescreening is desirable. In vitro assays can be carried out on the polymer directly; however, extracts of the polymer are also used to evaluate the cytotoxicity of leachable materials (5). While implantation studies are useful for evaluating chronic tissue reactions, cell culture assays are generally useful in testing for acute cellular reactions. Furthermore, the growing sophistication of cell culture methods has led to serious consideration of replacing some in vivo biocompatibility tests with tissue culture tests (2).

Evaluation of the biocompatibility of polymers via tissue culture techniques is based on analysis of cellular growth, division, enzyme levels, and synthesis of important macromolecules. One method (17) involves growing cells on a Millipore filter, which is then placed on agar with the cell side down. Test substances are placed on the filter and incubated for a predetermined period of time. The cell layer is then assayed for an enzyme such as succinate dehydrogenase. A zone of inhibited enzyme indicates that the cells were damaged and/or the enzyme was inhibited. This is a test for biocompatibility that heretofore has not been widely used owing to the difficulties of identifying macromolecules specifically from cells.

Two other improved cell culture techniques involve the use of standardized cell lines. In the first method, test materials are sterilized and placed directly on cell monolayers. After incubation, the cells are stained and the area of detached cells is measured. In the second method, 1% agar is spread over the monolayer and the test materials are then placed on the agar. Areas of cell deterioration are measured beneath the agar using an inverted cell culture microscope (18). In addition, cellular growth rates may be evaluated in response to test materials. These methods have been used to evaluate highly toxic polymers such as PVC and less toxic polymers such as silicone rubber, ester polyurethane, polyethylene, and polyethylene terephthalate (18). This study was then expanded to include primary cell types such as human lymphocytes, polymorphonuclear leukocytes, mouse embryos, and mouse peritoneal macrophages (19). In the later study, biochemical assays of the cellular synthesis of DNA, protein, and ATP were correlated with the toxicity ranking of materials. It was shown that this ranking was independent of the cell culture system used. In rats, in vitro tests were more sensitive to differences in material composition than histological evaluations of subcutaneous implants after 90 days.

A systematic study of the biocompatibility of polyamides, polyesters, polyethers, polysulfonamides, polysulfonate, polyphosphonate, polyimide, polyamide-imides, and polyester-amide was accomplished

Table 1   Biocompatibility Studies of Polymers Used
in Transdermal Devices

Polymer	References
Silicone polymers	39, 40, 42, 46, 48–52
Polyethylene	53–58
Polypropylene	43, 59
Polyvinyl chloride	45, 60, 61
Polyvinylidene fluoride	9
Polymethyl methacrylate	7
Polyurethane	47
Hydrogels	49, 63–65
Collagen	66–70

by cell culture methods (20). These methods involved plating cells
directly onto the polymer films. After incubation, the cells were
stained and the total cellular protein extracted and quantitatively
analyzed. The introduction of nitro- or chloro- groups into the
polymers reduced cell attachment, and these differences were noted.
However, the relatively crude measurements of cell growth in the
study did not allow fine distinctions to be made between the polymers.
    Table 1 lists various polymers used in transdermal devices and
references discussing biocompatibility studies done on each polymer.

III. CELLULAR RESPONSE TO POLYMERS

The most obvious indication of the extent of interaction between
foreign material and body tissues is the cellular response in the immediate vicinity of the implant. When a foreign material interacts
with tissues, a specific sequence of reaction occurs. In the acute
or early stage there is hyperemia, exudation of fluid, and immigra-
tion of neutrophils from the local circulation. Varying populations
of eosinophils, plasma cells, and lymphocytes may also appear. A
chronic tissue response occurs later and may be characterized by
the appearance of monocytes, which may differentiate into macrophages and multinuclear giant cells (21). Multinuclear giant cells
are created by the fusion of young monocytes with mature macrophages (22). These cells are capable of phagocytosis and may in-
gest bacteria, foreign particles, damaged cells, noncellular debris

such as fibrin, and denatured protein. Fibroblasts present in surrounding tissues may then initiate the synthesis of a collagenous matrix around the material. The resulting complex of foreign material, monocytes, macrophages, and multinuclear giant cells surrounded by collagenous fibers constitutes a chronic tissue response, or the foreign body reaction (23). When the material induces a systemic response, a physiological process may be altered or pathological changes may be produced at distant sites. Chronic tissue reactions may be evaluated through hematological studies, urinalysis, biopsies, or autopsy.

Many additives used in the manufacture of polymers have the potential to induce an allergic or tumorigenic response. Clinical cases of allergic responses to manufactured polymers are few, however, and little is known about the possible allergic reactions to materials which have prolonged contact with tissues. Polymeric materials can present potential carcinogenic activity if there is a carcinogenic substance in the material or if a carcinogenic agent is generated through polymer degradation. Although the concentration of unreacted monomers and additives used to manufacture polymeric materials is extremely low, the hazard for systemic toxicity or carcinogenesis cannot be ignored. It should be noted, however, that while tumor growth in animal models exposed to various polymers is well documented (24–26), actual evidence for a polymeric material producing a tumor in humans has not been substantiated (27).

IV. POLYMER DEGRADATION

It is assumed by the designers of transdermal devices that the polymers comprising structural or adhesive components remain intact and do not permeate the epidermis. However, most polymers are susceptible to degradation by one or more mechanisms. For polymers consisting of a carbon–carbon backbone (Table 2), the mechanism of degradation is via free-radical depolymerization. This type of degradation can be initiated by heat, oxidation, mechanical energy, or electromagnetic radiation (28–31). When the polymer backbone contains atoms other than carbon, such as oxygen, nitrogen, sulfur, or silicon, degradation can occur by either hydrolytic mechanisms or free-radical depolymerization. Examples of polymers particularly susceptible to hydrolytic degradation are those containing ester or amide bonds.

In the presence of free radicals, polymers containing double bonds, disulfide cross-links, or hydrocarbon chains may degrade. This occurs most readily with polymers that are produced by a free-radical mechanism.

The net result of this reaction is the breakage of a covalent bond with the formation of two active radical centers. This chain scission will occur preferentially in amorphous regions of crystalline

Table 2   Repeat Units of Typical Synthetic Polymers

Polymer	Repeat unit
Polyethylene	$\left[\text{CH}_2\right]_n$
Polytetrafluoroethylene	$\left[\text{CF}_2\right]_n$
Polyethylene terephthalate	$\left[\overset{O}{\overset{\|}{C}}\text{—}\bigcirc\text{—}\overset{O}{\overset{\|}{C}}\text{OCH}_2\text{CH}_2\text{O}\right]_n$
Polyvinyl chloride	$\left[\begin{smallmatrix}H&H\\C&-C\\H&Cl\end{smallmatrix}\right]_n$
Polyvinylidene fluoride	$\left[\begin{smallmatrix}H&F\\C&-C\\H&F\end{smallmatrix}\right]_n$
Polymethyl methacrylate	$\left[\begin{smallmatrix}H&CH_3\\C&-C\\H&C-O-CH_3\\&O\end{smallmatrix}\right]_n$
Poly(2-hydroxyethyl methacrylate) (HEMA—hydrogel)	$\left[\text{CH}_2\text{—}\overset{CH_3}{\underset{\underset{O}{C-CH_2CH_2OH}}{C}}\right]_n$
Polydimethyl siloxane	$\left[\overset{CH_3}{\underset{CH_3}{\text{Si}}}\text{—O}\right]_n$
Polysulfone	$\left[\bigcirc\text{—O—}\bigcirc\text{—}\overset{O}{\underset{O}{S}}\right]_n$
Polyamide	$\left[\overset{O}{\overset{\|}{C}}\text{—NH}\right]_n$
Polyurethane	$\left[\text{O-}\overset{O}{\overset{\|}{C}}\text{—NH}\right]_n$
Polyester	$\left[\overset{O}{\overset{\|}{C}}\text{—O}\right]_n$

polymers, and although the two radical centers may recombine, they usually propagate. Propagation usually occurs in such a fashion that the active center is transferred two carbon atoms down the chain and monomer is eliminated.

Hydrolytic degradation of condensation polymers is catalyzed by heat, acid, base, or enzymes. Degradation of a polyester is a typical example of hydrolytic breakdown of a condensation polymer. The ester bond is cleaved by reaction with water to form an acid and an alcohol end groups.

Enzymatic hydrolysis is a special case of the simple hydrolytic mechanism, where the polymer has a particular bond or series of bonds which is available for enzymatic cleavage (32,33). Enzymes are substrate specific and normally are not thought of as being capable of catalyzing the degradation of the redundant synthetic polymer backbone. However, there is now evidence (34–36) to suggest that enzymes may indeed be able to influence the degradation of synthetic polymers. It is thought that enzymes may reduce the activation energy of degradation that normally takes place at high temperatures to a point where in the presence of ultraviolet light or oxygen, hydrolysis may take place in a physiological environment. Other studies (37,38) have shown that bacteria may also be capable of degrading at least some synthetic polymers. The biological effects of breakdown products of polymers to be used in transdermal drug delivery also must be considered in any biocompatibility assessment.

V. CONCLUSIONS

This chapter has briefly discussed the assessment of skin biocompatibility. It has been established that biocompatibility studies must go beyond acute dermal toxicity tests and should include implantation studies as well as cell culture tests to evaluate cytotoxic effects of the material, leachable components, and degradation products. The long-term benefits of using transdermal delivery systems must always be balanced against any potential toxic effects induced by polymers within the system.

REFERENCES

1. P. M. Galletti and T. W. Boretos, Report on the consensus development conference on clinical applications of biomaterials, *J. Biomed. Mater. Res.*, 17: 539 (1983).
2. N. B. Graham and D. A. Wood, Polymeric inserts and implants for the controlled release of drugs, in *Macromolecular Biomaterials* (G. W. Hastings and P. Ducheyne, eds.), CRC Press, Boca Raton, FL, 1984, p. 181.

3. Y. W. Chien, Novel Drug Delivery Systems: Fundamentals, Development and Concepts, Biomedical Assessments, Dekker, New York, 1982, p. 149.
4. R. E. Marchant, K. M. Miller, and J. M. Anderson, In vivo leukocyte interactions with Biomer, J. Biomed. Mat. Res., 18: 1169 (1984).
5. J. Autian, Toxicological aspects of implantable plastics used in medical and paramedical applications, in Fundamental Aspects of Biocompatibility (D. F. Williams, ed.), CRC Press, Boca Raton, FL, 1981, p. 63.
6. W. R. Sewell, J. Wiland, and N. C. Bradford, A new method of comparing ovine catgut with sutures of bovine catgut in 3 species, Surg. Gynecol. Obstet., 100: 483 (1955).
7. S. J. Gourlay, R. M. Rice, A. F. Hegyeli, C. W. R. Wade, J. G. Dillon, H. Jaffe, and R. K. Kulkarni, Biocompatibility testing of polymers: In vivo implantation studies, J. Biomed. Mater. Res., 12: 219 (1978).
8. R. E. Marchant, J. M. Anderson, and E. O. Dillingham, Inflammatory response to polyethylene and to a cytotoxic polyvinylchloride, J. Biomed. Mater. Res., 20: 37 (1986).
9. R. Aoshima, Y. Kanda, A. Takada, and A. Yamashita, Sulfonated poly(vinylidene fluoride) as a biomaterial: Immobilization of urokinase and biocompatibility, J. Biomed. Mater. Res., 16: 289 (1982).
10. R. L. Bronaugh and H. I. Maibach, Evaluation of skin irritation: Correlations between animals and humans, in Safety and Efficacy of Topical Drugs and Cosmetics (A. M. Klingman and J. J. Leyden, eds.), Grune and Stratton, New York, 1982, p. 51.
11. L. Phillips, M. Steinberg, H. I. Maibach, and W. A. Akers, A comparison of rabbit and human skin response to certain irritants, Toxicol. Appl. Pharmacol., 21: 369 (1972).
12. F. N. Marzulli and H. I. Maibach, The rabbit as a model for evaluating skin irritants: A comparison of results obtained on animals and man using repeated skin exposures, Cosmet. Toxicol., 13: 533 (1975).
13. R. J. Feldmann and H. I. Maibach, Regional variation in percutaneous absorption of ^{14}C-cortisol in man, J. Invest. Dermatol., 48: 181 (1967).
14. M. J. Bartek, M. A. La Buddle, and H. I. Maibach, Skin permeability in vivo: Comparison in rat, rabbit, pig and man, J. Invest. Dermatol., 58: 114 (1972).
15. R. L. Bronaugh, R. F. Stewart, and E. R. Cogdon, Methods of in vitro percutaneous absorption studies. II. Animal models for human skin, Toxicol. Appl. Pharmacol., 62: 481 (1982).
16. G. V. Foster, Animal models for assessment of systemic effects from topically applied substances, in Safety and Efficiency of

Topical Drugs and Cosmetics (A. M. Kligman and J. J. Leyden, eds.), Grune and Stratton, New York, 1982, p. 99.

17. A Wennberg, G. Hasselgren, and L. Tronsted, A method for toxicity screening of biomaterials using cells cultured on Millipore filters, *J. Biomed. Mater. Res.*, *13*: 109 (1979).

18. H. J. Johnson, S. J. Northup, P. A. Seagraves, P. J. Garvin, and R. F. Wallin, Biocompatibility test procedures for materials evaluation in vitro. I. Comparative test system sensitivity, *J. Biomed. Mater. Res.*, *17*: 571 (1983).

19. H. J. Johnson, S. J. Northup, P. A. Seagraves, M. Atallah, P. J. Garvin, L. Lin, and T. D. Darby, Objective method of toxicity assessment, *J. Biomed. Mater. Res.*, *19*: 489 (1985).

20. Y. Imai, A. Watanabe, and E. Masuhara, Structure–biocompatibility relationship of condensation polymers, *J. Biomed. Mater. Res.*, *17*: 905 (1983).

21. W. Mohr and C. J. Kirkpatrick, Biocompatibility of polymers, *Aktuel. Probl. Chir. Ortho.*, *26*: 18 (1985).

22. M. Mariano and W. G. Spector, The formation and properties of macrophage polykaryons (inflammatory giant cells), *J. Pathol.*, *113*: 1 (1974).

23. D. O. Adams, The granulomatous inflammatory response. *Am. J. Pathol.*, *84*: 164 (1976).

24. B. S. Oppenheimer, E. T. Oppenheimer, A. P. Stout, M. Wilhite, and I. Danishefsky, The latent period in carcinogenesis by plastics in rats and its relation to the presarcomatous state, *Cancer*, *11*: 204 (1958).

25. F. C. Turner, Sarcomas at sites of subcutaneously implanted Bakelite disks in rats, *J. Natl. Canc. Inst.*, *2*: 81 (1941).

26. F. Bischoff and G. Bryson, Carcinogenesis through solid-state surfaces, *Prog. Exp. Tumor Res.*, *5*: 85 (1964).

27. W. Burns, S. Kanhouwa, L. Tillman, N. Saini, and J. B. Herrmann, Fibrosarcoma occurring at the site of a plastic vascular graft, *Cancer*, *29*: 66 (1972).

28. R. L. Simha and L. A. Wall, Kinetics of chain depolymerization, *J. Phys. Chem.*, *56*: 707 (1952).

29. S. L. Madorsky, Thermal degradation of organic polymers, in *Polymer Reviews*, Vol. 7, Wiley, New York, 1964, Chapters 3 and 4.

30. D. K. Backman and K. L. Devries, Formation of free radicals during machining and fracture of polymers, *J. Polym. Sci.*, *A7*: 2125 (1969).

31. A. Chapiro, *Radiation Chemistry of Polymeric High Polymers*, Wiley, New York, 1962.

32. D. F. Williams, Corrosion of implant materials, *Annu. Rev. Mater. Sci.*, *6*: 237 (1976).

33. D. F. Williams, Effects of cellular enzymes on polymers, *Proceedings of the Conference on Plastics Medicine and Surgery*, Plastics and Rubber Institute, London, 1979, p. 5.
34. S. N. Levine, Survey of biomedical materials and some relevant problems, *Ann. N.Y. Acad. Sci.*, *146*: 3 (1968).
35. J. B. Mermann, R. J. Kelly, and G. A. Higgins, Polyglycolic acid sutures, *Arch. Surg.*, *100*: 486 (1970).
36. T. N. Salthouse and B. F. Matlaga, Polyglactin 910 suture absorption and the role of cellular enzymes, *Surg. Gynecol. Obstet.*, *142*: 544 (1976).
37. F. Rodriques, The prospects for biodegradation plastics, *Chemtech*, *1*: 409 (1971).
38. S. A. Bradley, P. Engler, and S. H. Carr, Microbial degradation of polymer solids. II. Comparison of fungal attack in cellophane and amylose films, *Appl. Polym. Symp.*, *22*: 269 (1973).
39. M. S. Lucas and D. J. Moore, Tissue culture and histologic study of a new elastomer, *J. Prosthet. Dent.*, *42*: 447 (1979).
40. P. A. J. van Vuuren, A. J. Ligthelm, and M. R. Ferreira, Evaluation of the biocompatibility of five elastomeric impression materials, *J. Dent. Assoc. S. Africa*, *37*: 863 (1982).
41. A. B. Swanson, R. M. Nalbandian, T. J. Zmugg, S. Jaeger, B. K. Mupin, and G. Swanson, Silicone implants in dogs, *Clin. Orthop. Rel. Res.*, *184*: 293 (1984).
42. T. K. Issa, M. A. Bahgat, and F. H. Linthicum, Jr., Tissue reaction to prosthetic materials in human temporal bones, *Am. J. Otol.*, *5*: 40 (1983).
43. D. J. Apple, N. Mamalis, S. E. Brady, K. Loftfield, D. Kavka-Van Norman, and R. J. Olson, Biocompatibility of implant materials: A review and scanning electron microscopic study, *Am. Intra-Ocular Implant Soc. J.*, *10*: 53 (1984).
44. R. T. Green, R. L. Knoll, and B. H. Vale, Evaluation of tissue response to hydrogel composite materials, *Scanning Electron Microsc.*, *11*: 871 (1979).
45. J. A. Taylor, R. A. Abodeely, and R. L. Fuson, Rapid screening of biomedical polymers by two methods of tissue culture, *Trans. Am. Soc. Artif. Intern. Organs.*, *19*: 175 (1973).
46. M. M. Abdelnnabi, D. J. Moore, and J. S. Sakumura, In vitro comparison study of MDX-4-4210 and polydimethyl siloxane silicone materials, *J. Prosthet. Dent.*, *51*: 523 (1984).
47. D. J. Lyman, D. W. Hill, R. K. Stirk, C. Adamson, and B. R. Mooney, The interaction of tissue cells with polymer surfaces. *Trans. Am. Soc. Artif. Intern. Organs*, *18*: 19 (1972).
48. P. Vondracek and B. Dolezel, Biostability of medical elastomers: A review, *Biomaterials*, *5*: 209 (1984).

49. B. H. Vale and R. T. Greer, Ex vivo shunt testing of hydrogel–silicone composite materials, *J. Biomed. Mater. Res.*, *16*: 171 (1982).

50. R. A. White, F. M. Hirose, R. W. Sproat, R. S. Lawrence, and R. J. Nelson, Histopathologic observations after short-term implementation of two porous elastomers in dogs, *Biomaterials*, *2*: 171 (1981).

51. T. Devanathan and K. A. Young, Effect of postcuring on hemocompatibility of silicone rubber, *Biomater. Med. Dev. Artif. Organs*, *9*: 225 (1981).

52. R. Rudolph and J. Abraham, Tissue effects of new silicone mammary-type implants in rabbits, *Ann. Plast. Surg.*, *4*: 14 (1980).

53. T. Palva and J. Makinen, Histopathological observations on polyethylene-type materials in chronic ear surgery, *J. Biomed. Mater. Res.*, *17*: 129 (1983).

54. P. Roschger, E. M. Hoerl, H. Stachelberger, and H. Plank, Jr., Detection of aluminum oxide and polyethylene wear particles from joint endoprostheses using cathodoluminescence and X-ray analysis in SEM, *J. Biomed. Mater. Res.*, *14*: 765 (1980).

55. M. Spector, S. L. Harmon, and A. Kreuther, Characteristics of tissue growth into proplast and porous polyethylene implants in bone, *J. Biomed. Mater. Res.*, *13*: 677 (1979).

56. J. P. Deemer and P. J. Tsaknis, The effects of overfilled polyethylene tube intraosseous implants in rats, *Oral Surg. Oral Med. Oral Pathol.*, *48*: 358 (1979).

57. W. Remagen and E. Morscher, Histological results with cement-free implanted hip sockets of polyethylene, *Arch. Orthop. Trauma Surg.*, *103*: 145 (1984).

58. J. R. Atkinson and R. Z. Cicek, Silane crosslinked polyethylene for prosthetic applications. II. Creep and wear behavior and a preliminary moulding test, *Biomaterials*, *5*: 326 (1984).

59. P. H. Mook, P. Wong, C. R. Wildevuur, P. J. Mayes, and J. D. Gaylor, Comparative performance of microporous polypropylene membrane lungs for CO_2 removal at low blood flow rates, *Trans. Am. Soc. Artif. Intern. Organs*, *29*: 215 (1983).

60. R. Sharma and P. Vasudevan, Biocompatibility screening of poly(vinyl chloride) implants, *Biomaterials*, *3*: 109 (1982).

61. J. M. Monroe, R. C. Ligana, and M. C. Williams, Hemolytic properties of special materials exposed to a shear flow and plasma changes with shear, *Biomater. Med. Dev. Artif. Organs*, *8*: 103 (1980).

62. G. F. Klomp, H. Hashiguchi, P. C. Ursell, Y. Takeda, T. Taguchi, and W. H. Dobelle, Macroporous hydrogel membranes for a hybrid artificial pancreas. II. Biocompatibility, *J. Biomed. Mater. Res.*, *17*: 865 (1983).

63. H. R. Dickinson, A. Hiltner, D. F. Gibbons, and J. M. Anderson, Biodegradation of a poly(alpha-amino acid) hydrogel. I. In vivo, *J. Biomed. Mater. Res.*, *15*: 577 (1981).
64. R. Langer, H. Brem, and D. Tapper, Biocompatibility of polymeric delivery systems for macromolecules, *J. Biomed. Mater. Res.*, *15*: 267 (1981).
65. R. Marchant, A. Hiltner, C. Hamlin, A. Rabinovitch, R. Slobodkin, and J. M. Anderson, In vivo biocompatibility studies. I. The cage implant system and a biodegradable hydrogel, *J. Biomed. Mater. Res.*, *17*: 301 (1983).
66. M. Chvapil, R. L. Kronenthal, and W. van Winkle, Medical and surgical applications of collagen, *Int. Rev. Connect. Tissue Res.*, *6*: 1 (1973).
67. C. J. Doillon, C. Whyne, R. A. Berg, R. M. Olson, and F. H. Silver, Fibroblast–collagen sponge interactions and the spatial deposition of newly synthesized collagen fibers in vitro and in vivo, *Scanning Electron Microsc.*, *11*: 1313 (1984).
68. T. Elsdale and J. Bard, Collagen substrate for studies on cell behavior, *J. Cell Biol.*, *54*: 626 (1972).
69. A. W. Klein, Implantation techniques for injectable collagen, *J. Am. Acad. Dermatol.*, *9*: 224 (1983).
70. P. G. Shakespeare and R. W. Griffiths, Dermal collagen implants in man, *Lancet*, *1*: 795 (April 1980).

6

Design and Calibration of In Vitro Permeation Apparatus

KAKUJI TOJO / Rutgers—The State University of New Jersey, Piscataway, New Jersey

I. INTRODUCTION

The development of transdermal drug delivery systems using polymeric materials to control the delivery of drugs has been receiving more and more attention in the pharmaceutical and allied industries. Numerous scientific papers have been published on transdermal drug delivery in the past 10 years. The rates of drug permeation across the skin have been measured using different kinds of in vitro skin permeation apparatus. However, the rates of drug release and/or permeation reported often vary from one laboratory to another, which creates some difficulty in making a meaningful comparison of the data generated in different laboratories, despite many significant advances in the development of analytical methods for the determination of drug concentration.

Because the permeation, diffusion, and partitioning of drugs are often influenced by the hydrodynamic characteristics of the in vitro system used, which affect heat and mass transfer, the flow pattern in the system must be precisely controlled. The variation in release and/or permeation rates among laboratories can be considered to be primarily the results of variations in system design among the in vitro apparatuses, which could produce differences in the hydrodynamics among the systems used. Unfortunately, the hydrodynamic characteristics of membrane permeation apparatuses designed for transdermal drug delivery studies frequently are overlooked and have not been fully investigated yet. Furthermore, many research groups tend to use their own in vitro designs; some systems yield excellent mixing efficiency, and others may provide poor mixing conditions. In the latter cases, the rates of drug release and skin permeation may be significantly distorted by the presence of both hydrodynamic and thermal diffusion layers on the surface of the drug delivery device or skin.

Ideally, an in vitro system for transdermal drug delivery studies should be designed in such way that the intrinsic rate of release or permeation, which is theoretically independent of the in vitro design, can be accurately determined. The most straightforward means of eliminating diffusional resistance in the hydrodynamic boundary layer and obtaining the intrinsic rate profile is simply to increase the rate of stirring in the apparatus until the drug flux reaches a constant level, and then to perform the measurement at that particular stirring rate or higher. However, this approach is not always practical, since it may be limited by high solution viscosity, the mechanical strength of the membrane, and/or high lipophilicity of the drugs.

Only an in vitro skin permeation system with precisely defined hydrodynamic and thermal characteristics can provide a reliable and reproducible means for the determination of drug release and skin permeation rates. Once the hydrodynamics of the in vitro apparatus has been well calibrated, the apparent rate of release or permeation so obtained in an experiment can be corrected for the effect of hydrodynamic diffusion layer, and the intrinsic rate of release or permeation can then be determined.

For transdermal drug delivery, it is well known that the main resistance to drug transport resides in the skin, that is, diffusion through the stratum corneum. If an in vitro apparatus has poor mixing conditions, the release rate from the transdermal drug delivery system, which is usually much greater than the skin permeation rate, may be strongly distorted by the diffusion boundary layer. In this case, the in vitro release rate may become relatively close to the in vivo permeation rate, and it will be believed erroneously that the rate of drug delivery is controlled by the transdermal drug delivery system, not by the skin permeation. On the other hand, a well-designed in vitro apparatus can assure that the mechanism of drug delivery is truly from the transdermal drug delivery system (Fig. 1).

A survey of the literature has indicated that a number of in vitro apparatuses with different system designs have been used in transdermal drug delivery studies for the determination of drug release and/or skin permeation kinetics. A detailed review of all the systems is certainly not the objective of this chapter. Rather, we discuss

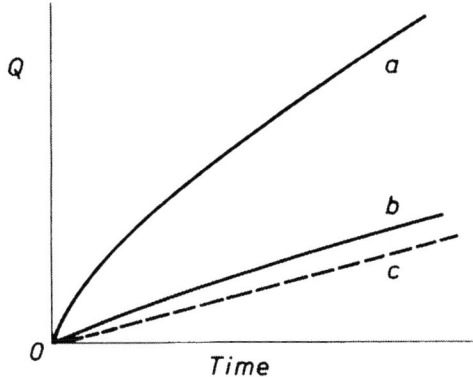

Figure 1   Release and permeation profiles for skin-limited transdermal drug delivery. Curve a, release under good mixing condition; curve b, release under poor mixing conditions; curve c,
permeation under in vivo conditions.

fundamental aspects of the design of in vitro skin permeation apparatuses, analyze the hydrodynamic characteristics of various
in vitro membrane permeation systems, and illustrate the procedure
for determining the intrinsic rate of permeation, which is independent of the system design.

II. DESIGN OF IN VITRO SKIN PERMEATION
    APPARATUS

Various types of in vitro apparatus for measuring drug permeation
profiles across the skin have been reported in the literature (1-5).
They can be broadly classified into two categories as shown in
Table 1. Several designs are illustrated in Figure 2.
    For studying the release profiles of drugs from a transdermal
drug delivery system, the effect of the hydrodynamic diffusion layer
(existing on the drug-releasing surface) on the rate of drug release
must be carefully investigated. Generally speaking, the mechanism
of agitation in the in vitro diffusion cell should be designed to maintain a hydrodynamic condition such that the thickness of the diffusion boundary layer is at a minimum, while the primary convective
flow toward the drug-releasing surface also is minimized. It is,
therefore, more desirable to have the in vitro diffusion cell designed
in such way that the agitation element will rotate at a plane parallel
to the drug-releasing surface (Fig. 2a, c-d). If this is not the

Table 1   Classification of In Vitro Membrane Permeation Systems

---

Physical design of diffusion cell

   Horizontal type (Figs. 2a, 2b)

   Vertical type (Figs. 2c, 2d, 2e)

   Flow-through type (Figs. 2f, 2g)

Method of sampling and measurement

   Continuing system

      Fluid circulation system (Fig. 2f)

      Noncirculation system (Fig. 2g)

   Intermittent system: rotating agitation systems (Figs. 2a-2e)

---

case, the intensity of agitation must be controlled within an appropriate range.

   On the other hand, the effect of the hydrodynamic diffusion layer on the rate of skin permeation may not be substantial, since the principal resistance to drug transport in the transdermal delivery system is often the drug permeation process through the stratum corneum. This is because the diffusivity of a drug across the stratum corneum normally ranges from 10^{-8} to 10^{-13} cm^2/sec, as

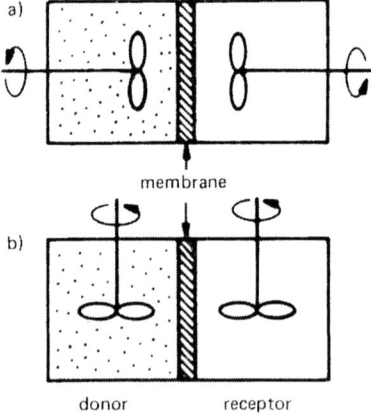

Figure 2   In vitro membrane permeation systems.   (a, b) horizontal type; (c, d, e) vertical type; (f, g) flow-through type.

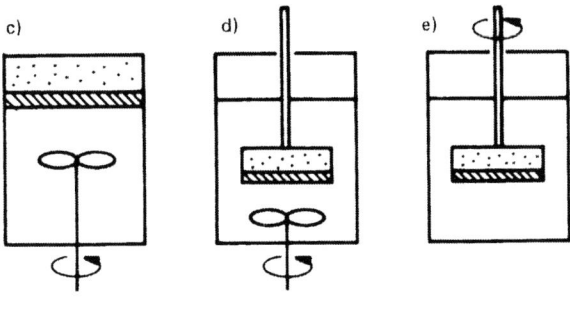

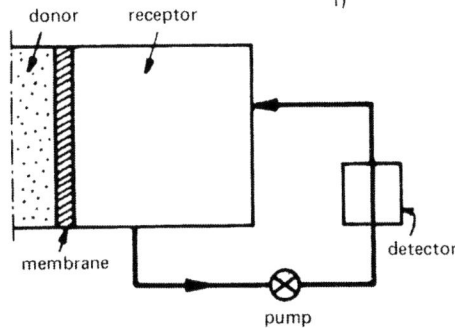

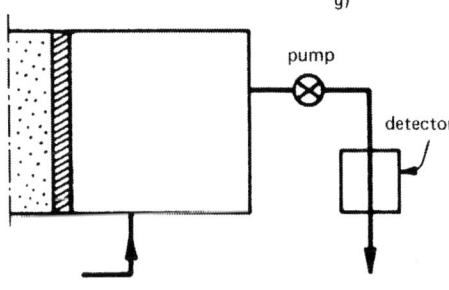

Figure 2 (continued)

compared to the intrinsic diffusivity of 10^{-5} to 10^{-6} cm^2/sec in the elution medium. Therefore, the agitation in this skin-limited permeation study is often important only for maintaining uniform temperature and drug distribution throughout the in vitro skin permeation cell. However, if the barrier function of the stratum corneum is markedly reduced, as in the case of increased skin permeability, the effect of the diffusion layer on the rate of skin permeation could become rather significant.

Several designs of in vitro membrane permeation apparatus, whose hydrodynamic characteristics have been fully investigated, are shown in Figure 3 and discussed in the sections that follow.

A. Horizontal-Type Skin Permeation System, Small Cell Volume

The skin permeation system (Fig. 3a) developed by Valia and Chien (6) has been extensively used for studying the skin permeation kinetics of drugs, using either human cadaver skin or freshly excised animal skin. This cell design (the V–C cell) has a solution compartment of relatively small volume (3.5 ml) in each half-cell for maximal analytical sensitivity, and a rather small membrane area (0.64 cm^2) to accommodate the skin specimen available. Both the donor and receptor solutions are agitated, under a totally enclosed system, by a matched set of star-head magnets (diameter, 8 mm), which are rotated at a synchronous speed of 600 rpm at a fixed position in the stirring platforms by a specially designed driving unit positioned directly underneath the cells. The temperature of the system can be controlled at isothermal or nonisothermal conditions by circulating thermostated water through the water jacket surrounding the solution compartment. The hydrodynamics of this skin permeation system was characterized by Tojo et al. (7).

B. Horizontal-Type Membrane Permeation System, Large Solution Volume

The second horizontal membrane permeation system is also composed of one pair of donor and receptor compartments in mirror image (Fig. 3b), in which the fluid is agitated by a matched set of bar-shaped magnets (2.54 cm long). The magnets are driven by a pair of synchronous motors located directly underneath the cells to rotate at a synchronous but variable rate in a specially designed stirring platform. Each pair of half-cells has a large effective membrane area for permeation (13.9 cm^2). Each compartment can hold a volume of 140–250 ml of solution. The rotation speed of the magnets can be controlled at a constant level of 60–1000 rpm. Samples may be withdrawn for analysis from a sampling port at various intervals. The

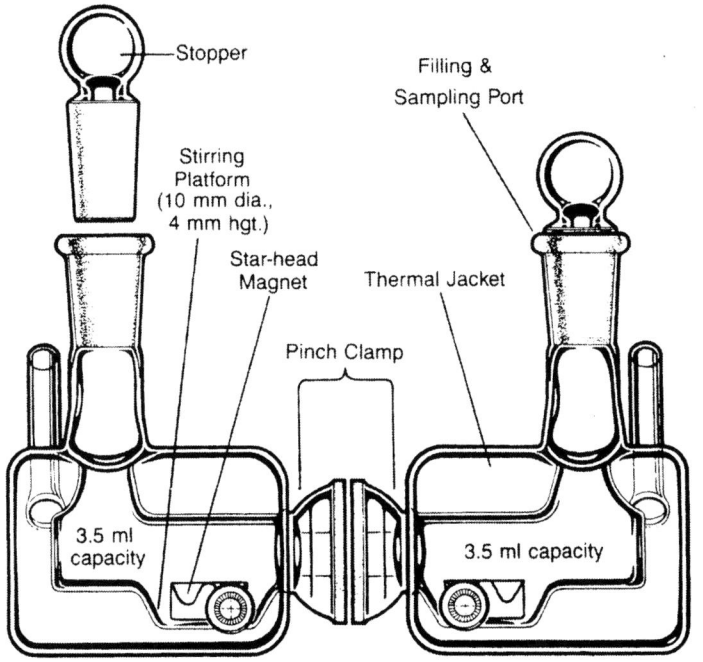

DONOR (Left) HALF-CELL   RECEPTOR (Right) HALF-CELL

(a)

Figure 3   In vitro membrane permeation systems with fully-investigated hydrodynamic characteristics. (a) Valia–Chien (V–C) skin permeation cell. (b) Ghannam–Chien (G–C) membrane permeation cell. (c) Franz diffusion cell. (d) Keshany–Chien (K–C) skin permeation cell. (e) Jhawer–Lord (J–L) rotating-disc system.

donor and receptor compartments are both jacketed and thermostated by an external circulating bath to maintain isothermal conditions, or if desired, the temperature in either donor or receptor compartment can be programmed to simulate any environmental variations. This diffusion cell (the G–C cell) was developed by Ghannam and Chien and its hydrodynamics has been fully calibrated by Tojo et al. (8).

C. Franz Diffusion Cell

The vertical-type skin permeation system (Fig. 3c) developed by Franz and commercialized by Crown Glass has been frequently used for studying the kinetics of percutaneous absorption (9–11). The

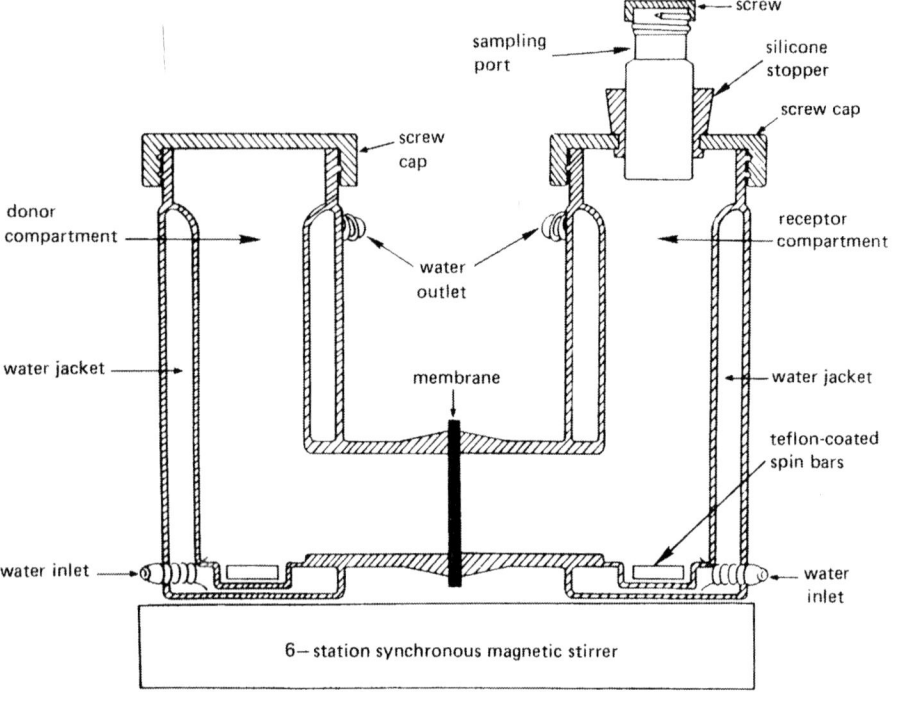

(b)

DONOR COMPARTMENT
(cell cap)

AIR

SAMPLING PORT

TRANSDERMAL SYSTEM

SKIN

WATER OUT

RECEPTOR COMPARTMENT
(cell body)

WATER JACKET

37°C WATER IN

STIRRING BAR

(c)

Figure 3   (continued)

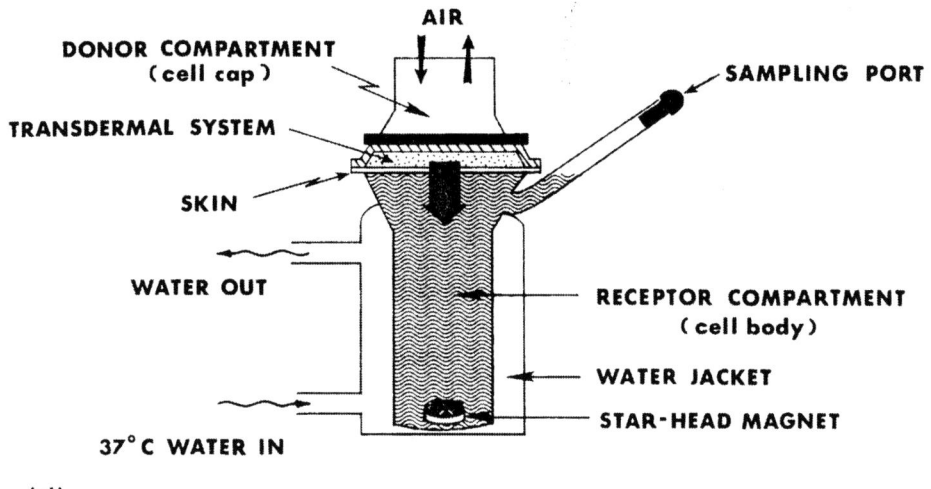

(d)

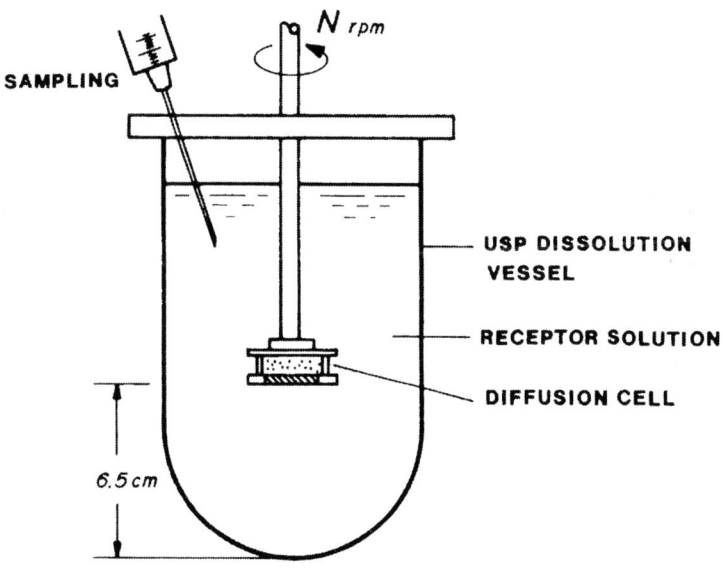

(e)

Figure 3   (continued)

cell has a receptor compartment with an effective volume of approximately 10–12 ml and an effective surface area for permeation varying from 1.57 to 4.71 cm^2. The solution in the receptor compartment is stirred by a rod-shaped magnet driven by a 3-W synchronous motor. The stirring magnet rotates at a speed of 600 rpm in a low-viscosity receptor solution such as saline solution. The temperature in the bulk of the solution can be maintained at a constant level by circulating thermostated water through the water jacket surrounding the receptor compartment. However, the temperature near the upper opening, at which the skin will be positioned, varies as the surrounding temperature varies. The observed variation in receptor solution temperature results because the donor compartment is not thermally controlled. The hydrodynamic characteristics of the Franz diffusion cell recently were established (12).

D. Modified Franz Diffusion Cell

Another vertical-type skin permeation cell (Fig. 3d) was recently developed in response to the observation that the Franz cell (Fig. 3c) has rather poor solution hydrodynamics as a result of inefficient mixing. The results are a significant temperature gradient in the diffusion cell and an inhomogeneous drug concentration in the receptor solution. Recognizing these deficiencies, Keshary and Chien (13) set forth to modify the Franz diffusion cell to improve its efficiency of fluid mixing. The modified cell (the K–C cell) has an effective receptor solution volume of 12 ml and a skin surface area of 3.14 cm^2. The receptor solution is stirred by a star-head magnet rotating at a constant speed of 600 rpm by the same driving unit originally designed for Franz diffusion cell. The hydrodynamic characteristics of the modified Franz cell were recently investigated (12).

E. Rotating-Disc-Type Membrane Permeation Cell

One of the advantages of the rotating-disc cell is that the hydrodynamic diffusion boundary layer on the surface of the rotating disc has been well established theoretically (14).

If the rotating disc is assumed to be sufficiently large that the edge effects are negligible, the thickness of diffusion boundary layer is given by:

$$\delta = 1.61 \left(\frac{D_f \rho}{\mu} \right)^{1/3} \left(\frac{\mu}{\rho \omega} \right)^{1/2} \tag{1}$$

where D_f is the drug diffusivity in the fluid, ρ is the density of the fluid, μ is the viscosity of the fluid, ω is the angular velocity ($= \pi N d$).

In the rotating-disc diffusion cell, if the disc is not large enough, the flow pattern in the cell is easily influenced by the wall of the vessel. Then the diffusion layer determined experimentally is usually thicker than that calculated from Eq. (1) due to the dissipation of additional energy on the vessel wall (15). Therefore, Eq. (1) should not be used a priori for estimating the diffusion boundary layer thickness existing on the surface of the rotating disc.

Recently, Jhawar and Lordi (16) developed a rotating-disc-type membrane permeation cell (the J–L cell) for studying the release of drug from suppositories (Fig. 3e). The rotating disc has an effective membrane area of 12.6 cm^2 and can be used together with the one-liter USP dissolution vessel as the receptor compartment. The hydrodynamic characteristics of this diffusion cell were recently investigated (17).

III. METHOD FOR CHARACTERIZING THE HYDRODYNAMICS OF IN VITRO SYSTEMS

The dissolution process of solid drug in various elution media can be used to evaluate the thickness of the hydrodynamic diffusion layer in an in vitro membrane permeation cell. The benzoic acid disc has been frequently used as the calibration agent for this purpose, since its physicochemical properties, such as diffusivity and solubility, are well established. A thin benzoic acid disc of suitable size and thickness is mounted on each unit of membrane permeation cell between the donor and receptor compartments (Fig. 4). With the benzoic acid disc in place, aqueous solution containing various volume fractions of a solubilizer, such as polyethylene glycol 400 (PEG 400), is charged into one of the compartments as the dissolution medium, while the other compartment remains empty. At predetermined time intervals, samples are withdrawn from the dissolution medium for the assay of benzoic acid concentration. If the in vitro cell is a flow-through system as shown in Figure 5, the concentration of benzoic acid in the solution can be monitored continuously. The physical properties of benzoic acid in various aqueous PEG 400 solutions are summarized in Table 2.

Assuming that perfect mixing conditions are maintained for the bulk solution in the receptor comparment and that plug flow is achieved in the circulation tubing, we obtain a mass balance equation for the concentration of benzoic acid in the receptor solution:

$$V\frac{dC(t)}{dt} = kA[C_s - C(t)] + F\left[C\left(t - \frac{V_p}{F}\right) - C(t)\right] \tag{2}$$

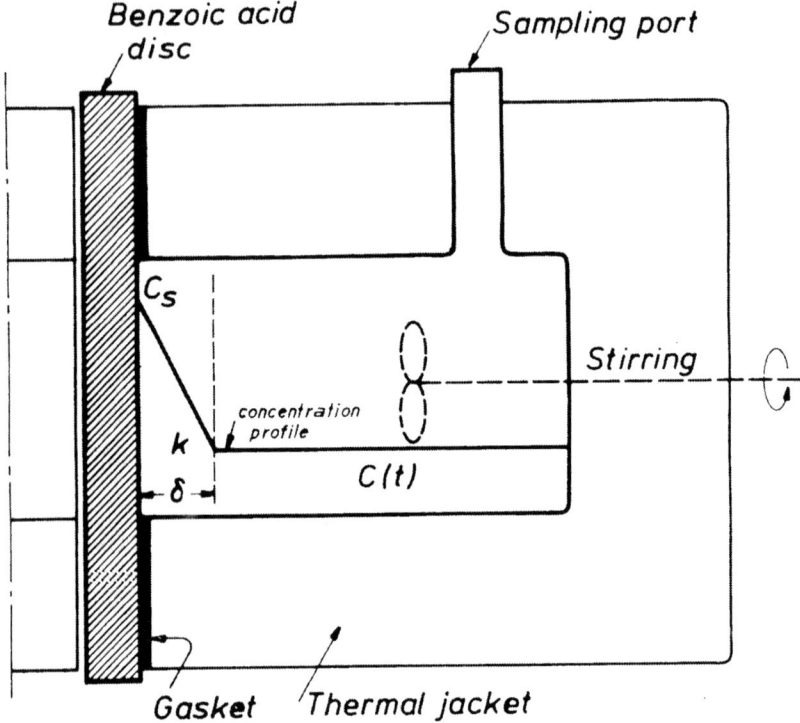

Figure 4 Calibration of the hydrodynamic characteristics in an in vitro membrane permeation system using a benzoic acid dissolution process. The solid line in the receptor compartment shows the concentration profile of benzoic acid on the basis of film theory. C_S = saturated concentration, $C(t)$ = bulk concentration at time t, k = mass transfer coefficient, δ = thickness of diffusion boundary layer.

By expanding the $C(t - V_p/F) - C(t)$ term in the Taylor series and truncating it at the square term, Eq. (2) can be rewritten for the mass transfer coefficient k as follows (18):

$$k = \frac{1}{C_S - C}\left[\frac{V + V_p}{A}\frac{dC}{dt} - \frac{V_p^2}{2FA}\frac{d^2C}{dt^2}\right] \tag{3}$$

where V and V_p are, respectively, the volume of the receptor compartment and the volume of the circulation tubing; C_S and C are the equilibrium solubility and the concentration of benzoic acid in the

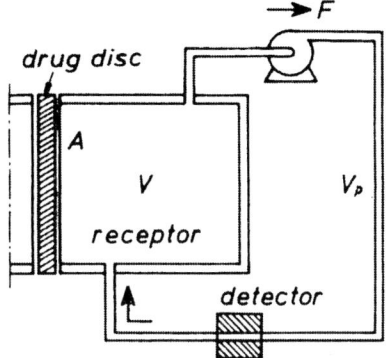

Figure 5 Benzoic acid dissolution method for evaluation of the diffusion boundary layer in flow-through systems by continuous measurement of benzoic acid concentration in the medium. A = effective surface area of benzoic acid disc for dissolution, F = flow rate, V = volume of receptor compartment, V_p = volume of circulation tubing.

receptor solution at time t; A is the effective surface area for drug dissolution, k is the mass transfer coefficient, and F is the flow rate of the solution in the circulation tubing for continuous measurement. To obtain the derivatives, dC/dt and d^2C/dt^2 in Eq. (3), which can be estimated from the transient response curve of the benzoic acid concentration change, third-order forward differences, based on the Gregory-Newton interpolating polynomials, can be used (19). If the volume of the receptor compartment (V) is much larger than the volume of the circulation tubing (V_p) or if the in vitro system is not equipped with circulation tubing, Eq. (3) can be simplified and the mass transfer coefficient determined by:

$$k = \frac{1}{C_s - C} \frac{V}{A} \frac{dC}{dt}$$

$$= \frac{V}{At} \ln\left[\frac{C_s - C_i}{C_s - C}\right] \tag{4}$$

where C_i is the initial drug concentration in the receptor solution. Equation (4) is also applicable to the in vitro systems outlined in Figures 3a-d.

The mass transfer coefficient (k) is related by the following dimensionless equation to the Sherwood number (Sh), the Reynolds number (Re), and the Schmidt number (Sc) (20,21):

Table 2 Physical Properties of Benzoic Acid in Aqueous
Polyethylene Glycol 400 Solutions

Physical properties	Volume fraction of PEG 400			
	0	10%	20%	40%
PEG 400 solution				
Density (g/ml)				
(10-37°C)	0.99	1.00	1.02	1.04
Viscosity (g/cm-sec)				
10°C	0.013	0.031	0.050	0.120
20°C	0.010	0.016	0.027	0.070
37°C	0.007	0.010	0.018	0.046
Benzoic acid				
Equilibrium solubility (mg/ml)				
10°C	2.25	3.59	5.09	19.80
20°C	2.64	4.23	7.53	22.60
37°C	4.39	7.85	15.36	54.20
Diffusivity (cm^2/sec × 10^5)				
10°C	0.70	0.30	0.18	0.076
20°C	0.98	0.60	0.37	0.14
37°C	1.45	0.99	0.55	0.22

$$Sh = const\ Re^m\ Sc^n \tag{5}$$

where

$$Sh = \frac{kd}{D_f} \tag{6}$$

$$Re = \frac{du\rho}{\mu} \tag{7}$$

$$Sc = \frac{\mu}{\rho D_f} \tag{8}$$

and d is the length of the agitator, μ and ρ are the viscosity and density of the solution, respectively; and u is the characteristic velocity of the fluid motion, which is frequently defined as the tip speed of the agitator ($N \times d$). The exponents m and n in Eq. (5) are empirical constants, which depend on the type of in vitro system used.

For the rotating-disc-type membrane permeation cell with an idealized laminar flow pattern surrounding the disc, the correlation equation for mass transfer coefficient was treated by Levich (14) and is described by:

$$Sh = 1.557 \left(\frac{Nd^2 \rho}{\mu} \right)^{1/2} \left(\frac{\mu}{\rho D_f} \right)^{1/3} \tag{9}$$

As mentioned earlier, the constants for the rotating-disc permeation cell used in drug release or permeation studies may be smaller than the theoretical value given by Eq. (9).

Once the dimensionless relationship has been fully established, it can be used to estimate the effect of the diffusion boundary layer on the rate of drug release or membrane permeation. Furthermore, similar dimensionless equation, which is similar to the ones for mass transfer (Eqs. 8, 9), can also be derived to evaluate the temperature profile near the membrane surface, since there is a similarity between the heat transfer and the mass transfer processes on the basis of the theory of similitude (22). The effect of the thermal diffusion layer has been analyzed and found to be one of the most important phenomena in transdermal drug delivery (23).

IV. CORRELATION EQUATION FOR MASS TRANSFER COEFFICIENT

The values of the mass transfer coefficient (k) determined from the benzoic acid dissolution experiments are correlated using the dimensionless relationship of Eq. (5). The exponent n on the Schmidt number was found to be 1/3 (8). The same number frequently has been found to be acceptable in solid–liquid mass transfer operations (24,25).

The mass transfer coefficients obtained in various membrane permeation systems (Fig. 3) were plotted as $\log(Sh/Sc^{1/3})$ versus $\log(Re)$ in Figure 6. The correlation equations obtained for these in vitro systems are summarized in Table 3.

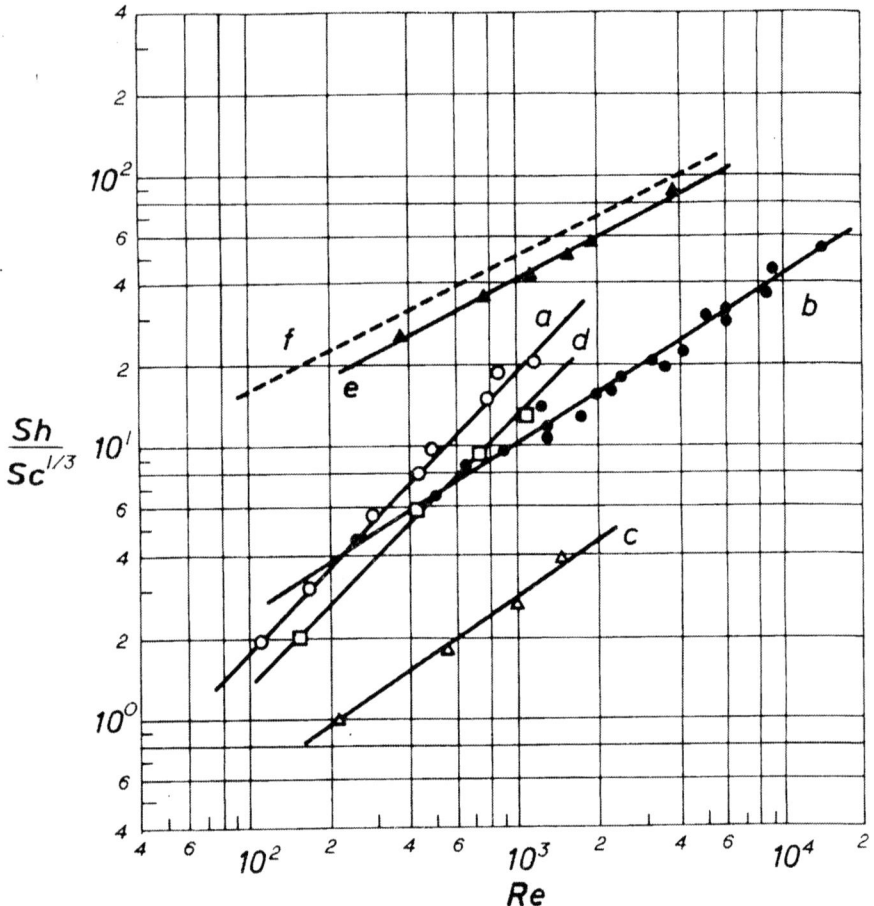

Figure 6   Correlation of mass transfer coefficients for various
in vitro membrane permeation systems.   Curve a, V–C cell (Fig. 3a);
curve b, G–C cell (Fig. 3b); curve c, Franz cell (Fig. 3c); curve
d, K–C cell (Fig. 3d); curve e, J–L cell (Fig. 3e); curve f, ideal
rotating-disc device (Eq. 9).

Table 3 Correlation Equations for the Mass Transfer Coefficient of Various In Vitro Membrane Permeation Systems

Membrane permeation system	Correlation equation
V-C cell (Fig. 3a)	$Sh = 0.0124 \, Re^{1.03} \, Sc^{1/3}$ for $100 < Re < 1000$, $20-40°C$
G-C cell (Fig. 3b)	$Sh = 0.234 \, Re^{0.57} \, Sc^{1/3}$ for $100 < Re < 10,000$, $10-40°C$
	$Sh = 0.154 \, Re^{0.61} \, Sc^{1/3}$ for $300 < Re < 20,000$, $37°C$
Franz cell (Fig. 3c)	$Sh = 0.026 \, Re^{0.68} \, Sc^{1/3}$ for $500 < Re < 2000$, $37°C$
K-C cell (Fig. 3d)	$Sh = 0.0146 \, Re^{0.98} \, Sc^{1/3}$ for $100 < Re < 2000$, $37°C$
J-L cell (Fig. 3e)	$Sh = 1.163 \, Re^{0.51} \, Sc^{1/3}$ for $400 < Re < 4000$, $37°C$

By using the correlation equations in Table 3, the mass transfer coefficient and the thickness of the hydrodynamic diffusion layer (= d/Sh) for any drug-solution system can be determined if the values of diffusivity (D_f), density (ρ), and viscosity (μ) are known or available. The effect of the diffusion boundary layer on the rate of drug permeation can also be analyzed by solving the governing equation (mass balance equation), after it has been subjected to the appropriate boundary conditions (which depend on the hydrodynamic characteristics of the in vitro system) and initial conditions. The intrinsic rate of permeation, which is useful in establishing a reliable in vitro–in vivo correlation, can then be determined for such a drug-solvent system.

V. EFFECT OF THE DIFFUSION BOUNDARY LAYER ON DRUG PERMEATION

A. Membrane-Moderated Drug Delivery

If a pseudo-steady state is established and the drug permeation across a two-layer membrane (composite of a synthetic membrane on biological membrane, like the skin) is under perfect sink conditions (i.e., $C_0 = 0$) as shown in Figure 7, the steady-state rate of permeation across a unit surface area of the membrane can be represented by the following equation:

$$\frac{dQ}{dt} = k_d(C_d - C_m) = \frac{D_m}{\ell_m}(K_m C_m - C_1) = \frac{D_1}{\ell_1}(K_1 C_1 - C_1')$$

$$= \frac{D_2}{\ell_2}(C_2' - K_2 C_2) = k_r(C_2 - C_0) \cong k_r C_2 \tag{10}$$

where

C_1, C_1', C_2, C_2', C_m = drug concentrations

C_d = drug solubility in the donor solution

D_1 = diffusivity of drug through membrane layer 1

D_2 = diffusivity of drug through membrane layer 2

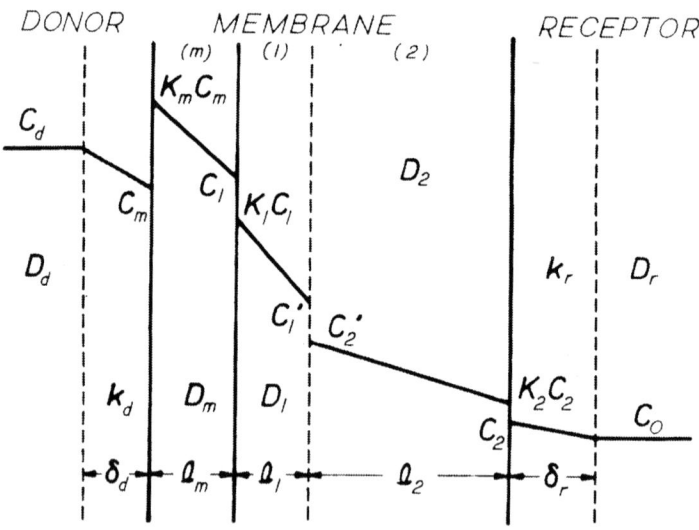

Figure 7   Steady-state drug concentration profile in the two-layer membrane and in the solution: membrane-moderated skin permeation study.

D_m = diffusivity of drug through membrane layer m

K_1 = partition coefficient between membrane layer m and membrane layer 1

K_2 = partition coefficient between the receptor phase and membrane layer 2

K_m = partition coefficient between the donor phase and membrane layer m

k_d = mass transfer coefficient in the donor-side boundary layer

k_r = mass transfer coefficient in the receptor-side boundary layer

ℓ_1 = thickness of membrane layer 1

ℓ_2 = thickness of membrane layer 2

ℓ_m = thickness of membrane layer m

Rearranging, Eq. (10) yields:

$$\frac{dQ}{dt} = \frac{C_d}{\dfrac{1}{k_d} + \dfrac{\ell_m}{D_m K_m} + \dfrac{\ell_1}{D_1 K_1}\dfrac{1}{K_m} + \dfrac{\ell_2}{D_2 K_2}\dfrac{C_d}{C_r} + \dfrac{1}{k_r}\dfrac{C_d}{C_r}} \tag{11}$$

where the donominator consists of the sum of diffusional resistances due to the donor-side boundary layer, the membranes, and the receptor-side boundary layer.

If the solutions in the donor and receptor compartments are both subjected to vigorous mixing such that the diffusional resistance in the diffusion boundary layers becomes negligibly small, Eq. (11) is reduced to:

$$\left(\frac{dQ}{dt}\right)_i = \frac{C_d}{\dfrac{\ell_m}{D_m K_m} + \dfrac{\ell_1}{D_1 K_1}\dfrac{1}{K_m} + \dfrac{\ell_2}{D_2 K_2}\dfrac{C_d}{C_r}} \tag{12}$$

which defines the intrinsic rate of permeation, $(dQ/dt)_i$.

The ratio of the permeation rate with the effect of the diffusion boundary layer to the permeation rate without this effect, $(dQ/dt)/dQ/dt)_i$, is then given by:

$$\gamma_r = \frac{dQ/dt}{dQ/dt_i} = 1 - \frac{\alpha + \beta}{Sh_r}\frac{dQ/dt}{D_r C_d/d} \tag{13}$$

where $\alpha = k_r/k_d = (Sh_r/Sh_d)(D_r/D_d)$, $\beta = C_d/C_r$, and D_r and D_d are the drug diffusivities in the receptor and donor solutions, respectively. If the diffusivity is not available, it can be estimated by the following empirical relationship:

$$\frac{D_u}{D_k} = \left(\frac{M_u}{M_k}\right)^{-p} \tag{14}$$

where M is the molecular weight of a drug, and subscripts u and k stand for unknown and known drugs, respectively. The exponent p in Eq. (14) depends on the molecular weight of the drug. For molecules with a molecular weight less than 1000, p has a value of $1/2$, while for a larger molecule, the p value is $1/3$ (26-28). The effect of molecular weight on diffusivity and p value is shown in Figure 8.

The intrinsic rate of membrane permeation $(dQ/dt)_i$ can then be calculated from the experimental value of (dQ/dt) by:

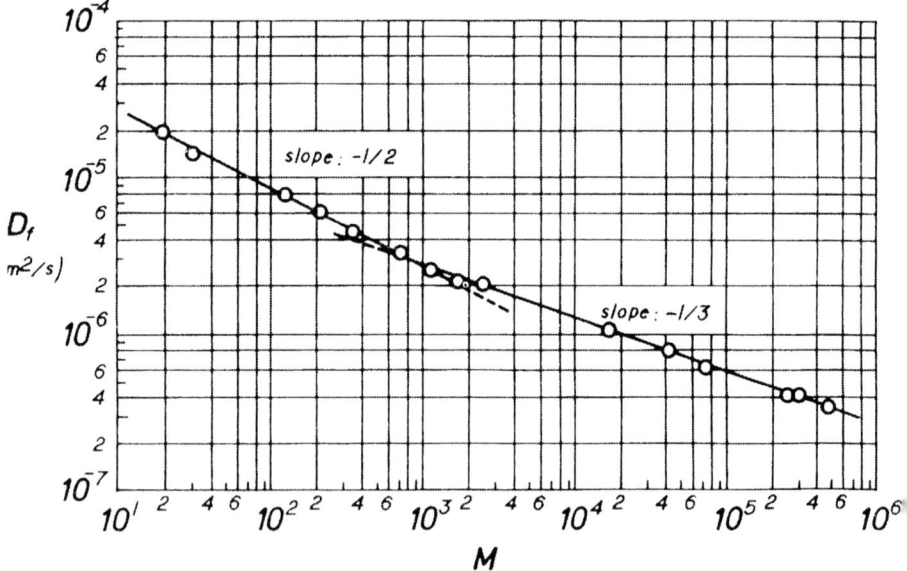

Figure 8   Effect of drug molecular weight (M) on its aqueous diffusivity (D_f).

$$\left(\frac{dQ}{dt}\right)_i = \left(\frac{dQ}{dt}\right)\frac{1}{\gamma_r}$$ (15)

if the value of γ_r is known or predetermined by Eq. (13).
Figure 9 shows the effect of partition coefficient on the relation
of γ_r to Sh when the same elution medium and the same agitation
intensity are used in both the donor and receptor compartments
(8). The data suggest that it is essential to take hydrodynamics
into account for proper analysis of the experimental data obtained
in membrane permeation studies. For a hydrophilic drug with a
partition coefficient of 0.05, for example, a Sherwood number of
only 30 would be sufficient to assure a γ_r value of 1, whereas for
a lipophilic drug with a relatively high partition coefficient of 50,
a Sherwood number of 3×10^4 would be needed to assure the same
γ_r value. Since Sherwood number is proportional to Reynolds number with the exponent in the range of 0.5 to 1.0, the agitation
speed in the solution required for a drug with K = 50 should be
more than 10^5 times greater than that for a drug with K $\doteq$ 0.05, to
assure the same hydrodynamic conditions (or intrinsic permeation
rate). This is, of course, impossible to achieve.

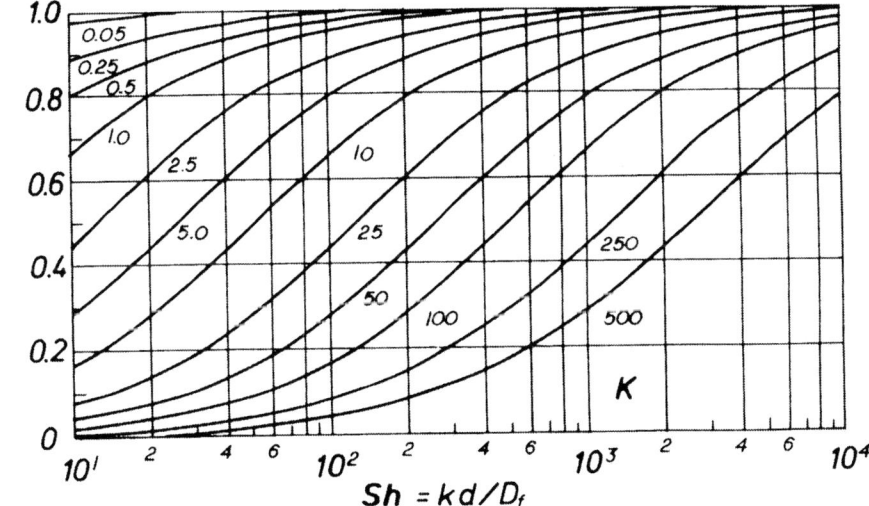

Figure 9   Effect of Sherwood number (Sh) on the ratio (γ_r) of the
apparent rate of drug permeation over the intrinsic rate of permea-
tion [γ_r = (dQ/dt)/(dQ/dt)$_i$]: D_p/D_r = 0.01, d/ℓ = 254, $\alpha + \beta$ = 2.
The values on the curves denote the respective magnitudes of the
partition coefficient K.

The time lag is also influenced by the hydrodynamics in the membrane permeation cell. Since the time lag value is frequently measured for the determination of membrane diffusivity (29), the effect of the hydrodynamic diffusion layer on time lag must be corrected if one wants to determine intrinsic diffusivity. A simple evaluation method for the calculation of intrinsic diffusivity was recently porposed by Tojo et al. (30) based on the three-layer model.

B. Matrix-Diffusion-Controlled Drug Delivery

Under the pseudo-steady-state and sink conditions, the rate of drug permeation from the matrix-diffusion-controlled drug delivery system across the two-layer membrane (Fig. 10) can be represented by (31):

$$\frac{dQ}{dt} = D_p \frac{C_p - C_1}{X} = \left(A - \frac{C_p + C_1}{2}\right)\frac{dX}{dt} = D_1 \frac{K_1 C_1 - C_1'}{\ell_1}$$

$$= D_2 \frac{C_2' - K_2 C_2}{\ell_2} = k_r(C_2 - C_0) \cong k_r C_2 \tag{16}$$

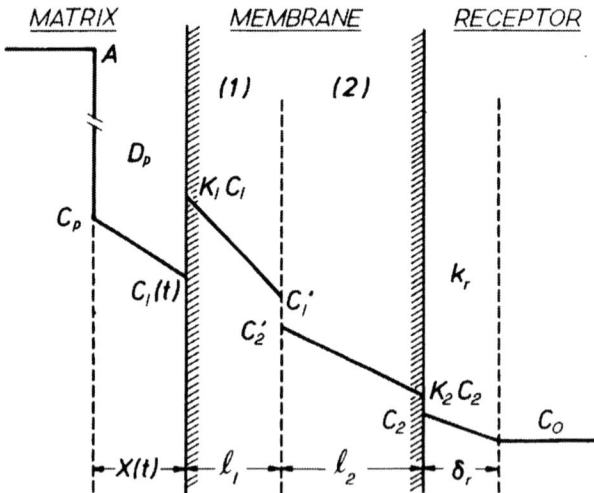

Figure 10 Drug concentration profile in the matrix-diffusion-controlled type of drug delivery system based on the pseudo-steady-state condition.

where

$$A = \text{drug loading dose}$$

$$C_1, C_1', C_2, C_2' = \text{drug concentrations on the boundaries (Fig. 10)}$$

$$C_p = \text{drug solubility in the polymer matrix of the delivery system}$$

$$X = \text{diffusion front of the drug in the matrix (Fig. 10)}$$

The third term in Eq. (16) can be approximated by $(A - C_p/2)$ dX/dt, since excess drug is loaded in the matrix-type drug delivery system $(A \gg C_p > C_1)$.
Solving Eq. (16) gives:

$$\frac{dQ}{dt} = D_p C_p \left[\frac{2C_p D_p t}{A - C_p/2} + \left(\frac{b}{a}\right)^2 \right]^{-1/2} \tag{17}$$

where

$$a = \frac{k_m}{D_p} \tag{18}$$

$$b = \frac{\beta k_r \ell_2}{K_2 D_2} + \frac{K_2}{K_1} + \frac{k_r \ell_1}{K_1 D_1} \tag{19}$$

Integration of Eq. (17) gives the cumulative amount of drug released, Q, as follows:

$$Q = \int_0^t \left(\frac{dQ}{dt}\right) dt$$

$$= \left(A - \frac{C_p}{2}\right) \left\{ \left[\frac{2C_p D_p t}{A - C_p/2} + \left(\frac{b}{a}\right)^2 \right]^{1/2} - \frac{b}{a} \right\} \tag{20}$$

The ratio γ_m of cumulative amount of drug released with the diffusion barriers to the cumulative amount released without the barriers (i.e., the composite of the membrane, like skin and the diffusion boundary layer), is given as:

$$\gamma_m = \frac{Q}{Q_i} = \left[1 - \frac{Q/t}{C_r}(R_1 + R_2 + R_3)\right]^{1/2} \tag{21}$$

where Q_i is the intrinsic cumulative amount of drug released, which is defined by:

$$Q_i = [(2A - C_p)D_p C_p t]^{1/2} \tag{22}$$

and

$$R_1 = \frac{\ell_1}{K_1 D_1} \tag{23}$$

$$R_2 = \frac{\ell_2}{K_2 D_2} \tag{24}$$

$$R_3 = \frac{K_2}{K_1} \frac{C_r}{C_d} \frac{1}{k_r} \tag{25}$$

If there is no membrane on the surface of the drug-releasing surface (Fig. 10), Eq. (21) can be simplified to (32):

$$\gamma_m = \left[1 - \frac{Q/t}{C_r} \frac{1}{k_r}\right]^{1/2} \tag{26}$$

If the following condition is satisfied:

$$\frac{k_r^2 t}{K^2} \gg \frac{D_p}{2}\left(\frac{A}{C_p} - \frac{1}{2}\right) \tag{27}$$

where K is the partition coefficient [$= C(\text{matrix})/C(\text{solution})$].

The cumulative amount of drug released in the absence of membrane can be approximated by (32):

$$Q = [(2A - C_p)D_p C_p t]^{1/2} - \frac{(A - C_p/2)KD_p}{k_r} \tag{28}$$

Equation (28) indicates that the intrinsic rate of release from a matrix-type drug delivery system can be determined from the slope of experimental plots of Q versus $\sqrt{t}$ under the conditions of Eq. (27).

For a unilayer membrane, such as viable skin (without stratum corneum) only, Eq. (21) can be reduced to:

$$\gamma_m = \left[1 - \frac{Q/t}{C_r} \frac{l_2}{D_2 K_2} + \frac{1}{k_r} \right]^{1/2} \tag{29}$$

The intrinsic cumulative amount of drug released, Q_i, at the time t, is then given by:

$$Q_i = \frac{Q}{\gamma_m} \tag{30}$$

where the mass transfer coefficient needed for the determination of γ_m can be calculated from the correlation equations for the in vitro apparatus listed in Table 3.

VI. CALCULATION OF INTRINSIC RATE OF PERMEATION

A. Example 1

The experiment of testosterone permeation through a silicone (PDMS) membrane was carried out at 37°C under the following conditions:

1. G–C membrane permeation cell (Fig. 3b)
   Donor: saturated drug solution in water
   Receptor: water without drug
   Rotating speed of magnet: 425 rpm
   Drug solubility in water: 25 μg/ml
   Drug diffusivity in water: 6.54×10^{-6} cm^2/sec
2. V–C skin permeation cell (Fig. 3a)
   Donor: saturated drug solution in 40% PEG 400 solution
   Receptor: 40% PEG 400 solution without drug
   Drug solubility in 40% PEG 400 solution: 508 μg/ml
   Drug diffusivity in 40% PEG 400 solution: 0.98×10^{-6} cm^2/sec

The apparent steady-state rates of permeation for testosterone were 7.75 μg/cm^2/hr in the G–C cell (8) and 9.20 μg/cm^2/hr in the V–C cell (33), respectively.

The intrinsic permeation rate of testosterone through the silicone membrane can be calculated as follows:

Solution

(1) G–C membrane permeation cell:

$$Re = \frac{Nd^2\rho}{\mu} = \frac{(425/60)(2.54^2)(0.993)}{0.0069} = 6577$$

$$Sc = \frac{\mu}{\rho D_f} = \frac{0.0069}{(0.993)(6.54 \times 10^{-6})} = 1062$$

$$Sh = 0.154 \, Re^{0.61} \, Sc^{1/3} = 0.154(6577)^{0.61}(1062)^{1/3}$$

$$= 334$$

The correction factor γ_r can be calculated from Eq. (13):

$$\gamma_r = 1 - \frac{\alpha + \beta}{Sh_r} \frac{dQ/dt}{D_f C_d/d} = 1 - \frac{1+1}{334} \frac{7.75/3600}{(6.54 \times 10^{-6})25/2.54}$$

$$= 0.800$$

By Eq. (15), the intrinsic rate of permeation can be determined as follows:

$$\left(\frac{dQ}{dt}\right)_i = \frac{dQ/dt}{\gamma_r} = \frac{7.75}{0.80} = 9.69 \; \mu g/cm^2/hr$$

(2) V–C skin permeation cell:

$$Re = \frac{(600/60)(0.80^2)(1.047)}{0.046} = 145.7$$

$$Sc = \frac{0.046}{(1.047)(0.98 \times 10^{-6})} = 4.48 \times 10^4$$

$$Sh = 0.0157(145.7)^{1.03}(4.48 \times 10^4)^{1/3} = 94$$

$$\gamma_r = 1 - \frac{1+1}{94} \frac{(9.20/3600)}{(0.98 \times 10^{-6})(508)/0.8} = 0.913$$

$$\left(\frac{dQ}{dt}\right)_i = \frac{9.20}{0.913} = 10.1 \; \mu g/cm^2/hr$$

It is interesting to note that the intrinsic rate of permeation obtained in the different membrane permeation systems is almost identical (9.69 $\mu g/cm^2/hr$ in the G–C cell versus 10.1 $\mu g/cm^2/hr$ in the V–C cell). If the apparent permeation data were compared directly, it might be erroneously concluded that the permeation rate obtained in the 40% PEG 400 solution is greater than that in the water and that the difference is due to the solubility increase in the donor solution as a result of adding 40% PEG 400.

For a more lipophilic drug such as progesterone, the steady-state permeation rate is expected to be much more influenced by the diffusion boundary layer formed in the membrane permeation apparatus (34).

B. Example 2

The permeation of progesterone through hairless mouse skin was carried out in a V–C skin permeation cell under the following experimental conditions:

Donor: saturated solution in 40% PEG 400 solution
Receptor: 40% PEG 400 solution without drug
Drug solubility in 40% PEG 400 solution: 208 $\mu g/ml$
Drug diffusivity in 40% PEG 400 solution: 0.98×10^{-6} cm^2/sec

The steady-state rates of permeation across the intact skin and the stripped skin (without the stratum corneum) were 2.2 and 3.5 $\mu g/cm^2/hr$, respectively (34).

Calculate the intrinsic permeation rate of progesterone across the whole skin and stripped skin of hairless mouse.

Solution

$$Re = \frac{(10)(0.80^2)(1.047)}{0.046} = 145.7$$

$$Sc = \frac{0.046}{(1.047)(0.98 \times 10^{-6})} = 4.48 \times 10^4$$

$$Sh = 0.0157(145.7)^{1.03}(4.48 \times 10^4)^{1/3} = 94$$

$$\gamma_r = 1 - \frac{1+1}{94}\frac{2.2/3600}{(0.98 \times 10^{-6})(108)/0.80} = 0.949 \text{ (whole skin)}$$

$$\gamma_r = 1 - \frac{1+1}{94}\frac{3.5/3600}{(0.98 \times 10^{-6})(208)/0.80} = 0.919 \text{ (stripped skin)}$$

$$\left(\frac{dQ}{dt}\right)_i = \frac{2.2}{0.949} = 2.32 \ \mu g/cm^2/hr \ \text{(whole skin)}$$

$$\left(\frac{dQ}{dt}\right)_i = \frac{3.5}{0.919} = 3.81 \ \mu g/cm^2/hr \ \text{(stripped skin)}$$

The effect of the diffusion boundary layer on the rate of skin permeation is usually not very remarkable, because the principal resistance to drug transport often resides in the drug diffusion across the skin. However, if the barrier function of the skin is reduced as the result of applying skin permeation enhancer and/or the prodrug approach, the effect of the diffusion boundary layer on the rate of skin permeation could become significant and should be taken into consideration.

VII. EFFECT OF TEMPERATURE ON DRUG PERMEATION

The rate of drug delivery from a transdermal delivery system is often subjected to the effects of environmental temperature. Thus the temperature in an in vitro skin permeation system must be controlled precisely to maintain a target temperature. Otherwise, the release and/or permeation data may be significantly distorted due to poor control of system temperature. Temperature control is particularly critical for vertical-type skin permeation apparatuses, such as the Franz cell, since the donor temperature is not thermostated and is therefore subject to variations in environmental temperature. So, a temperature gradient may be developed beneath the delivery system and/or skin in the receptor solution.

Figure 11 shows the effect of the variation in system temperature on the rate of steroid permeation across hairless mouse skin (35) and across PDMS membrane (36). Apparently, the rate of drug permeation is markedly influenced by the system temperature. Therefore, the thermal diffusion layer in an in vitro system must be characterized in addition to the mass diffusion layer. The thickness of the thermal diffusion layer can be estimated also using the dimensionless correlation equations discussed earlier for the mass transfer coefficient on the basis of the theory of similitude between mass transfer and heat transfer (22).

If a temperature gradient is formed across the membrane, thermal diffusion takes place in addition to ordinary molecular diffusion. This effect, the so-called Soret effect, was found to have only a negligible influence on drug transport across the membrane under conditions normally encountered in transdermal drug delivery (35,37).

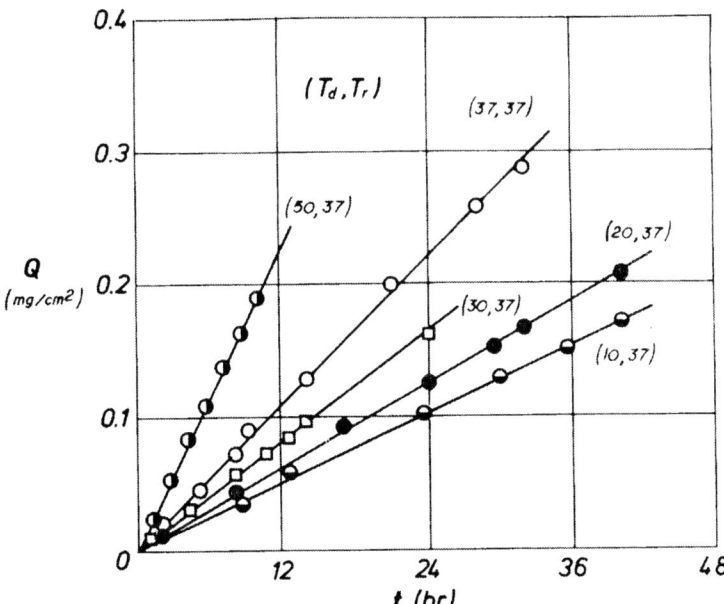

(a)

Figure 11 Effect of system temperature on the rate of drug permeation: numbers in parentheses represent T_d (temperature in the donor solution and T_r (temperature in the receptor solution. (a) Testosterone permeation through a PDMS membrane 0.013 cm thick in a G-C cell (Fig. 3*b*). (b) Progesterone permeation through the whole abdominal skin of a hairless mouse in a V-C cell (Fig. 3*a*).

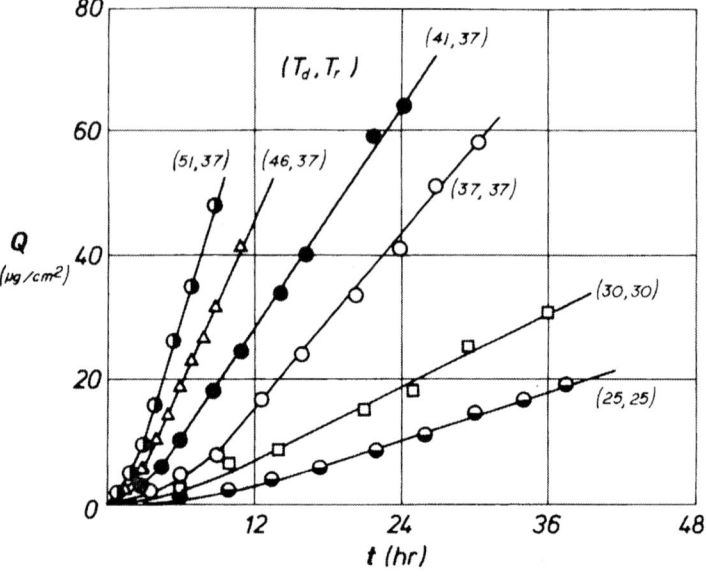

(b)

Figure 11   (continued)

VIII. CONCLUSION

The hydrodynamic characteristics of several in vitro membrane permeation systems were presented for estimating the effect of the diffusion
boundary layer on the rate of drug permeation. The methods for
correcting the effect of the diffusion boundary layer and for determining the intrinsic rate of permeation were illustrated for both membrane-
moderated and matrix-diffusion-controlled drug delivery systems.
The approach used to calculate the intrinsic rate of drug permeation
from the apparent permeation data, discussed in this chapter, would
be useful for gaining a fundamental understanding of the mechanism
of drug permeation for transdermal drug delivery systems. Since
only the in vitro permeation apparatus with precisely defined hydrodynamic characteristics will allow the determination of the real mechanism of drug permeation, not distorted by variations in diffusion cell
design, the hydrodynamic characteristics of an in vitro system must
be determined before carrying out any permeation experiments.

ACKNOWLEDGMENTS

The author wishes to acknowledge Drs. Y. Sun, M. Ghannam, P. Keshary, and Mr. J. A. Masi for sharing their experimental findings. The author is also grateful to Dr. Y. W. Chien for his valuable comments.

REFERENCES

1. H. Durheim, G. L. Flynn, W. I. Higuchi, and C. R. Behl, *J. Pharm. Sci.*, *69*: 781 (1980).
2. R. J. Scheuplein, *J. Invest. Dermatol.*, *45*: 334 (1965).
3. A. S. Michaels, S. K. Chandrasekaran, and J. E. Shaw, *AIChE J.*, *21*: 985 (1975).
4. E. R. Garrett and P. B. Chemburkar, *J. Pharm. Sci.*, *57*: 944 (1968).
5. S. A. Akhter and B. W. Barry, *J. Pharm. Pharmacol.*, *37*: 27 (1985).
6. Y. W. Chien and K. H. Valia, *Drug Dev. Ind. Pharm.*, *10*: 575 (1984).
7. K. Tojo, J. A. Masi, and Y. W. Chien, *Ind. Eng. Chem. Fundam.*, *24*: 368 (1985).
8. K. Tojo, Y. Sun, M. Ghannam, and Y. W. Chien, *AIChE J.*, *31*: 741 (1985).
9. T. J. Franz, *J. Invest. Dermatol.*, *64*: 190 (1975).
10. D. S.-l. Chow, I. Kaka, and T. I. Wang, *J. Pharm. Sci.*, *73*: 1794 (1984).
11. B. Mollgaard and A. Hoelgaard, *Int. J. Pharm.*, *15*: 185 (1983).
12. K. Tojo, Y. Sun, M. Ghannam, J. A. Masi, P. R. Keshary, and Y. W. Chien, Abstract of APhA/APS 37th National Meeting, Philadelphia, October 1984, IPT no. 10.
13. P. R. Keshary and Y. W. Chien, *Drug Dev. Ind. Pharm.*, *10*: 883 (1984).
14. V. G. Levich, *Physicochemical Hydrodynamics*, Prentice-Hall, Englewood Cliffs, NJ, 1962, Chapter II.
15. C. V. King and S. S. Brodie, *J. Am. Chem. Soc.*, *59*: 1375 (1957).
16. R. C. Jhawar, Ph.D. thesis, Rutgers University, College of Pharmacy, 1984.
17. R. C. Jhawar, K. Tojo, and N. G. Lordi (in preparation).
18. K. Tojo and K. Miyanami, *Chem. Eng. J.*, *24*: 89 (1982).
19. R. W. Southworth and S. L. Deleeuw, *Digital Computation and Numerical Methods*, McGraw-Hill, New York, 1965, p. 363.
20. T. G. Kaufmann and E. F. Leonard, *AIChE J.*, *14*: 110 (1968).
21. C. K. Colton and K. A. Smith, *AIChE J.*, *18*: 958 (1972).
22. D. A. Frank-Kamenetskii, *Diffusion and Heat Transfer in Chemical Kinetics*, Plenum Press, New York, 1969, Chapter I.

23. K. Tojo, Y. Sun, M. Ghannam, and Y. W. Chien, *J. Chem. Eng. Jpn.* (submitted for publication).
24. J. T. Davies, *Turbulence Phenomena*, Academic Press, New York, 1972, Chapter 3.
25. R. B. Bird, W. E. Stewart, and E. N. Lightfoot, *Transport Phenomena*, Wiley, New York, 1960, Chapter 19.
26. A. Einstein, *Investigation on the Theory of Brownian Movement* (1905); reprint, Dover, New York, 1956.
27. R. W. Baker and H. K. Lonsdale, in *Controlled Release of Biologically Active Agents* (A. C. Tranquary and R. E. Lacey, eds.), Plenum Press, New York, 1974.
28. J. Drobnik, P. Spacek, and O. Wichterle, *J. Biomed. Mater. Res.*, *8*: 45 (1974).
29. H. A. Daynes, *Proc. R. Soc. London*, *A97*: 286 (1920).
30. K. Tojo, Y. Sun, M. Ghannam, and Y. W. Chien, *Drug Dev. Ind. Pharm.*, *11*: 1363 (1985).
31. K. Tojo, P. R. Keshary, and Y. W. Chien, *Chem. Eng. J. Biochem. Eng. Section*, *32*: B57 (1986).
32. K. Tojo, *J. Pharm. Sci.*, *74*: 685 (1985).
33. K. Tojo, Y. Sun, and Y. W. Chien, unpublished data.
34. K. Tojo, M. Ghannam, Y. Sun, and Y. W. Chien, *J. Cont. Release*, *1*: 197 (1985).
35. K. Tojo, C. C. Chiang, and Y. W. Chien, Abstract of APhA/APS 39th National Meeting, Minneapolis, October 1985, Basic no. 87.
36. M. M. Ghannam, K. Tojo, and Y. W. Chien, Abstract of APhA/APS 39th National Meeting, Minneapolis, October 1985, Basic no. 72.
37. Y. Sun, M. Ghannam, K. Tojo, and Y. W. Chien, Abstract of APhA/APS 39th National Meeting, Minneapolis, October 1985, Basic no. 75.

7

In Vitro Evaluations of Transdermal Drug Delivery

YIH-CHAIN HUANG / Rutgers—The State University of New Jersey, Piscataway, New Jersey

I. INTRODUCTION

The successful development of scopolamine- and nitroglycerin-releasing transdermal therapeutic systems (TTS) has triggered a great deal of interest in transdermal drug delivery research among pharmaceutical scientists.

Once a drug candidate has been identified (based on its physico-chemical, pharmacokinetic, and pharmacodynamic properties), many feasibility studies must be conducted to investigate the mechanisms of skin permeation of the drug itself before it can be developed into a TTS for systemic therapy.

One of the approaches commonly used in the design and development of a TTS is the study, in vitro first, of the permeation kinetics of the drug across excised skin. When the basic information governing controlled drug delivery through the skin becomes available, the development processes move forward into in vivo evaluations in humans, using the optimal formulation developed in the in vitro study (Chapter 6).

The methodology used in the in vitro study is relatively easy to follow and generally affords the investigator better control over the experimental conditions than is possible in vivo. Since the percutaneous absorption of a drug can be studied without the complications arising from the disposition of the drug in the body, the analytical assay is usually easier in an in vitro study as compared to work on

a living organism. Information such as the time needed to attain
steady-state permeation and the permeation flux at steady state can
be obtained from in vitro studies and used to optimize the formulation
design of a TTS before it becomes the subject of a more expensive
in vivo study in humans.

Skin has a complex structure. It consists of three diffusional
layers: the stratum corneum, the viable epidermis, and the dermis.
Even though each layer may have a different diffusion constant (1),
it is generally considered valid to use excised skin in in vitro studies
because: (a) the stratum corneum, which is a physiologically inactive tissue, is the principal barrier to the permeation of a drug,
and (b) diffusion through the stratum corneum is a passive process
(2).

In in vitro studies, excised skin is mounted in skin permeation
cells. Although human cadaver skin may be the logical choice as the
skin model if the final product will be used in humans, it is not
easily available to most investigators. Among the animal skins commonly used in in vitro studies, hairless mouse skin is generally
favored, partly because no potentially detrimental hair-removing
procedure is required; also it is relatively easy to obtain hairless
mice of a specific age or sex group, and skin specimens can be excised just prior to the permeation study. Good correlations between
permeation data across hairless mouse skin and human cadaver skin
have been reported (3-5).

Reviews on the relevance of animal models and in vitro-in vivo
comparisons are available in the literature (6-8).

Various skin permeation systems have been designed and used in
in vitro studies. However, because of the differences in cell design,
it is usually difficult to compare the results reported from different
laboratories using different skin permeation systems (Chapter 6).
In our laboratories, three different types of skin permeation cell—
the Franz diffusion cell, the Keshary-Chien skin permeation cell (an
improved version of the Franz cell), and the Valia-Chien skin permeation cell—are routinely used in transdermal drug delivery research.

This chapter addresses the following areas, based on our observations from in vitro skin permeation studies:

1. Effect of therapeutic system design on skin permeation
2. Effect of diffusion cell design on skin permeation
3. Effect of skin uptake and metabolism on skin permeation

II. IN VITRO SKIN PERMEATION KINETICS

A. Effect of Therapeutic System Design

Three once-a-day nitroglycerin-releasing TTSs have been successfully developed and marketed in the United States since 1981 (Chapter

1). Because these systems were designed and developed independently, using different approaches, by three different manufacturers, there was a question about their interchangeability, (Chapter 2). Since comparative bioavailability data are not available, the Controlled Drug-Delivery Research Center established an in vitro skin permeation system to study and compare the controlled skin permeation kinetics of nitroglycerin delivered by these nitroglycerin systems under the same experimental conditions. A more recently developed nitroglycerin TTS, the Deponit system, was also included in this investigation.

1. Experimental

Nitroglycerin-TTS: Nitrodisc system (16 mg/8 cm^2, Searle Pharmaceuticals), Nitro-Dur system (51 mg/10 cm^2, Key Pharmaceuticals), Transderm-Nitro system (25 mg/10 cm^2, Ciba Pharmaceutical Co.), and Deponit system (16 mg/16 cm^2, Pharma-Schwarz/Lohmann, Monheim, Germany) were tested as received.

Skin Preparation: A piece (3.5 cm × 3.5 cm) of full-thickness abdominal skin was freshly excised from a male hairless mouse, HRS/J strain, 5–7 weeks old (Jackson Laboratories, Bar Harbor, ME). The dermal side of the excised skin sample was carefully cleaned to remove any adhering subcutaneous tissue and blood vessels.

Elution Solution: The elution medium, freshly prepared from saline solution to contain 20% (w/w) polyethylene glycol 400 as the cosolvent to maintain a sink condition, was used as the receptor solution.

2. Skin Permeation and Release Kinetics Studies

The in vitro skin permeation system used was described earlier (9). The skin sample was assembled on Franz diffusion cells with its dermal side soaked overnight in the elution solution. After withdrawing all the elution solution, the nitroglycerin TTSs were applied to the stratum corneum surface; fresh elution solution was added, and the skin permeation studies were initiated. At predetermined times, 1 ml of sample solution was collected and the concentration of nitroglycerin in the sample solution was then analyzed by a high-pressure liquid chromatography (HPLC) method. The volume of solution withdrawn at each sampling time was immediately replaced with fresh elution solution to maintain constant solution volume and good contact with the dermal surface.

The release kinetics of nitroglycerin from these TTSs were also studied following the same procedure, except that no skin sample used. In the release studies, the total content of the receptor compartment was replaced with fresh elution solution at each sampling time to maintain the sink conditions required. The temperature of

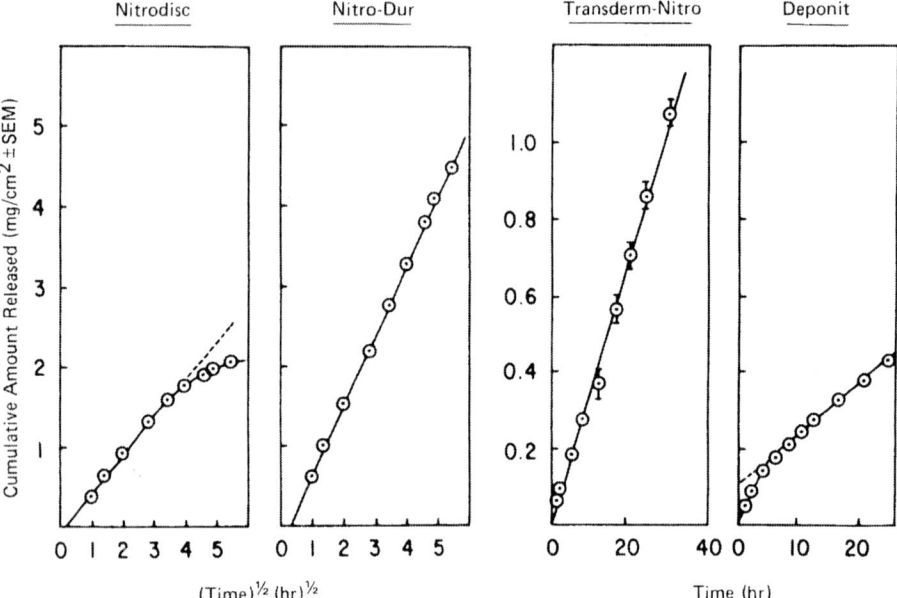

Figure 1 Release profiles of nitroglycerin from four commercially available transdermal therapeutic systems into saline solution (containing 20% w/w polyethylene glycol 400 to maintain sink conditions) at 37°C. The mean rates (or fluxes) of release are 498.5 $\mu g/cm^2/hr^{1/2}$ (Nitrodisc); 841.6 $\mu g/cm^2/hr^{1/2}$ (Nitro-Dur); 35.1 $\mu g/cm^2/hr$ (Transderm-Nitro), and 13.5 $\mu g/cm^2/hr$ (Deponit). Each data point stands for the mean ±1 standard error of four determinations.

the receptor compartment was maintained at 37°C by a circulating water bath, while the donor compartment was kept at ambient to simulate clinical conditions. For each formulation, at least four experiments were performed in each run of drug release and skin permeation studies.

3. Results and Discussion

The release and skin permeation profiles of nitroglycerin from these systems are shown in Figures 1 and 2, respectively. Apparently, both the Deponit and Transderm-Nitro systems release nitroglycerin at a constant rate, whereas the release of nitroglycerin from the Nitrodisc and Nitro-Dur systems can be better described by a Q versus $\sqrt{t}$ relationship (Fig. 1). However, the permeation

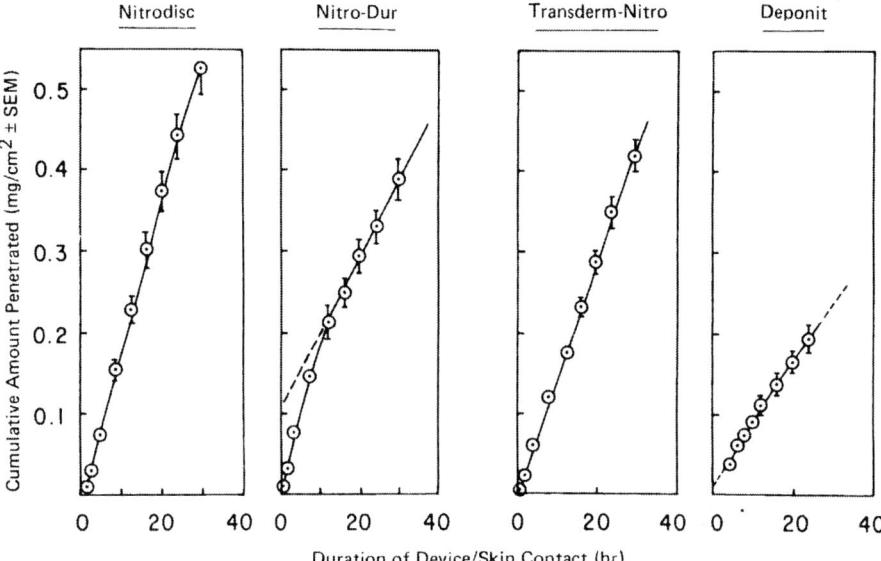

Figure 2   Skin permeation profiles of nitroglycerin from four commercially available transdermal therapeutic systems through the abdominal skin of hairless mouse. The mean rates of skin permeation
are 17.7 μg/cm^2/hr (Nitrodisc, N = 8), 17.0 [< 12 hr] and 10.3
[> 12 hr] μg/cm^2/hr (Nitro-Dur, N = 8), 14.1 μg/cm^2/hr (Transderm-
Nitro, N = 12), and 7.3 μg/cm^2/hr (Deponit, N = 4).

of nitroglycerin through the skin, following the release from the
TTS, seemed all to result in a constant rate profile in all cases
(Fig. 2).

Overall, the data (Table 1) indicated that even though the mechanism and the rate of release might be substantially different, the
rates of permeation of nitroglycerin across hairless mouse skin were
not greatly different among the transdermal therapeutic systems
evaluated (10.3–17.7 μg/cm^2/hr), except that for the Deponit system (7.3 μg/cm^2/hr). The slower rate of skin permeation of nitroglycerin from the Deponit system may be partially the result of its
lower loading dose (16 mg/16 cm^2) as compared to 16 mg/8 cm^2 in
the Nitrodisc system, 51 mg/10 cm^2 in the Nitro-Dur system, and
25 mg/10 cm^2 in the Transderm-Nitro system. The low loading dose
of nitroglycerin in the Deponit system may also account for the lower
release rate of nitroglycerin observed (13.5 μg/cm^2/hr).

The total nitroglycerin doses delivered through the hairless
mouse abdominal skin after 24-hr application by each of these systems

Table 1 Comparison of Drug-Release Kinetics and Skin Permeation Profiles[a] of Nitroglycerin from Four Nitroglycerin-Releasing Transdermal Therapeutic Systems

	Loading dose (mg)	Surface area (cm^2)	Flux or rate of release[b] (µg/cm^2)	Rate of skin permeation (µg/cm^2/hr)
Nitrodisc	16	8	498.5 ($\pm$13.9)hr$^{-\frac{1}{2}}$	17.7 ($\pm$1.0)[c]
Nitro-Dur	51	10	841.6 ($\pm$9.5)hr$^{-\frac{1}{2}}$	17.0 ($\pm$1.0)[c] [< 12 hr] 10.3 ($\pm$0.7)[c] [> 12 hr]
Transderm-Nitro	25	10	35.1 ($\pm$1.5)hr^{-1}	14.1 ($\pm$0.7)[d]
Deponit	16	16	13.5 ($\pm$0.5)hr^{-1}	7.3 ($\pm$0.7)[b]

[a] Mean $\pm$SEM.
[b] N = 4.
[c] N = 8.
[d] N = 12.

were fairly close in magnitude, mean values ranging from 3.28 to
3.41 mg, except for the Deponit system, which gave the dose of
2.80 mg at 24 hr. These in vitro data compare favorably with the
projected daily dose of 5 mg/24 hr.

We have also evaluated the new once-a-week transdermal antihypertensive system Catapres-TTS, using the same in vitro skin
permeation system. Catapres-TTS (7.5 mg clonidine/10.5 cm^2;
Boehringer Ingelheim Ltd.) was tested as received. Clonidine concentrations were also determined by an HPLC method.

The release and skin permeation profiles of clonidine from
Catapres-TTS are shown in Figure 3. After an initial burst,

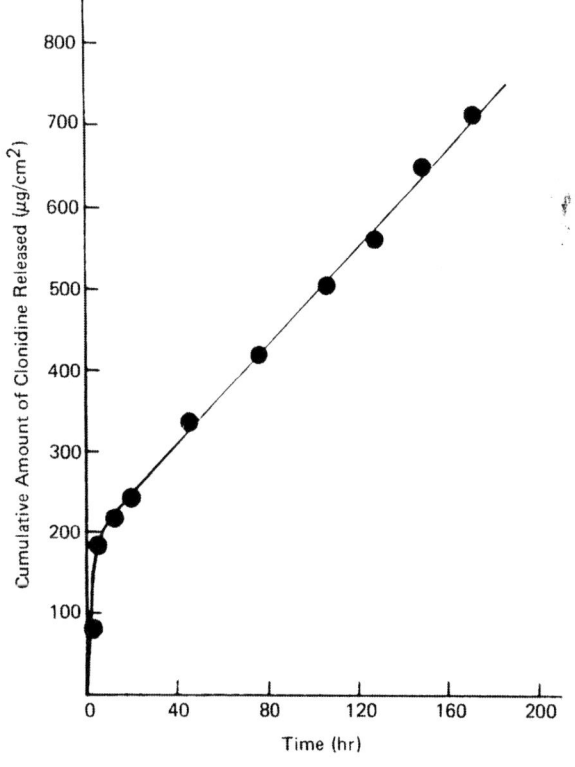

(a)

Figure 3 Release and skin permeation profiles of clonidine from
Catapres-TTS. The mean release rate is 3.02 µg/cm^2/hr (N = 6).
The mean rate of skin permeation is 2.43 µg/cm^2/hr with a permeation
lag time of 3.5 hr (N = 6).

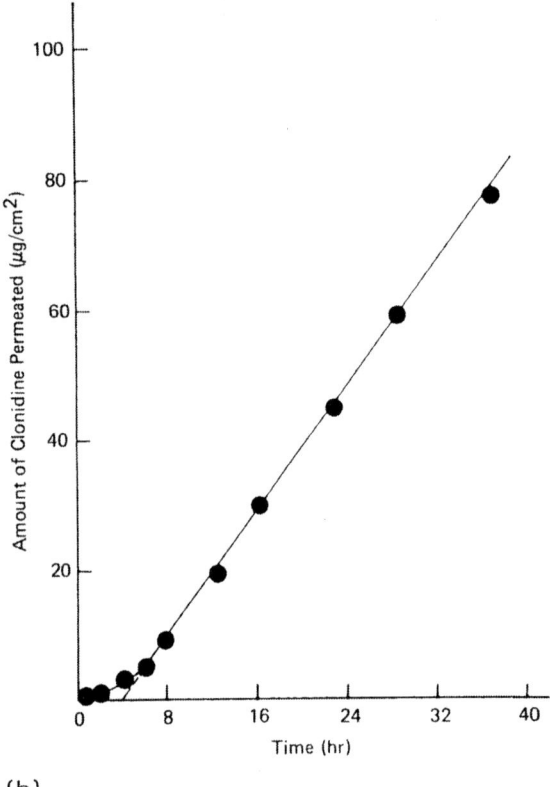

(b)

Figure 3   (continued)

clonidine was released at a constant rate of 3.02 μg/cm²/hr for nearly a week (Fig. 3a). This release pattern is expected because Catapres-TTS is a membrane-permeation-controlled drug delivery system, and drug release is regulated by a rate-controlling membrane. The initial burst observed could be the result of the immediate release of drug already accumulating in the adhesive polymer layer.

The skin permeation results indicated that clonidine penetrates through hairless mouse skin at a constant rate profile. The steady-state permeation rate was 2.43 μg/cm²/hr, with a permeation lag time of 3.5 hr. This skin permeation rate represents about 80% of the release rate for clonidine in an elution medium under sink conditions. A similar value (75%) was also reported based on the permeation rate observed in human cadaver skin and the release rate of clonidine into an infinite sink of water (10). These results suggest that hairless mouse skin is a rather good skin model for studying the rate of clonidine permeation through human cadaver skin in vitro. The in vivo skin permeation rate of clonidine from Catapres-TTS in humans was estimated to be 1.13 $\mu g/cm^2/hr$ calculated based on the data on the steady-state plasma level (11) and the total body clearance of clonidine reported (12). Therefore, the rate of skin permeation of clonidine obtained from hairless mouse skin in the present study represents approximately twice of that reported in human skin.

B. Effect of Diffusion Cell Design

A hydrodynamically sound design for the diffusion cell is essential in securing meaningful data from in vitro studies (Chapter 6). Selection of the diffusion cell system to be used is critical in the study of the fundamentals of skin permeation. During the course of transdermal drug delivery research, we noted several deficiencies in the design of the Franz diffusion cell, namely: in the solution hydrodynamics, in the mixing efficiency, and in the temperature control. A new finite-dosing diffusion cell was thus developed aiming to improve the hydrodynamic conditions of the original Franz diffusion cell. Figure 4 illustrates the basic structural differences between the Franz diffusion cell and the improved one, the Keshary–Chien diffusion cell.

The Keshary–Chien cell was carefully calibrated (13). The hydrodynamic conditions of the new cell were found to be much improved over the original Franz diffusion apparatus. Table 2 lists the improvements.

We evaluated the performance of these two diffusion cells by studying the release rates and skin permeation kinetics of four nitroglycerin-releasing transdermal therapeutic systems.

1. Experimental

The nitroglycerin TTS, the skin preparation, the elution solution, and the procedure used in this study are identical to those outlined earlier.

2. Results and Discussion

The release and skin permeation rates from four nitroglycerin TTSs evaluated in both diffusion cells are summarized in Table 3. The release and skin permeation rates of nitroglycerin from the Nitro-Dur system, a matrix-diffusion-type TTS and from the Transderm-Nitro system, a membrane-permeation-type TTS, are depicted in Figures 5 and 6, respectively. By using the Keshary–Chien cell, an improved version of the Franz diffusion cell, we observed an

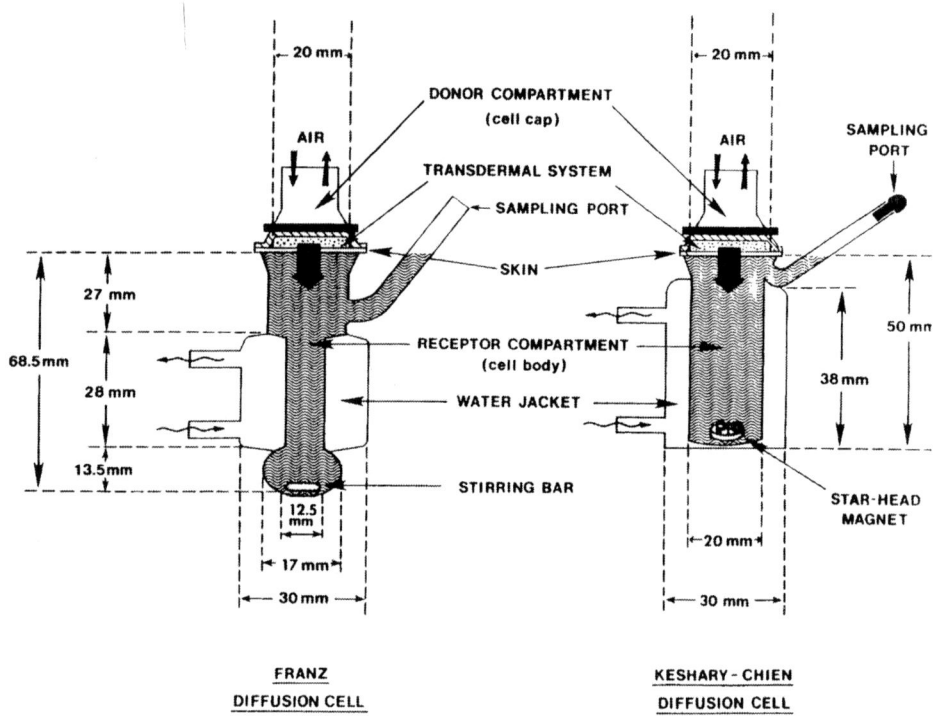

Figure 4   Diagrammatic illustration and comparison of the Franz diffusion cell and the Keshary–Chien skin permeation cell.   (From Ref. 13.)

increase in the release rate of nitroglycerin ranging from 130% (the Nitrodisc system) to 270% (the Transderm-Nitro system) and an increase of the skin permeation rate ranging from 153% (the Deponit system) to 261% (the Nitrodisc system).   These increases, from the systems releasing nitroglycerin by different mechanisms, could be attributed to the improvements in the hydrodynamic conditions in the Keshary–Chien cell (Chapter 6).   These improvements result in a thinner hydrodynamic boundary layer, more efficient solution mixing, and better temperature control in the cell (Table 2).   These data suggest that the Keshary–Chien cell is more suitable for studying the fundamentals and mechanisms of drug release and skin permeation.   Meaningful data may be derived with relatively less effect from the boundary layer.   This new improved finite-dosing cell has been used in the investigation of the mechanism of nitroglycerin skin permeation (14).

Table 2   Comparison of the Hydrodynamic Conditions Between the Franz Diffusion Cell and Keshary–Chien Cell

Physicochemical parameters	Franz cell	Keshary–Chien cell
Thickness of hydrodynamic boundary layer for diffusion of:		
Benzoic acid	337 μm	101 μm
Nitroglycerin	304 μm	108 μm
Mass transfer coefficient (cm/sec × 10^4)		
Benzoic acid	1.63	5.42
Nitroglycerin	1.32	3.73
Temperature control		
Time to reach an equilibrium temperature (from 21°C)		
At skin surface	20 min (33.2°C)[a]	15 min (36.8°C)[a]
In the receptor solution (at the surface)	15 min (31.2°C)[a]	10 min (36.7°C)[a]
Mixing efficiency		
Time to reach an equilibrium concentration	9.8 min	2.5 min

[a]The equilibrium temperature reached (target temperature = 37°C).

Table 3 Comparison of the Rates of Release and Skin Permeation[a] of Nitroglycerin Through the Abdominal Skin of Hairless Mouse from Four Transdermal Delivery Systems Used with the Keshary-Chien and the Franz Diffusion Cell Designs

System	Skin permeation rate ($\mu g/cm^2/hr$)		Release rate ($\mu g/cm^2/hr$)[b]	
	Franz cell	Keshary-Chien cell	Franz cell	Keshary-Chien cell
Deponit	7.3 ± 0.7[b]	11.2 ± 0.9[b]	13.5 ± 0.5	18.0 ± 0.5
Transderm-Nitro	14.1 ± 0.7[c]	23.6 ± 1.5[b]	35.1 ± 1.5	94.6 ± 2.1
Nitro-Dur	17.0 ± 1.0[d]	31.1 ± 1.0[b]	841.6 ± 9.5[e]	1303.2 ± 9.4[e]
Nitrodisc	17.7 ± 1.0[d]	44.7 ± 2.3[d]	498.5 ± 13.9[e]	552.4 ± 25.7[e]

[a] Mean ± SEM.
[b] N = 4.
[c] N = 12.
[d] N = 8.
[e] In $\mu g/cm^2/hr^{\frac{1}{2}}$.

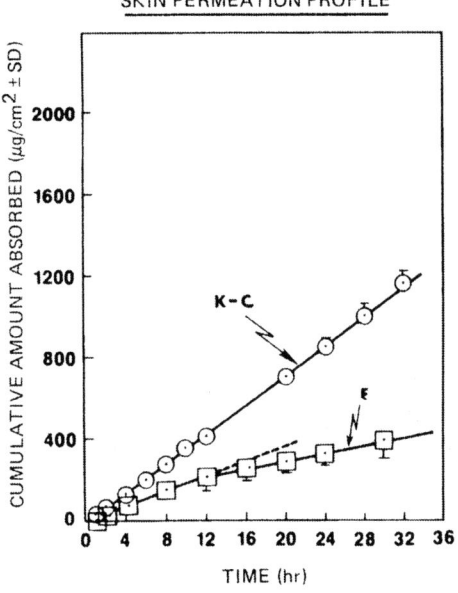

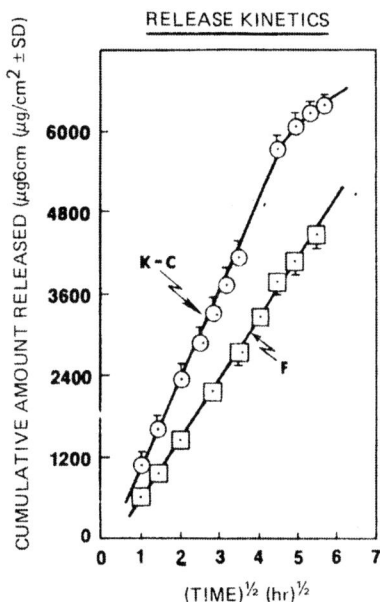

Figure 5 Comparison of skin permeation (through hairless mouse skin) and release profiles of nitroglycerin from the matrix-diffusion-controlled Nitro-Dur system evaluated by the Keshary–Chien (K–C) and Franz (F) diffusion cell designs. Greater rates of skin permeation and release of nitroglycerin were yielded with the K–C system than with the (F) cell. (From Ref. 13.)

C. Effect of Skin Uptake and Metabolism

The skin is no longer considered as merely an inert covering of the body. It has been shown that skin possesses some ability to metabolize drugs (15,16). The contribution of skin metabolism to the elimination of a drug from the body may be relatively small as compared to that in the liver (16) when a drug is administered systemically (i.e., by a nontransdermal route). Nevertheless, skin could become an important organ for metabolism when a drug is applied directly to the skin surface, since by this route, every molecule that becomes systemically available must penetrate through the metabolic-activity-rich region in the epidermis. Therefore, the skin may act as an important organ for first-pass elimination. And, depending on the pharmacological activity of the metabolite formed, the metabolic reaction occurring in the skin could affect the therapeutic activity of a drug applied to the skin (16). Alternatively,

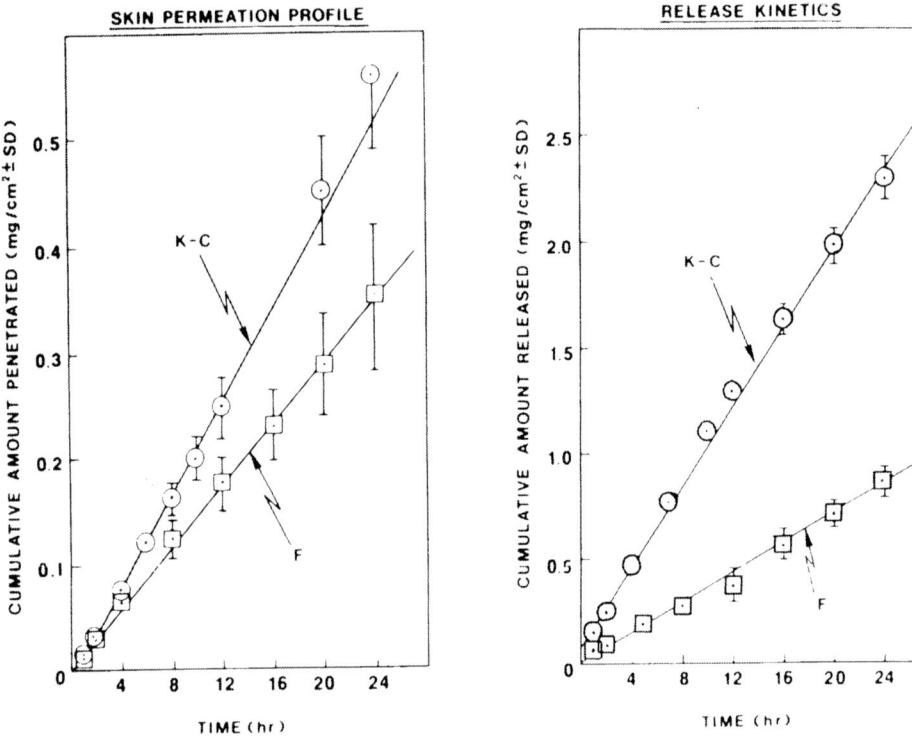

Figure 6 Comparison of skin permeation (through the hairless mouse skin) and release profiles of nitroglycerin from the membrane-permeation-controlled Transderm-Nitro system evaluated by the Keshary–Chien and Franz diffusion cell designs. Greater rates of skin permeation and release of nitroglycerin were produced with the K–C system than with the (F) cell. (From Ref. 13.)

we may also take advantage of this metabolic conversion in the skin to improve the transdermal bioavailability of a poorly permeated drug by applying its prodrug or derivative, if the prodrug offers better physicochemical properties for percutaneous absorption (such as improved lipophilicity) as compared to the parent drug. Once the prodrug has traveled down to the epidermis region, it will be metabolized, and the active drug will be formed and delivered into systemic circulation (17–19). This "prodrug" approach has been the focus of research in the design and development of transdermally active drugs (20–22). Since permeation and bioavailability of a drug at the site of application are prerequisites to any possible metabolic reactions in the skin, it is conceivable that factors affecting the skin permeation of a drug would also influence the metabolism of a drug in the skin. The Controlled Drug-Delivery Research Center used estradiol and estradiol esters as model drugs to study skin permeation and metabolism in hairless mouse skin, using a newly developed horizontal-type cell, the Valia–Chien cell.

1. Experimental

The Valia–Chien (V–C) skin permeation system (Fig. 7) was designed for long-term skin permeation study. The design and calibration of the V–C permeation cell were described earlier (23).

Study of Skin Uptake and Metabolism of Estradiol: A piece (3 cm × 3 cm) of full-thickness skin or stripped skin freshly excised from a hairless mouse, 5–7 weeks old, was mounted between the two compartments of each V–C permeation cell in such a way that either the stratum corneum or the dermis faced the drug solution and the other side of the skin was protected with impermeable aluminum foil

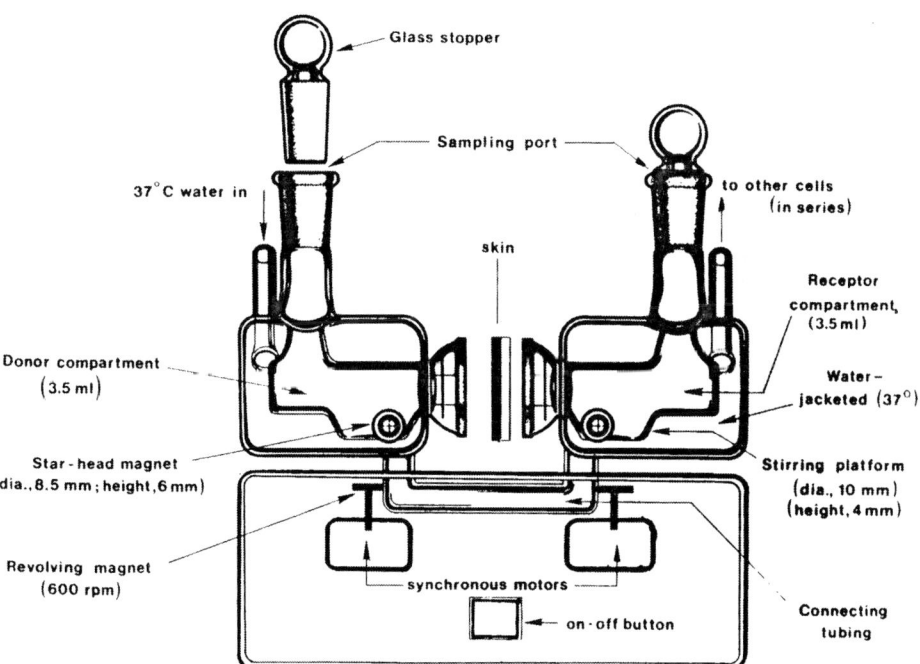

Figure 7   Diagrammatic illustration for a unit of the Valia–Chien skin permeation system.   (From Ref. 22.)

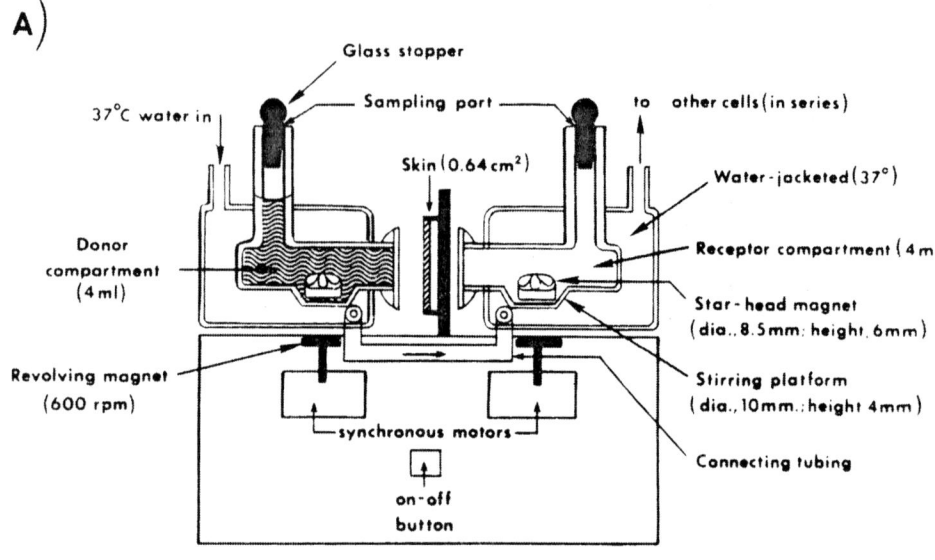

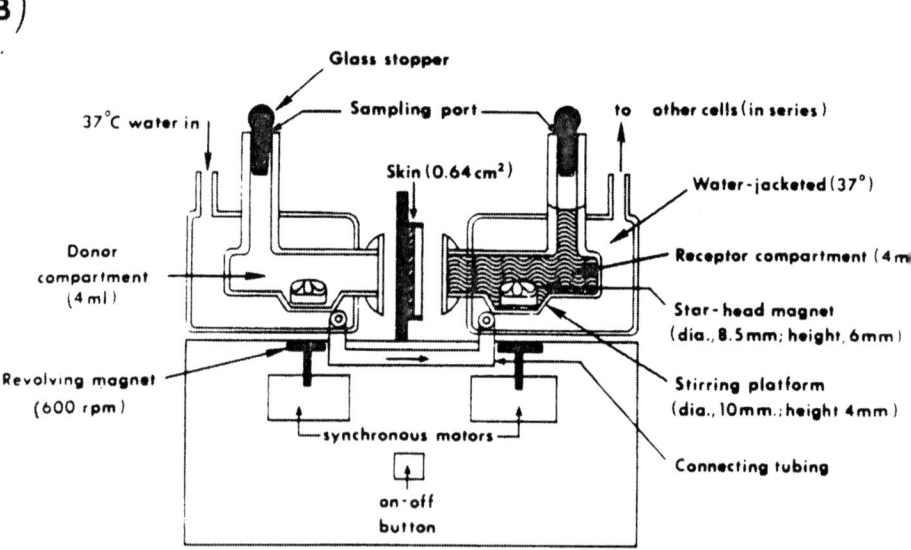

Figure 8 The experimental setup for the skin uptake and metabolism experiments: (A) from the stratum corneum side and (B) from the dermal side. (From Ref. 24.)

(Fig. 8). The compartment with the skin surface uncovered was filled with a saturated solution of estradiol in normal saline and the compartment with the skin surface covered with aluminum foil remained empty. Both compartments were maintained isothermally at 37°C. Samples were withdrawn from the solution compartment at predetermined times and assayed, by an HPLC method, for estradiol and any possible metabolites.

Study of Skin Uptake and Metabolism of Estradiol Esters: A piece of full-thickness skin was mounted between the two compartments of each V–C permeation cell in such a way that the dermis faced the drug solution and the stratum corneum was protected with impermeable aluminum foil. The compartment facing the dermal side was filled with a saturated solution of estradiol ester in 40% (v/v) PEG 400/normal saline; the other compartment was kept empty. Both compartments were maintained at 37°C. Samples were withdrawn from the solution compartment at predetermined times and assayed for estradiol ester and any possible metabolites (e.g., estradiol) by an HPLC method.

2. Results and Discussion

Figures 9 and 10 show the disappearance of estradiol and the formation of its metabolite estrone, after the application of a saturated solution of estradiol in normal saline onto the stratum corneum side of a piece of full-thickness skin or stripped skin from female hairless mice. These data demonstrated that hairless mouse skin is capable of converting estradiol into estrone and that the stratum corneum seems to be a rate-limiting factor in the reaction. For example, in the skin from the female hairless mouse the rate of disappearance of estradiol increased when the stratum corneum was removed by stripping: 0.2280 μM/hr (< 12 hr), 0.6967 μM/hr (12–21 hr) for stripped skin versus 0.1079 μM/hr for the full-thickness skin. The appearance of the metabolite estrone in the solution compartment was also faster in the stripped skin: 30 min for estrone to appear in the stripped skin versus 38.5 hr in the full-thickness skin; estrone was formed faster in the stripped skin (0.1245 μM/hr at 0–12 hr; 0.5289 μM/hr at 12–21 hr) than in the skin with stratum corneum (0.0505 μM/hr).

Table 4 summarizes the formation of estradiol following the application of various estradiol esters in the V–C skin permeation cell. The rate of appearance of estradiol was found to decrease in the order of diacetate > valerate > heptanoate > cypionate > acetate. There was nearly a fivefold increase in the rate of estradiol formation when the alkyl chain length of the esters increased from acetate to valerate. However, further increases in the chain length from valerate to heptanoate resulted in reduction in the rate of formation of estradiol (20). It is also interesting to note that the fluxes of estradiol from estradiol valerate and estradiol heptanoate were two

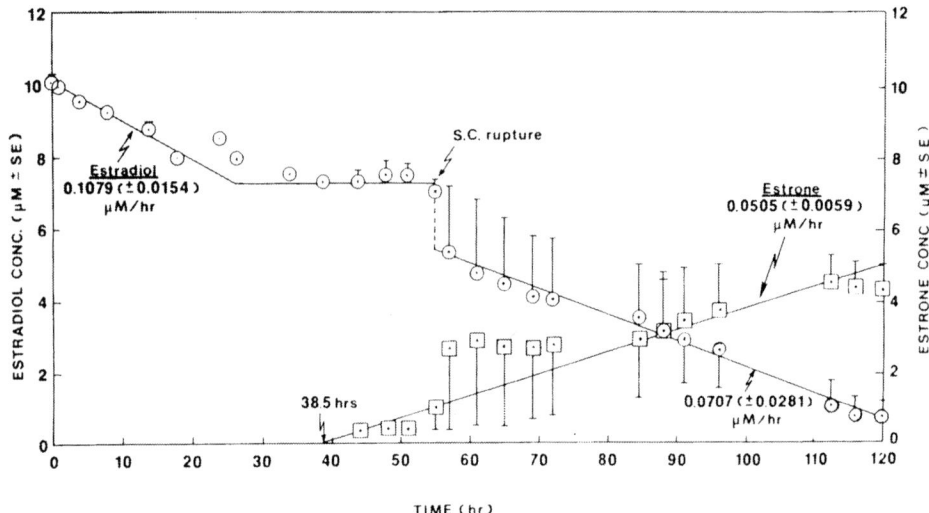

Figure 9   Time course for the uptake of estradiol by the stratum corneum (S.C.) of female hairless mouse abdominal skin and the formation of estrone.   Each data point represents the mean and one standard error of three determinations.   (From Ref. 24.)

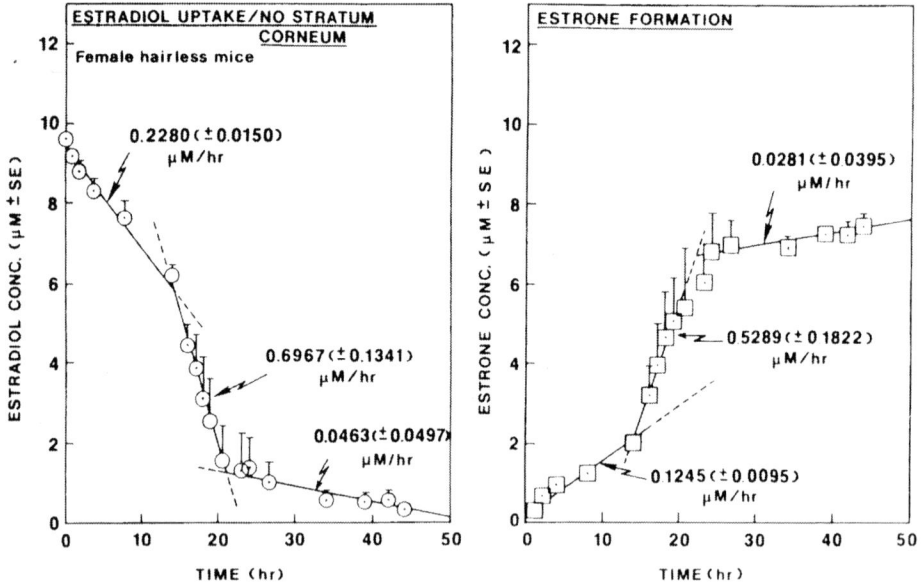

Figure 10   Time course for the uptake of estradiol by stripped female hairless mouse abdominal skin and the formation of estrone. Each data point represents the mean and one standard error of three determinations.   (From Ref. 24.)

Table 4   Rate of Appearance of Estradiol Following the
Application of Estradiol and Various Estradiol Esters

Estrogenic steroids	Rate of estradiol appearance (μmol/cm^2/sec $\times$ 10^8)
Estradiol	7.87 ± 0.73
Estradiol acetate	4.79 ± 0.46
Estradiol valerate	22.91 ± 0.74
Estradiol heptanoate	13.32 ± 2.09
Estradiol cypionate	5.97 ± 0.38
Estradiol diacetate	81.90 ± 8.91

to three times the flux from estradiol itself. The data generated
have provided the basic information for the development of a transdermal bioactivated hormone delivery system (22).

III. CONCLUSION

In vitro skin permeation studies have been extensively used in the
design and development of transdermal therapeutic systems. The
fundamentals and mechanisms governing the permeation of a drug
through skin can be derived from in vitro studies using a well-
designed (and calibrated) skin permeation system. The advantages
of using in vitro techniques to evaluate the performance of marketed
transdermal therapeutic systems also have been demonstrated. Although an in vitro-in vivo correlation has yet to be established, the
use of hairless mouse skin in studying the cutaneous metabolism of
drugs or the bioconversion of a prodrug seems to be promising.

ACKNOWLEDGMENTS

The author wishes to thank Professors Yie W. Chien and Kakuji Tojo
for their valuable comments. Acknowledgments also go to Drs. P. R.
Keshary, K. H. Valia, and Mr. T. Y. Chien for providing their
experimental findings and to Ms. M. Boslet for manuscript preparation.

REFERENCES

1. R. J. Scheuplein, *Curr. Probl. Dermatol.*, 7: 172–186 (1978).
2. R. T. Tregear, *Physical Functions of the Skin*, Academic Press,
   New York, 1966.

3. H. Durrheim, G. L. Flynn, W. I. Higuchi, and C. R. Behl, J. Pharm. Sci., 69: 781–786 (1980).

4. R. B. Stoughton, Animal models for in vitro percutaneous absorption, in Animal Models in Dermatology (H. I. Maibach, ed.), Churchill–Livingston, Edinburgh, 1975.

5. R. L. Bronaugh, R. F. Stewart, and E. R. Congdon, Toxicol. Appl. Pharmacol., 62: 481–488 (1982).

6. T. J. Franz, J. Invest. Dermatol., 64: 190–195 (1975).

7. R. C. Wester and P. K. Noonan, Int. J. Pharm., 7: 99–110 (1980).

8. R. L. Bronaugh and H. I. Maibach, In vitro percutaneous absorption, in Dermatotoxicology (F. N. Marzulli and H. I. Maibach, eds.), Hemisphere, Washington, DC, 1983.

9. Y. W. Chien, P. R. Keshary, Y. C. Huang, and P. P. Sarpotdar, J. Pharm. Sci., 72: 968–970 (1983).

10. J. E. Shaw, R. M. Gale, D. J. Enscore, and L. C. Chu, Proceedings of the 10th International Symposium on "Controlled Release of Bioactive Materials," San Francisco, 1983, Controlled Release Society, Inc., Lincolnshire, IL, pp. 320–326.

11. J. E. Shaw, Am. Heart J., 108: 217–223 (1984).

12. D. S. Davies, L. M. H. Wing, J. L. Reid, E. Neile, P. Tippett, and C. T. Dollery, Clin. Pharmacol. Ther., 21: 593–601 (1977).

13. P. R. Keshary and Y. W. Chien, Drug. Dev. Ind. Pharm., 10: 883–913 (1984).

14. P. R. Keshary, Y. C. Huang, and Y. W. Chien, Drug Dev. Ind. Pharm., 11: 1213–1253 (1985).

15. A. Pannatier, P. Jenner, B. Testa, and J. C. Etter, Drug Metab. Rev., 8: 319–343 (1978).

16. U. Täuber, Metabolism of drugs on and in the skin, in Dermal and Transdermal Absorption (R. Brandau and B. H. Lippold, eds.), Wissenschaftliche Verlagsgesellschaft, Stuttgart, 1982, pp. 133–151.

17. T. Loftsson and N. Bodor, J. Pharm. Sci., 70: 756–758 (1981).

18. B. Mølgaard, A. Hoelgaard, and H. Bundgaard, Int. J. Pharm., 12: 153–162 (1982).

19. C. D. Yu, J. L. Fox, N. F. H. Ho, and W. I. Higuchi, J. Pharm. Sci., 68: 1341–1346 (1979).

20. K. H. Valia, K. Tojo, and Y. W. Chien, Drug. Dev. Ind. Pharm., 11: 1133–1174 (1985).

21. K. Tojo, K. H. Valia, G. Chotani, and Y. W. Chien, Drug. Dev. Ind. Pharm., 11: 1175–1194 (1985).

22. Y. W. Chien, K. H. Valia, and U. B. Doshi, Drug. Dev. Ind. Pharm., 11: 1195–1212 (1985).

23. Y. W. Chien and K. H. Valia, Drug. Dev. Ind. Pharm., 10: 575–599 (1984).

24. K. H. Valia and Y. W. Chien, Drug Dev. Ind. Pharm., 10: 991–1015 (1984).

8

In Vivo Evaluations of Transdermal Drug Delivery

RICHARD H. GUY, JONATHAN HADGRAFT,* ROBERT S. HINZ, KATHLEEN V. ROSKOS, and DANIEL A. W. BUCKS / University of California at San Francisco, San Francisco, California

I. INTRODUCTION

In the development of a transdermal drug delivery (TDD) system, several crucial questions need to be answered. Most, if not all, of these demands are identified elsewhere in this book. Specifically, for the purposes of this chapter, though, only two basic questions must be addressed:

1. Does the drug proposed for transdermal delivery penetrate skin in vivo and, if so, to what extent?
2. How is a useful indicator of in vivo skin penetration obtained and, hence, how feasible is the transdermal route of drug administration?

Clearly, the answer to the first question may begin to resolve the objective of the second. However, the experimental system chosen to respond to question 2 may, if improperly selected, provide a

---

*Present affiliation: The Welsh School of Pharmacy, U.W.I.S.T., Cardiff, Wales, United Kingdom.

misleading guide to the initial unknown. Thus, the fundamental questions pertaining to in vivo evaluations of TDD are inextricably linked. What options are available, then, for the estimation of the potential of TDD in vivo? Two obvious, prime, candidates can be identified.

1. Measure skin penetration and subsequent biodisposition in an intact animal model.
2. Evaluate percutaneous absorption directly in human volunteers.

A third, simpler, but perhaps less readily acceptable alternative is:

3. Formulate a biophysical model for TDD and, after validation, use the simulation to predict the feasibility of drug administration via the skin.

Each of these three possibilities will be considered in this chapter. None of the approaches, needless to say, is problem-free, but all, when employed carefully in full knowledge of their likely limitations, can prove instructive and valuable.

As we will indicate, a definitive response to "What is the best method to evaluate TDD in vivo?" cannot, at this time, be made. Eventually, the development of a TDD system requires extensive pharmacokinetic and pharmacodynamic characterization in vivo in humans. These determinations can be performed and have already been documented (1-14) for the TDD devices currently on the market. Nevertheless, it cannot be stated too frequently that, although these systems are being safely and effectively used for therapeutic benefit, our knowledge of the process, by which the delivered drug gains systemic access (viz., percutaneous absorption) is incomplete. Among the unresolved issues, which should be borne in mind when one considers the results of an in vivo experiment, are the following:

1. How does the barrier function of human skin change with increasing age? Despite a number of studies (15-19), which have shown how the permeability of neonate skin differs from that of adults, almost no comparative information is available from the opposite end of the age spectrum. Since TDD is suited to chronic drug therapy, a requirement most often exhibited by elderly patients, the effect of aging on percutaneous absorption is a highly pertinent unknown factor for in vivo evaluation.

2. What is the significance of skin metabolism? An often-cited advantage (20,21) of TDD is that the cutaneous route of drug input avoids the hepatic first-pass effect. However, the ability of the skin to metabolize penetrating compounds is established (22); indeed,

the potential utility of this biotransformation capacity (via a prodrug approach) has attracted significant interest (23). The *extent* of metabolism is not yet quantified, nor is it known whether the skin handles transporting drugs in the same way as the liver; for example, it appears that the 1,2- and 1,3-dinitrate metabolites of nitroglycerin are formed in different ratios depending on the route (sublingual versus topical) of parent drug administration (24). In addition, skin surface microflora are capable of topical drug degradation (25, 26). The occlusive environment beneath a TDD device may be expected to increase the significance of this potential metabolic pathway.

3. Do we understand how penetration enhancers function in vivo? Although our comprehension of absorption promotion is improving and various classes of adjuvant can now be identified (27–29), it remains unclear whether drugs of different physicochemical properties require enhancers of different types. The breadth of applicability of TDD is presently determined by the barrier function of skin. If we can safely, reversibly, and controllably increase cutaneous permeability with suitable formulation components, the possibilities for the dermal route of administration will expand considerably.

4. What is the relationship between a drug's structure and properties and its potential to elicit an irritant or allergic reaction in human skin? The provocation of an inflammatory cutaneous response by an externally applied chemical requires both percutaneous penetration and intradermal pharmacological effect. A large reaction could be caused either by a poorly absorbed but highly potent molecule or by a well-absorbed, low-activity moiety; that is, the magnitude of response does not unequivocally categorize the antagonist. The literature in this field lacks a standardized reporting approach, which makes the anticipation of problems difficult. As discussed elsewhere, structure–activity relationships are required (30), and steps toward their establishment have been initiated.

We now discuss, in turn, three discrete approaches to the in vivo evaluation of TDD: animal models, human experimentation, and kinetic modeling and prediction. Problems considered above, and other difficulties, will be addressed within the context of each attack. The order of the discussion is as stated; at present, in preformulation studies, animal experiments precede human testing. Although, logically, one might consider the theoretical simulation approach to be the initial feasibility test, its relative infancy as a viable means of TDD prediction requires that it be debated last in the sequence as a promising but as yet "experimental" tool.

II. ANIMAL MODELS

Although the most relevant data pertaining to TDD are obtained in humans, this desirable approach is not always possible, since considerable time and resources are required to conduct a safe and meaningful percutaneous absorption study in man. Consequently, one must be prepared to use an in vivo animal model. Although the range of species employed in previous work is very broad, there is no general agreement as to the "best," or most predictive, model for skin penetration work. Therefore, in addressing the suitability of an animal test system, the investigator should evaluate three basic considerations:

1. How does percutaneous absorption in different animals compare to or rank with that observed in man?
2. Which, if any, of the animal models provides the closest representation of penetration in humans for the widest range of tested compounds?
3. Are there new developments taking place that warrant careful monitoring in the immediate future?

The following discussion aims to respond to these questions. While it may not be possible, at present, to state exactly what should be done, it is suggested that the available literature both provides strong considerations as to those species whose use is questionable, and perhaps misleading, and offers a new approach that has demonstrated significant potential.

A. Rankings

The subject of in vivo animal models for percutaneous absorption has been reviewed recently (31,32). Only a brief discussion will be given here, therefore, with a few illustrative and representative examples. It is first appropriate to list the various species that have been used as experimental test systems either in vivo or in vitro. The following is a comprehensive, but not necessarily complete, compilation: mouse, rat, guinea pig, rabbit; hairless mouse, hairless rat, hairless dog; cat, dog, miniature pig, pig, horse, goat; squirrel monkey, rhesus monkey, chimpanzee (33–40). The diversity is striking and is manifested in the histological appearance of the skins from these different animals. It is clear that there have been studies in which an animal model has been chosen with no consideration whatsoever of the physiological/anatomical relevance of the "model" skin to that of man.

To rank the disparate animal types with respect to their ability to provide an acceptable prediction of in vivo skin absorption in man involves consideration of two groups of studies: (a) those in which percutaneous penetration of one or a few compounds is measured in several species (including human), and (b) those in which absorption of one or more chemicals is compared between the chosen animal model and man. The former category is obviously labor-intensive and is customarily exemplified by the work of Bartek et al. (34) (Fig. 1). These experiments utilized a standard radiochemical approach (41–46) (see below) for the measurement of percutaneous absorption. The different chemicals were applied to the animals' shaved backs. Each site of administration was protected with a nonocclusive guard. While the results are not sufficiently comprehensive to draw unequivocal conclusions, it is clear that the rat and the rabbit do not offer reliable estimations of human penetration. The pig, on the other hand, appears to provide a reasonable approximation to absorption in man. As a general rule, it may be suggested that animals with high follicular density are less likely to provide good predictions of in vivo transdermal delivery in human subjects. This observation is also supported by in vitro measurements (47,48); furthermore, the preparation of hairy skin for study (e.g., by shaving or depilation) may, in itself, damage the barrier function, resulting in a membrane of unusually low (and nonrepresentative) resistance.

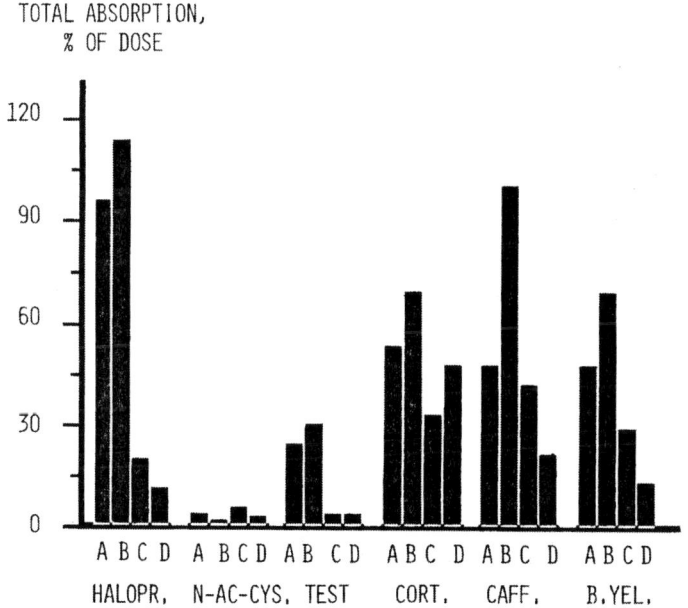

Figure 1   In vivo percutaneous absorption in various animals (A = rat, B = rabbit, C = pig) compared to that in man (D) for haloprogin, *N*-acetylcysteine, testosterone, cortisone, caffeine, and butter yellow. (Adapted from Ref. 34.)

Using the same procedures, Bartek and La Budde (35) later reported on the in vivo absorption of four pesticides in rabbit, pig, squirrel monkey, and man. Once again, penetration in the rabbit was very high (4–10 times greater than man). The squirrel monkey gave values for absorption that were as predictive as those from the pig, indicating that the lower primate may be an alternative representation for man. However, by far the most extensive in vivo comparison between a single animal and man (group b, in the preceding paragraph) has been performed with the rhesus monkey, details of which are now discussed.

B. The Rhesus Monkey

The laboratories of Maibach, Wester, et al. (49–59) have established the rhesus monkey as one of the most frequently cited "good" animal models for in vivo evaluation of TDD in man. As stated earlier, this area of research has been reviewed on a number of occasions (31,32) and only brief recapitulation is warranted here. Again, standard radiotracer methodology has been followed (41–46); the application site has generally been either the forearm or the abdomen. Compound is usually administered after light clipper shaving of the site to be treated. While the rhesus monkey is certainly "hairy," these typical sites of dosing are among the least well covered on the animal's body.

The compounds for which the rhesus–man comparison has been made include hydrocortisone, testosterone, benzoic acid, 2,4-dinitrochlorobenzene (DNCB), nitrobenzene, and a range of hair dyes (60–63). In some cases (hydrocortisone, testosterone, and benzoic acid), the comparisons have been performed following the administration of more than one topical dose (60) (Fig. 2). On the whole, as can be seen, the coincidence between rhesus penetration and percutaneous absorption in man is good. This agreement, as elsewhere, is based on "total" penetration (measured as % [14]C dose excreted) in a defined period of time, typically 5 or 7 days. True validation of the animal model requires the kinetic profiles of the chemical disposition to match; regrettably, this information is less often available in the published literature.

The nitroaromatic compounds also showed excellent correlation (61): for DNCB, human absorption was $53.1 \pm 6.2\%$ compared to $52.5 \pm 4.3\%$ in the rhesus; for nitrobenzene, the corresponding man and monkey values were $1.5 \pm 0.3\%$ and $4.2 \pm 0.5\%$, respectively. In addition, impressive coincidence between penetration across human and monkey skin in vitro was demonstrated for the same two compounds and three additional nitroaromatic derivatives (p-nitroaniline, 4-amino-2-nitrophenol, and 2-nitro-p-phenylenediamine).

Wolfram and Maibach (62,63) measured the in vivo percutaneous absorption of various hair dyes in rhesus and man. Agreement was

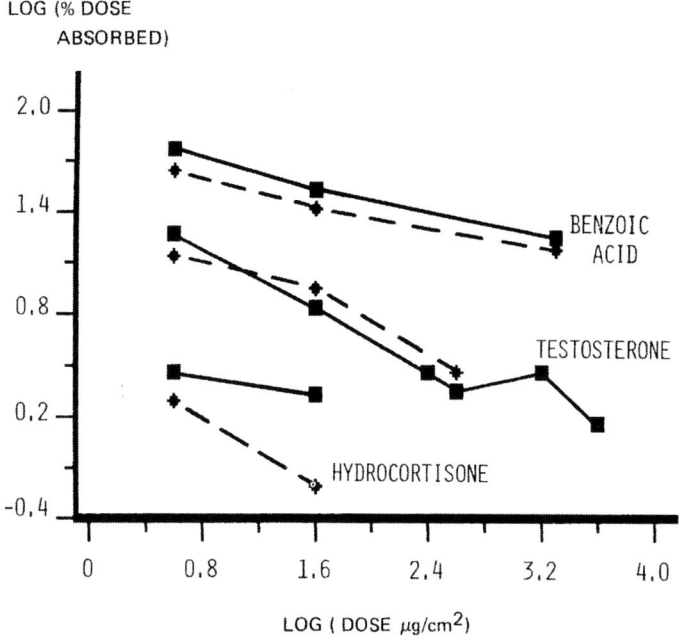

LOG (% DOSE
ABSORBED)

LOG (DOSE μg/cm²)

Figure 2   In vivo percutaneous absorption of hydrocortisone,
testosterone, and benzoic acid in rhesus monkeys (solid curves)
and in humans (dashed curves). (Adapted from Ref. 60.)

very close for resorcinol, p-phenylenediamine, and HC Blue No. 1
and was acceptable for 2,4-diaminoanisole and 2-nitro-p-phenylene-
diamine. Excretion half-lives of the topically administered radioactivity were also assessed in man and rhesus and were, on the
whole, similar (Table 1). Although the assay procedures used in
this work were identical to the studies described earlier in this
section, the site of application (the scalp) and the method of chemical administration (working the hair dye lotion into the hair and
scalp versus deposition of penetrant in acetone) were distinctly different. These investigations serve, therefore, as positive reinforce-
ment of the potential utility and representative nature of the rhesus
monkey as a model for human skin absorption (and, hence, TDD)
in vivo.

C. Recent Developments

Despite the persuasive evidence to support the rhesus monkey as an
excellent simulator for human percutaneous absorption, other

Table 1   Percutaneous Penetration of Hair Dyes in Rhesus Monkey and in Man[a]

Chemical	Species	% Dose absorbed (±SD)	Urinary excretion half-life (hr)
2,4-Diaminoanisole	Man	0.02 ± 0.01	18
	Rhesus	0.03	20
Resorcinol	Man	0.08 ± 0.03	31
	Rhesus	0.18 ± 0.03	31
4-Amino-2-hydroxytoluene	Man	0.20 ± 0.10	24
p-Phenylenediamine	Man	0.19 ± 0.06	16
	Rhesus	0.18 ± 0.06	22
2-Nitro-p-phenylenediamine	Man	0.14 ± 0.04	24
	Rhesus	0.55 ± 0.01	24
4-Amino-2-nitrophenol	Man	0.24 ± 0.08	10
HC Blue No. 1	Man	0.15 ± 0.12	18
	Rhesus	0.13 ± 0.03	40

[a]The number of subjects was 2 or 3 for the monkey studies, 3 or 5 in man.
Source: Adapted from Refs. 62 and 63.

alternatives are being continually sought. The cost, relative accessibility, and handling capabilities required for these primate experiments precludes, at this time, the general use of rhesus monkeys. A more recent additional complication centers on the emotional issue of the use of animals in research, in particular the employment of primates and "domestic" species. A detailed and impressive example of the search and identification of other in vivo possibilities has been reported recently by Reifenrath et al. (64,65).

These authors have evaluated four possible models for predicting skin penetration in man: the human-skin-grafted congenitally (nude) mouse ("man–mouse"), the pig-skin-grafted nude mouse ("pig–mouse"), the hairless dog, and the weanling Yorkshire pig. To each model, at a single dose (4 μg/cm²), were separately applied nine radiolabeled compounds, which had been previously tested in man. The chemicals were caffeine, benzoic acid, *N,N*-diethyl-*m*-toluamide; testosterone, progesterone, fluocinolone acetonide; lindane, parathion, and malathion. Percutaneous absorption was evaluated in the normal way by monitoring the excretion of radioactivity from the animal after dosing. To correct for incomplete excretion, a parenteral dose was also administered and the elimination monitored as before.

The results obtained from the nude mouse experiments are summarized in Figure 3. It can be seen that the mouse itself offers a negligible cutaneous barrier to chemical ingress; absorption for some compounds is almost as high as that seen following subcutaneous injection. The "man–mouse" and "pig–mouse," however, experience much lower penetration and are consistent. These observations can be highlighted by a consideration of Figure 4, which shows the marked

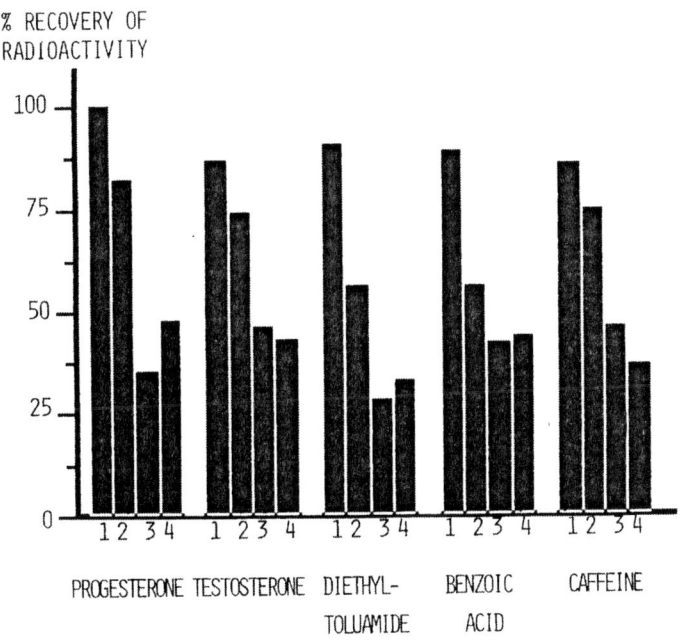

(a)

Figure 3 Absorption of nine chemicals following subcutaneous (1) and topical (2) administration to the nude mouse and topical application to the "man–mouse" (3) and "pig–mouse" (4). (Adapted from Ref. 65.)

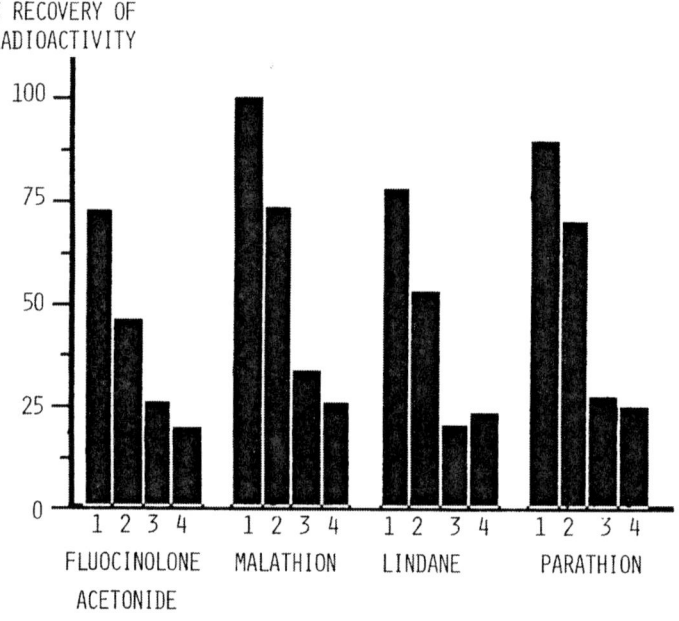

(b)

Figure 3   (continued)

change in the stratum corneum of a human-skin-grafted mouse at the
border of the xenograft. Whereas the nude mouse has only a minimal horny layer, the human skin demonstrates a particularly well-
formed and appreciable keratinized layer.

Comparison between percutaneous absorption in the "man–mouse"
with that previously reported in man (42,43,46) (Fig. 5) reveals a
reasonably linear correlation, with the grafted animal generally over-
estimating the human results. The other significant correlation was
that between human absorption and penetration in the weanling pig
(Fig. 6). The hairless dog and the "pig–mouse" proved to be less
representative models for human penetration.

When the percutaneous absorption ratio "man–mouse"/man is
plotted as a function of penetrant octanol/water partition coefficient
(Fig. 7), the deviation from unity increases with increasing hydro-
phobicity. It has been suggested that this effect occurs because the
xenograft uses split-thickness skin approximately 0.7 mm thick (i.e.,
skin from which a significant portion of the dermis has been removed).
It is conceivable that the graft procedure removes, therefore, part
of the skin membrane that controls absorption for more lipophilic

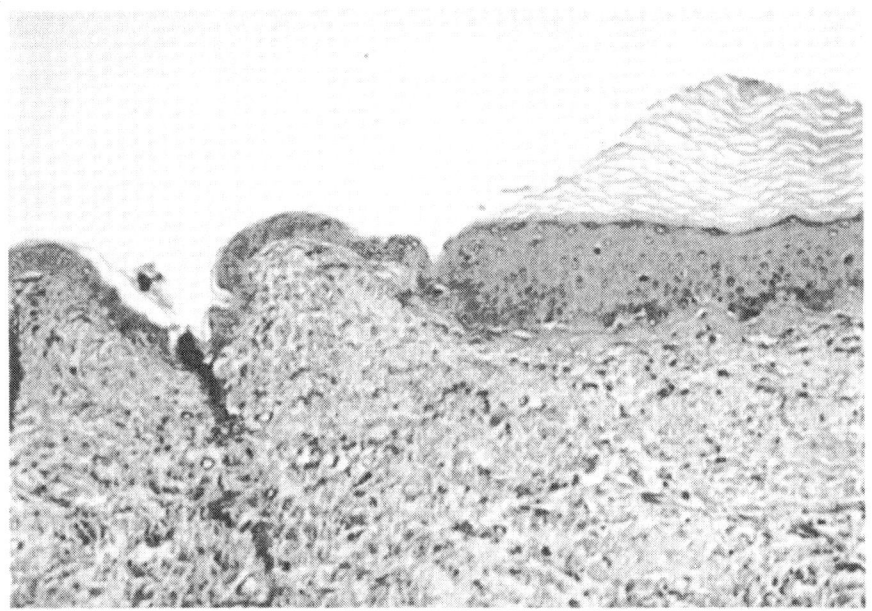

Figure 4   Micrograph of the border of a human skin xenograft onto the nude mouse. The marked difference between the stratum corneum layers is clear. Tissue processing has caused extensive swelling of the human horny layer.

substances. Unfortunately, "control" measurements (using full-thickness grafts) have not been reported because dermatoming of the tissue is necessary to ensure an acceptable surgical success rate (64,65).

D. Conclusions

The available information on in vivo animal models points to some very simple conclusions:

1. Small "hairy" animals (e.g., rat, rabbit) invariably yield penetration values much greater than those seen in man. Their usefulness as predictive models for human in vivo TDD is questionable.
2. The use of the rhesus monkey, if available, appears to be the most reliable and well-validated of the existing models for human skin penetration.

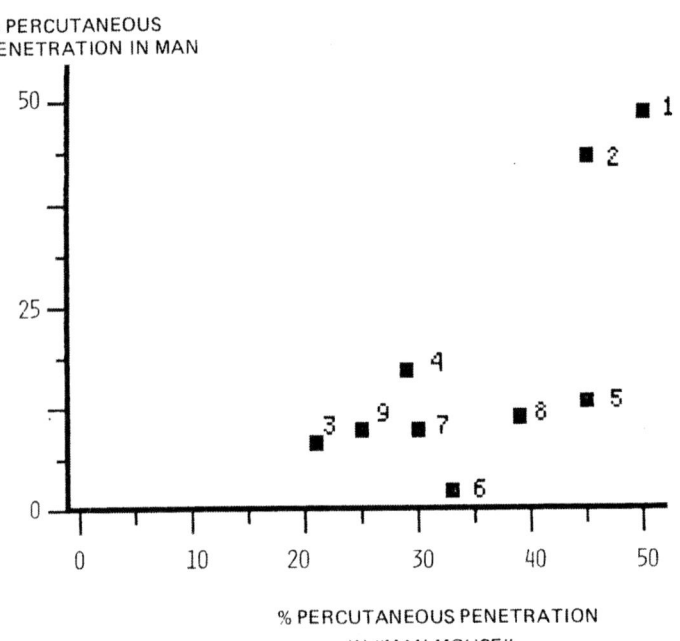

% PERCUTANEOUS
PENETRATION IN MAN

% PERCUTANEOUS PENETRATION
IN "MAN-MOUSE"

Figure 5   Percutaneous penetration in man (42,43) compared to that
in the human-skin-grafted nude mouse ("man–mouse") for caffeine
(1), benzoic acid (2), malathion (3), N,N-diethyl-m-toluamide (4),
testosterone (5), fluocinolone acetonide (6), parathion (7), progesterone (8), and lindane (9). (Adapted from Ref. 65.)

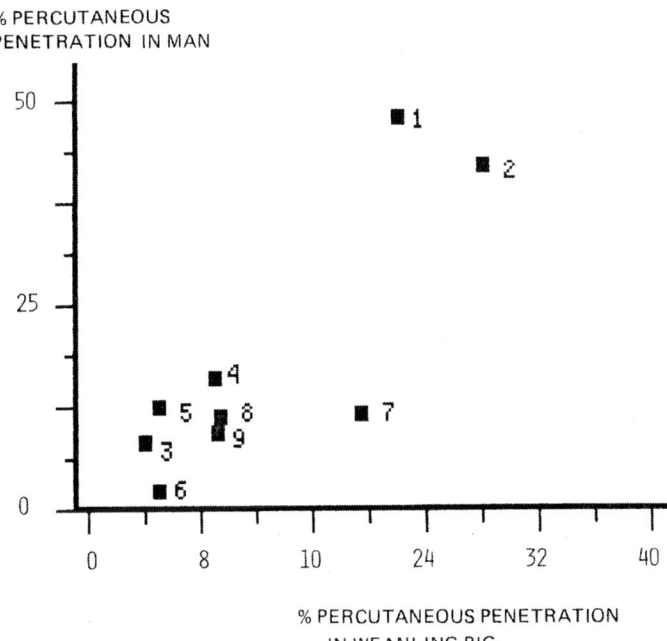

% PERCUTANEOUS
PENETRATION IN MAN

% PERCUTANEOUS PENETRATION
IN WEANLING PIG

Figure 6   Percutaneous penetration in man (42,43) compared to that in the weanling pig for caffeine (1), benzoic acid (2), malathion (3), *N,N*-diethyl-*m*-toluamide (4), testosterone (5), fluocinolone acetonide (6), parathion (7), progesterone (8), and lindane (9). (Adapted from Ref. 65.)

PA IN "MAN-MOUSE"

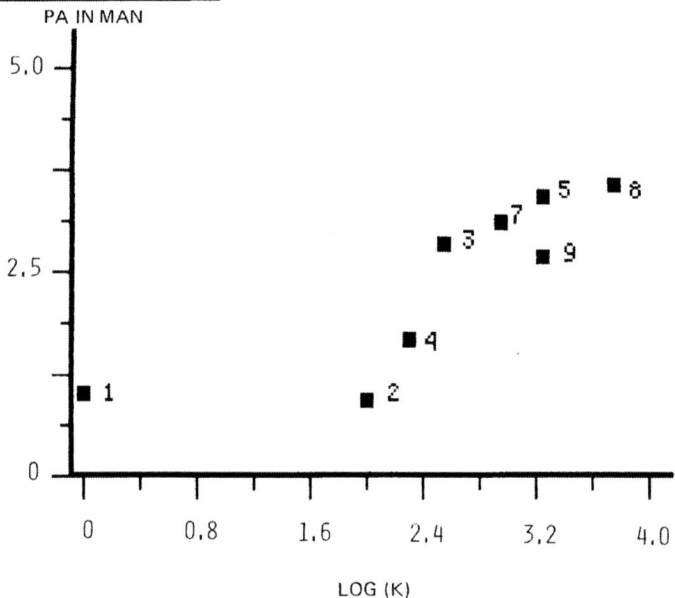

Figure 7   The ratio of percutaneous absorption (PA) in the "man-mouse" to that in man (42,43) plotted as a function of the octanol/ water partition coefficient (K) (103) for caffeine (1), benzoic acid (2), malathion (3), N,N-diethyl-m-toluamide (4), testosterone (5), parathion (7), progesterone (8), and lindane (9). (Adapted from Ref. 64.)

3. The weanling pig (although perhaps not the most convenient and readily available species either) and the human-skin-grafted nude mouse (again, an experimental animal requiring surgical skill and clean laboratory space) offer new, alternative models of much promise and potential.

III. HUMAN EXPERIMENTATION

Eventually, in the development of a TDD system, the drug must be applied to human subjects and pharmacokinetic and pharmacodynamic data must be collected; specific, sensitive assays for the parent drug and any active metabolites will have been developed, and a suitable pharmacological response, which can be quantified, will have been identified.

But does the drug penetrate human skin in vivo? This question will first be asked. Even though in vitro measurements and animal model experiments may be supportive of the likely penetration behavior of the compound in human subjects, a direct demonstration allows the decision to proceed to detailed kinetic and dynamic studies to be made with considerably more confidence. Equally, if several possible agents are under consideration for TDD, a human in vivo evaluation may facilitate the selection of the most promising candidate(s) much more quickly and convincingly than other experimental options.

How, then, can a meaningful in vivo evaluation be performed such that: (a) there is minimal risk to the human volunteers, and (b) predictive results can be generated within a reasonable time? In this section we consider this question in three parts by:

1. Describing the advantages, drawbacks, and predictability of the standard methodology, which has been used for nearly 20 years.
2. Considering two refinements (to the basic approach) that have been reported recently.
3. Examining (again, through studies currently in progress) whether there are age-related changes in skin that alter the barrier function sufficiently and imply, thereby, a closer consideration of subject selection for in vivo studies.

A. Standard In Vivo Methodology

Most of the in vivo human skin penetration data in the literature have been obtained using the procedures first described by Feldmann and Maibach (41–46). As mentioned above, these techniques have also been used in many animal studies. In brief, percutaneous absorption is determined by an indirect method of measuring radioactivity in excreta following topical application of the labeled drug. Generally, ^{14}C has been the radiolabel of choice. Although plasma levels of administered compound are perhaps most desirable, the low levels typically found in the blood after transdermal input preclude the routine use of specific chemical assay procedures. The use of an isotope and quantification in the urine (and feces) allows penetration to be measured following a very small, nonpharmacologically active dose of the chemical. In addition, the approach is applicable to any molecule into which a radiolabel can be incorporated at sufficient specific activity. Hence many more compounds have been evaluated for their in vivo penetration than would have been possible if routine analytical procedures had been sought and used.

Determination of absorption following topical administration in the manner described requires the investigator to know the amount of radioactivity retained in the body, or excreted by routes not assayed.

This necessitates measurement of elimination following parenteral (ideally intravenous) administration of the compound. The percentage of dose absorbed transdermally is then calculated from Eq. (1).

$$\begin{array}{c} \text{\% dose} \\ \text{absorbed} \end{array} = \frac{\begin{array}{c}\text{total radioactivity excreted} \\ \text{after topical administration}\end{array}}{\begin{array}{c}\text{total radioactivity excreted} \\ \text{after intravenous administration}\end{array}} \times 100 \qquad (1)$$

Obvious limitations are inherent in this simple methodology:

1. The radioactivity detected in the excreta is a mixture of parent chemical and metabolites.
2. The origin of the metabolites (e.g., that fraction generated in the skin during transdermal passage) is unknown.
3. Sophisticated kinetic analysis of the data on excretion rate versus time is therefore precluded.

From a practical standpoint, the procedure requires good subject compliance because excretion measurements must be made over several (typically 5-7) days. Most experiments have been performed with the application site unprotected and nonoccluded. In the published literature, reporting on this technique, therefore, there are no examples for which a successful mass balance between applied dose and (corrected) excretion levels has been possible.

However, one must qualify these criticisms by asking, What would be the state of our knowledge in the absence of the in vivo evaluations that have used this technique? The answer, quite simply, is: very limited. There have been a few studies in which chemical assays have been performed in blood and urine following topical administration, but the number is very small. Furthermore, the doses were of a therapeutic magnitude and the analysis procedures were invariably already in place. On the other hand, the radiotracer procedure has permitted a large human in vivo database to be established on a wide range of penetrants (e.g., steroids, pesticides, cosmetics, hair dyes) (42,43,46,61-63). This information, while subject to the foregoing limitations, currently offers the "benchmark" evaluation of skin penetration in man. Despite some recent provocative and challenging remarks (66) concerning the relative usefulness of in vitro over in vivo measurements of percutaneous absorption, there remain too many ill-defined parameters in in vitro methodology (67) for the arguments to be generally persuasive. Thus, although the standard procedure is certainly not without limitation, it has been, and continues to be, immensely valuable. Nevertheless, improvements are possible and unknowns persist; the remainder of this section will consider possible refinements and one important, and immediate, unresolved issue.

B. Refinements

1. *"Reservoir" Technique*

In three recently published papers (68-70), Rougier, Dupuis, and their colleagues have presented evidence (obtained in both hairless rat and man) for a relationship between so-called stratum corneum reservoir function and in vivo percutaneous absorption. The initial study (68) in the hairless rat compared (a) the total body distribution after 96 hr of 10 substances, having a wide range of physicochemical properties, following a 30 min-topical application in a 95:5 v/v ethanol/water vehicle, with (b) the corresponding amount of the same substances that could be found in the stratum corneum by tape-stripping after, again, a 30-min topical exposure. The penetrants were labeled with ^{14}C or ^{3}H and were analyzed by liquid scintillation counting. In terms of penetration, it was found that there was a factor of 50 between the best penetrant (benzoic acid) and the least absorbed compound (dexamethasone) (see Table 2). Comparison of these values with the levels measurable in the stratum corneum demonstrated high correlation (Fig. 8). Thus, a major implication of the work was that the simple, short exposure procedure followed by immediate tape-stripping would provide a facile prediction of in vivo penetration over a longer period.

A logical sequential step was then performed: evaluation of the technique in man (69). Following identical procedures, the experiment was conducted in human subjects using four different doses of benzoic acid delivered in an ethylene glycol vehicle containing 10% Triton-X-100. For comparative purposes, parallel control measurements were also made in the hairless rat. Benzoic acid was chosen because it penetrates human skin well and is almost totally excreted in the urine, thereby facilitating the determination of % dose absorbed. The results are summarized in Figure 9, which contains three important features. First, penetration in the rat is approximately twice that in man. Second, the stratum corneum content of benzoic acid in man after a 30 min-exposure is linearly related to the amount found to penetrate over the subsequent 4 days. Third, the linear relationship between these quantities, previously determined from the absorption of 10 very different substances in the hairless rat (68), is not significantly different from that which holds in man for benzoic acid over a 10-fold range in applied concentration. The results of this second study support, therefore, the initial conclusion obtained in the hairless rat and suggest, in addition, a commonality between predictive relationships in an animal model (the hairless rat) and man.

The most recent publication (70) from the same laboratory showed that there is no unique feature to the previously exclusive use of a 30-min skin contact time. In the hairless rat, using benzoic acid,

Table 2   Percutaneous Absorption Assessed by the "Reservoir" Technique[a]

Chemical[b]	Total penetration 96 hr after topical application ($nmol/cm^2 \pm SD$)	Amount in stratum corneum 0.5 hr after application ($nmol/cm^2 \pm SD$)
Benzoic acid	26.6 ± 0.7	17.6 ± 1.5
Benzoic acid[c]	79.3 ± 3.6	48.1 ± 5.1
Acetylsalicylic acid	6.7 ± 0.7	5.2 ± 0.6
Dihydroepiandrosterone	5.3 ± 0.2	2.0 ± 0.4
Sodium salicylate	5.0 ± 0.7	3.9 ± 0.3
Testosterone	4.3 ± 0.5	2.1 ± 0.2
Caffeine	3.7 ± 0.3	2.8 ± 0.3
Thiourea	3.2 ± 0.5	2.6 ± 0.3
D-Mannitol	2.6 ± 0.2	2.2 ± 0.4
Hydrocortisone	0.9 ± 0.1	0.9 ± 0.2
Dexamethasone	0.6 ± 0.1	0.4 ± 0.0

[a]Six animals were used per chemical.
[b]Topical dose was 200 $nmol/cm^2$ except as noted in note c.
[c]Dose = 450 $nmol/cm^2$.
Source: Adapted from Ref. 68.

nicotinic acid, aspirin, and theophylline, linear relationships between penetration, recovery, and application time have been established (Table 3). Exposure periods of 0.5, 2, 4, and 6 hr were investigated. The correlation between 4-day penetration and 30-min stratum corneum levels for the four compounds studied was not significantly different from those reported before for various compounds in the rat and for benzoic acid at different applied doses in man (68,69).

The persuasive nature of these combined results is indisputable. The apparent generality of the observations, and the coincidence between the data in hairless rat with those in man, offer well-validated predictive potential. However, limitations of the approach do exist and require discussion. First, the procedure yields a single time-point measurement that can provide only an estimation of total absorption: kinetic details of the rate and extent of absorption are

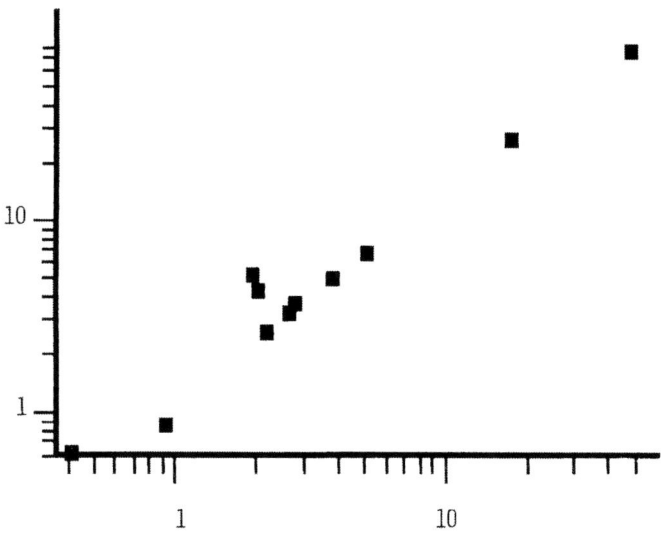

AMOUNT PENETRATED
IN 4 DAYS (NMOL/CM^2)

AMOUNT IN STRATUM CORNEUM
0.5 HR AFTER APPLICATION (NMOL/CM^2)

Figure 8   Total percutaneous penetration (nmol/cm^2) 4 days after topical application compared to amount (nmol/cm^2) in stratum corneum 30 min after administration for the compounds listed in Table 2. Linear regression of the data yields: y = 1.64x − 0.5, r = 0.998. (Adapted from Ref. 68.)

lost. Next, the technique is somewhat invasive, requiring stratum corneum removal by the tape-stripping process. Third, with only a 30-min application time, validation of the procedure has required the administration of large doses of radioactivity (so that absorption can be quantified by later tissue and body fluids analysis), which are probably unacceptable for routine studies in man. In addition, the brevity of the application period amplifies the uncertainty associated with the prediction estimation on the basis of the small difference between two large numbers. Modifications to the technique that would alleviate some of these shortcomings may be envisaged and an example follows. Nevertheless, in overall conclusion, it may be suggested that these experiments warrant cautious optimism and represent an encouraging advance.

AMOUNT PENETRATED
IN 4 DAYS (NMOL/CM^2)

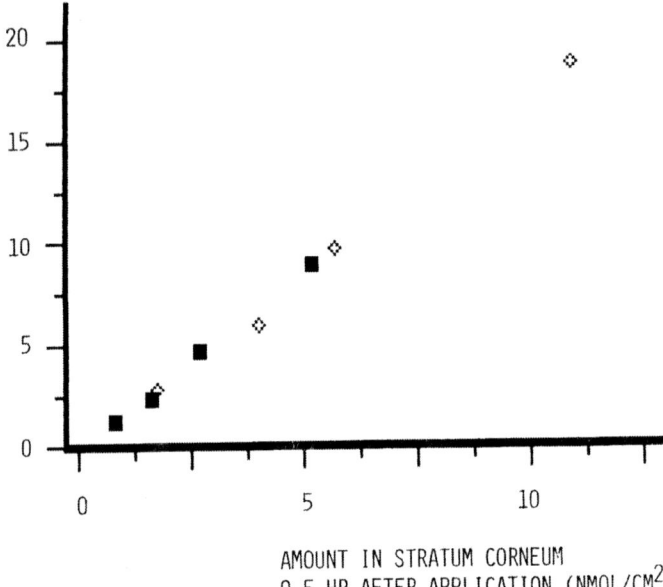

AMOUNT IN STRATUM CORNEUM
0.5 HR AFTER APPLICATION (NMOL/CM^2)

Figure 9   Correlation between total penetration of benzoic acid after 4 days with amounts recovered in the stratum corneum 30 min after application at 4 doses (125, 250, 500, and 1000 nmol/cm^2) in the rat (diamonds) and man (squares). Linear regression of the data points yields: $y = 1.83x - 0.52$, $r = 0.998$. (Adapted from Ref. 69.)

2. *"Mass Balance" Technique*

Recently, in our laboratory, a modification of the standard Feldmann and Maibach (41–46) in vivo approach has been explored. The procedure developed addresses some of the perceived "reservoir technique" limitations identified above. Experiments have so far been conducted with three steroidal penetrants: testosterone, estradiol, and hydrocortisone. The ^{14}C-labeled chemicals have been applied in acetone to the ventral forearm of male volunteers. Chemical and radioactivity doses were 4 µg/cm^2 and 1 µCi/cm^2, respectively; the area of application was 2.5 cm^2. After evaporation of the vehicle, the application site was covered with a polypropylene Hilltop chamber, which was affixed to the skin with adhesive tape.

Table 3   Influence of Application Time on the Assessment of Percutaneous Absorption by the "Reservoir" Technique[a]

Chemical[b]	Application time (hr)	Total penetration 96 hr after topical application (nmol/cm^2 ± SD)	Amount in stratum corneum 0.5 hr after application (nmol/cm^2 ± SD)
Theophylline	0.5	1.9 ± 0.1	2.5 ± 0.3
	2	7.0 ± 1.4	
	4	12.3 ± 1.2	
	6	25.1 ± 4.8	
Aspirin	0.5	8.1 ± 1.7	5.2 ± 0.6
	2	25.7 ± 1.9	
	4	53.6 ± 2.4	
	6	82.7 ± 14.0	
Nicotinic acid	0.5	15.7 ± 2.5	9.7 ± 0.9
	2	44.8 ± 11.7	
	4	123.5 ± 25.5	
	6	180.0 ± 61.5	
Benzoic acid	0.5	18.8 ± 2.6	10.5 ± 1.0
	2	78.6 ± 5.2	
	4	145.3 ± 12.7	
	6	185.2 ± 22.6	

[a]Five hairless rats were used per time point.
[b]Dose = 1000 nmol/cm^2.
Source: Adapted from Ref. 70.

The subjects collected their urine for 7 days postapplication; four fractions were collected on day 1 (0–4, 4–8, 8–12, and 12–24 hr), one per day, thereafter. After 24 hr, the occlusive chamber was removed and submitted to liquid scintillation counting. The application site was washed with a standardized procedure (soap solution, water, soap solution, water, water) and all washings were collected and assayed for residual surface chemical. For the remaining 6 days of the study, the administration site was again covered with a (new) chamber. An essentially identical protocol has also been performed following a multiple dosing regimen (71): daily topical doses of the same three compounds were administered over a 14-day period. The first and eighth doses were ^{14}C-labeled and urinary excretion for 7 days after each of the "hot" doses was followed. In this case, the 24-hr washing procedure was also performed daily, and a new chamber was provided on each occasion.

The results of these preliminary experiments are summarized in Figure 10, which plots the disposition of the ^{14}C-labeled chemical doses as a function of penetrant log (octanol/water) partition coefficient ($K_{o/w}$). It was found that the data from the single- and multiple-dose studies were indistinguishable and they have, therefore, been pooled. Surface wash recoveries for the multiple-administration regimen represent only those collected at 24 hr post-^{14}C administration; negligible radioactivity was present in the washings obtained on days 3–8 and 10–14. The data, as a whole, show that: (a) the sequestration of chemical by the polypropylene chamber is relatively constant and does not appear to be sensitive to $K_{o/w}$, (b) 24-hr surface wash recovery decreases linearly with increasing log $K_{o/w}$, (c) percutaneous absorption, determined as total (corrected) ^{14}C-urinary excretion level, increases linearly with increasing log $K_{o/w}$, (d) there appears to be a significant inverse correlation between surface wash recovery and percutaneous absorption, and (e) there is excellent mass balance between applied dose and postadministration disposition.

We believe, therefore, that this in vivo refinement is advantageous. The benign nature of the covering device and its apparent lack of specificity in binding are useful attributes. The ability to achieve mass balance in this type of experiment is an important improvement. The potential predictability of the surface wash measurement for percutaneous absorption and the correlation of these parameters with a physicochemical parameter of the penetrant is promising. Radiolabeled drug administration remains necessary, and kinetic data will be obtainable only if several small doses are applied at t = 0 and then removed at various times thereafter. Also, thus far, occlusion of the application site has been used. While this may be the most relevant situation for TDD, it will be interesting to observe whether the procedure is as effective if the dosing site is protected

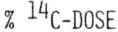 % ^{14}C-DOSE

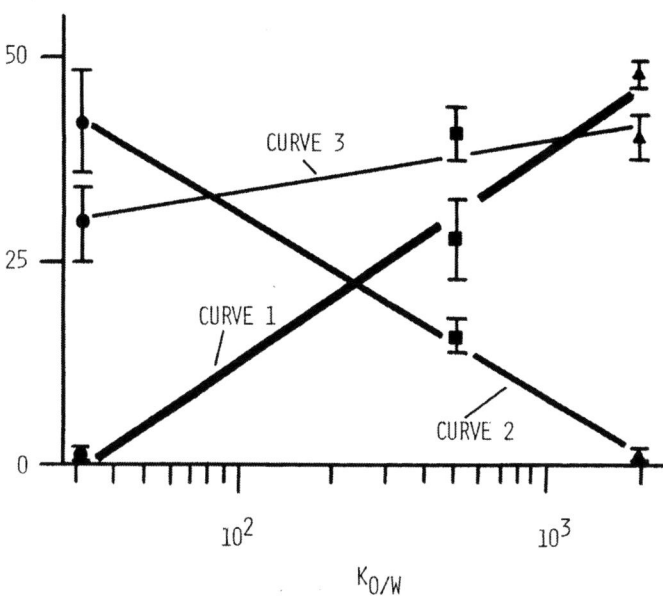

Figure 10   Disposition of testosterone (triangles), estradiol (squares), and hydrocortisone (circles), in vivo in man after topical application: curve 1, percutaneous absorption; curve 2, amount removed by washing; curve 3, chemical sequestered on polypropylene chamber. (Data presented at A. Ph. A. Academy of Pharmaceutical Sciences 39th National Meeting, Minneapolis, October, 1985, by D. A. W. Bucks, J. R. McMaster, H. I. Maibach, and R. H. Guy.)

rather than enclosed (e.g., with a ventilated chamber). It seems reasonable to speculate, however, that further validation of this approach with a wider variety and increased number of chemical species may establish a significantly improved technique for in vivo percutaneous absorption evaluation.

C. Effect of Aging on Skin Penetration

That human skin changes dramatically with increasing age is patently obvious on visual inspection. Physiological and biochemical changes within the tissue have been identified and investigated (72). However, we do not know whether, or how, the penetration barrier of the skin changes in the aged. At the opposite end of the age spectrum (i.e., in the neonate) some experimental data exist and have been recently reviewed (15–19). On the other hand, for the elderly, who represent the subject population most likely to take advantage of the benefits of TDD (long-term, chronic therapy offering excellent compliance and reduced side effects), the question of altered barrier function has been minimally studied.

The few investigations, which have been performed in vivo in man or in vitro on excised human skin, have produced inconsistent conclusions. Percutaneous absorption in vivo has been reported to be lower in aged subjects (73,74), yet, in vitro, penetration through skin excised from elderly cadavers was significantly higher than that through stratum corneum removed from young donors (73). Transepidermal water loss does not appear to change with age in adulthood (75). The role of microcirculation clearance as an integral part of percutaneous absorption has been investigated because of the perceived increasing comprimisation of dermal perfusion with advancing age (76,77). Removal rates of intradermally injected materials have been found to both increase and decrease as a function of age with no clear consensus evolving to explain the disparate observations. All too often, work in this field has been characterized by small subject populations, poorly defined procedural techniques, and experiment selections that preclude straightforward comparisons and unambiguous conclusions. A more detailed review of the literature has recently been compiled (78).

Presently, in our laboratory, a preliminary in vivo, percutaneous absorption study in two elderly populations ("young–old," 65–75 years; "old–old," >75 years) has been initiated. Four "model" penetrants (benzoic acid, hydrocortisone, estradiol, and testosterone), which demonstrate a wide range of penetrability characteristics and physicochemical properties, have been considered. Control data on "young" adults (18–35 years) have been published (42,43).

Using the standard radiochemical approach described earlier (41–46), the results collected in Table 4 have been obtained. For testosterone and estradiol, the two most lipophilic compounds, penetration in the three subject groups is essentially equivalent. In contrast, for hydrocortisone and benzoic acid, the less lipophilic and more water-soluble chemicals, absorption is significantly less in both elderly cohorts than in the young "controls." Thus, there appears to be good reason to suspect that percutaneous absorption does change with age and that the effect is sensitive to the physicochemical properties of the penetrant.

Why should the barrier function change toward compounds that are more hydrophilic than lipophilic? It is known that aged stratum corneum is considerably dryer than the young adult horny layer and that it contains a lower lipid content (72,75). A reduced presence of water implies that aged skin provides a less attractive environment

Table 4 Comparison of Percutaneous Absorption in "Young" and "Aged" Human Subjects[a]

Chemical	log K[a]	Cumulative % dose excreted in 5 days		
		Young	Young-old	Old-old
Testosterone[b]	3.31	13.2 ± 3.0 (n = 17)	10.6 ± 5.7 (n = 8)	15.2 ± 8.4 (n = 7)
Estradiol[b]	2.70	10.6 ± 4.9 (n = 3)	11.5 ± 3.5 (n = 6)	9.0 ± 5.6 (n = 6)
Hydrocortisone[c]	1.93	1.87 ± 1.6 (n = 15)	0.67 ± 0.58 (n = 8)	0.86 ± 0.50 (n = 9)
Benzoic acid[c]	1.87	42.6 ± 16.5 (n = 6)	27.5 ± 11.6 (n = 8)	23.1 ± 7.0 (n = 9)

[a]K = octanol/water partition coefficient (103).
[b]Penetration in the aged cohorts was not significantly different from that in the "young" group ($p > 0.05$).
[c]Penetration in the aged cohorts was significantly less than that in the "young" group ($p < 0.05$ or better).
Source: K. V. Roskos, R. S. Hinz, H. I. Maibach, and R. H. Guy, presented at the APhA Academy of Pharmaceutical Sciences 39th National Meeting, Minneapolis, October, 1985.

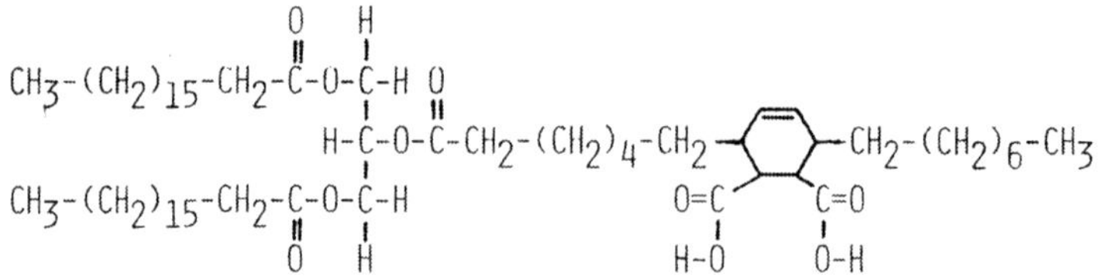

$$CH_3-(CH_2)_{15}-CH_2-\overset{\overset{\displaystyle O}{\|}}{C}-O-\overset{\overset{\displaystyle H}{|}}{C}-H \quad \overset{\displaystyle O}{\underset{\displaystyle \|}{}}$$

Chemical structure figure of the triglyceride Glyceridacid 100.

Figure 11   Chemical structure of the triglyceride Glyceridacid 100 (79–81).

to less lipophilic moieties. The diminished lipid content provides a reduced dissolution medium for chemicals administered to the skin surface. Such a change, one might predict, would differentiate against the absorption of compounds of relatively low lipid solubility—that is, agents with smaller rather than higher oil/water partition coefficients, namely, hydrocortisone and benzoic acid. A lowered water content and a smaller lipid capacity may not, however, affect stratum corneum uptake and passage of highly lipophilic molecules such as testosterone and estradiol.

Substantiation of these conclusions awaits further experiments with an expanded range of penetrants. In addition, close attention should be paid to recent investigations into a unique triglyceride skin softener (79–81) (Fig. 11). This agent shows a marked ability to improve the smoothness of the skin even at low water content and has potential, therefore, as a treatment for the relief of xerosis or dry skin in the elderly. While the mechanism of action remains speculative, X-ray data imply an important effect on the lipid structure within the horny layer. Specifically, a stabilization of the lamellar arrangement of intercellular lipids is supported.

Thus, probing the barrier function at both macroscopic and molecular levels as a function of age is now realistic. With the changing demographic pattern of Western civilization and the increasing awareness of the potential benefits that TDD can provide to elderly patients, the results of these rather new avenues of investigation are particularly important and pertinent to future geriatric chemotherapy.

IV.   KINETIC MODELING OF TRANSDERMAL DRUG DELIVERY

The objective of model development in TDD is to provide a predictive tool that may be used prospectively, at an early stage, in the screening of candidate drugs. A suitable simulation does not need to be exactly quantitative, nor is it reasonable to expect that exact coincidence between prediction and in vivo results can be routinely obtained. However, an acceptable model should identify high-priority compounds and should be able to indicate how "borderline" chemicals may be formulated to enable efficacious delivery via the skin. The simplest theoretical calculation involves application of the steady-state mass balance equation:

$$IN = Cl \cdot c_{ss} \qquad (2)$$

where IN ($\mu g/hr$) is the TDD input rate, Cl (cm^3/hr) is the drug clearance, and c_{ss} ($\mu g/ml$) is the target steady-state plasma concentration. If, for example, the TDD device was a "membrane-controlled" system (1-6,9,11-14), from which the drug was released with a zero-order kinetic rate constant k^0 ($\mu g/cm^2/hr$), then

$$IN = A \cdot k^0 \qquad (3)$$

where A is the area of the patch.

Equations (2) and (3) can be used to determine whether a feasible IN can be accomplished. For example, for the antihypertensive drug clonidine, a suitable target c_{ss} would be 0.75 ng/ml and the literature reports a clearance of about 1.2 L/hr for a 70-kg individual. It follows that:

$$IN = (1.2 \times 10^3) \; (0.75) \; ng/hr = 9 \; \mu g/hr$$

Hence, a 5-cm^2 device programmed to release clonidine at a little less than 2 $\mu g/cm^2/hr$ should provide a steady, pharmacologically efficacious level of drug. Such a system has indeed been developed (11-13), approved by the FDA, and is now marketed as Catapres-TTS by Boehringher-Ingelheim.

However, the predictive approach based on a steady-state calculation is deficient in two ways. First, the predicted A · k^0 product may not be feasible; that is, either an impossibly large area or input rate may be necessary to achieve the desired c_{ss}. Second, the calculation provides no indication of the time required to attain the target c_{ss}. For transdermal delivery, a classic estimation of this time based on the drug's biological half-life will often be inappropriate because percutaneous absorption is usually slower than the elimination process [i.e., "flip-flop" kinetics (82) pertain].

To resolve these difficulties, it is necessary to model the entire time course of transdermal delivery and, thus, it is essential to describe theoretically the kinetics of percutaneous absorption. As a first step, we identify the key physical events involved in the TDD process:

1. Transport within the delivery system
2. Drug partitioning from the device into the stratum corneum
3. Transport across the stratum corneum
4. Drug partitioning from the lipophilic stratum corneum into the (much more aqueous) viable epidermis
5. Transport across the viable epidermis
6. Uptake by the cutaneous capillaries (epidermal–dermal junction) and systemic distribution

Admittedly, this list does not include all possible interactions between drug and skin (83,84), but it does incorporate all the transport and partitioning steps necessary to move the drug from the device into the bloodstream. Transport (or diffusion) and partitioning are the key words here and must influence significantly the form of any effective model for TDD. The most rigorous approach to simulating this sequence of steps would involve, minimally, solution of Fick's second law of diffusion, with appropriate boundary conditions, for the device, the stratum corneum, and the viable epidermis. While this is theoretically feasible and has, in fact, been performed to various levels of sophistication (85–92), a complete treatment is mathematically complex, may require numerical solutions to the differential equations, and loses, as a result, a degree of insight and biophysical relevance.

An alternative approach involves the application of linear kinetics (93–102). While this methodology lacks rigorous purity, it does offer, we believe, an acceptable first approximation and it retains important physicochemical significance. Additionally, the model permits important, but experimentally inaccessible or intractable, questions to be addressed theoretically. Currently, the simulation has developed to the extent represented schematically in Figure 12. Details have been described fully in the literature (93,96–98,101,102) and only a brief recapitulation is given here. Input kinetics from the device are described by $f(k_{IN})$: for a so-called membrane-controlled patch, such as the clonidine-containing Catapres-TTS (11–13) (Fig. 13), $f(k_{IN})$ consists of a first-order component (k^I) accounting for drug release from the contact adhesive and a zero-order contribution (k^0) representing the membrane-determined flux of drug from the reservoir (1). The parameter k_r reflects the fact that there will be competition for drug between the patch and the stratum corneum. A well-designed patch will minimize k_r. However, it is clear that k_r will, for example, become progressively more significant for drugs of relatively low lipophilicity (log $K \leqslant 0$). Drug transport across stratum corneum and viable epidermis is characterized by two first-order rate constants, k_1 and k_2, respectively. These parameters are proportional to the corresponding diffusion coefficients across the two tissue layers and can be estimated from the drug molecular weight (M) via Eq. (4):

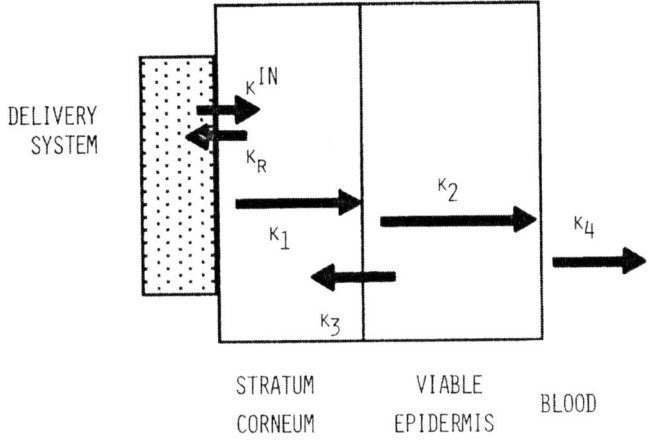

STRATUM CORNEUM   VIABLE EPIDERMIS   BLOOD

Figure 12   Kinetic model for transdermal drug delivery and percutaneous absorption (20,97,98,101,102).

$$k_i = C_i M^{-1/3} \qquad (i = 1, 2) \tag{4}$$

where C_i are known constants (97). The k_3 parameter reflects the relative rapidity with which the drug partitions from the stratum corneum to the viable tissue. Thus, for very lipophilic compounds, k_3 will be large and the transfer from stratum corneum to viable epidermis will be slow. The ratio k_3/k_2 measures, as a result, an "effective" stratum corneum/viable tissue partition coefficient for the drug and it has been empirically shown [by fitting in vivo percutaneous absorption data (97,98)] that

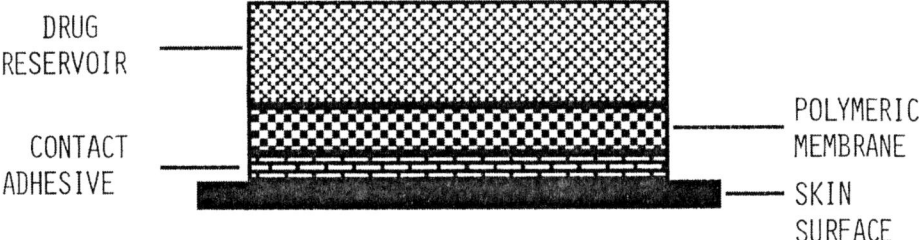

Figure 13   Schematic diagram of a membrane-moderated transdermal drug delivery system (9,20).

$$k_3/k_2 = K/5 \tag{5}$$

where K is the octanol/water partition coefficient of the drug. The empiricism of Eq. (5) should be emphasized—there is no a priori reason why a correlation of k_3/k_2 with K should exist. We suspect that other oil/water partition coefficients may be more appropriate; however, there is, of course, a very large database of log K (103), and this is the major reason for its use in this predictive approach. Last, k_4 (or a more complex function, if necessary) describes the drug's clearance from the systemic circulation. A prediction of k_4 is not possible; it must be measured following intravenous administration of the compound.

A series of differential equations describes the kinetics of the transdermal absorption process represented by Figure 12. These rate equations are easily solved to give the following expression for the drug concentration in blood (C_p) as a function of time (t) (98, 101,102):

$$C_p = f(k^I) + f(k^0) \tag{6}$$

where

$$f(k^I) = \frac{Mk^I k_1 k_2}{V} \left[\frac{\exp(-\alpha t)}{(\beta - \alpha)(\alpha - \omega)(\beta - \mu)} + \frac{\exp(-\beta t)}{(\alpha - \beta)(\beta - \omega)(\beta - \mu)} \right.$$
$$\left. + \frac{\exp(-\omega t)}{(\alpha - \omega)(\omega - \beta)(\omega - \mu)} + \frac{\exp(-\mu t)}{(\alpha - \mu)(\mu - \beta)(\mu - \omega)} \right] \tag{7}$$

and

$$f(k^0) = \frac{Ak^0 k_1 k_2}{V} \left[\frac{1}{\alpha \beta \epsilon} - \frac{\exp(-\alpha t)}{\alpha(\alpha - \beta)(\alpha - \epsilon)} - \frac{\exp(-\beta t)}{\beta(\beta - \alpha)(\beta - \epsilon)} \right.$$
$$\left. - \frac{\exp(-\epsilon t)}{\epsilon(\epsilon - \alpha)(\epsilon - \beta)} \right] \tag{8}$$

Equations (7) and (8) describe, respectively, the first-order and zero-order contributions to transdermal input from a device of the type illustrated in Figure 13, and

M = amount of drug in the "priming" contact adhesive

A = surface area of the device

$$\omega\mu = k^I k_1; \quad (\omega + \mu) = k^I + k_r + k_1$$

$$\alpha\beta = k_2 k_4; \quad (\alpha + \beta) = k_2 + k_3 + k_4$$

$$\epsilon = k_1 + k_r$$

Predictions of the C_p versus t profile following transdermal delivery have been successfully performed for nitroglycerin and clonidine using appropriate values for the parameters required (Table 5) (101,102). These simulations have been discussed extensively in previous publications (20,101,102), and Figure 14 summarizes the correlation between theory and human in vivo experiment. The agreement is good and shows that physicochemical characterization of transcutaneous kinetics, in conjunction with device release rate(s) and limited pharmacokinetic data, can be employed successfully to model and to predict TDD. More recently (104–106), plasma levels of estradiol, scopolamine, and timolol following TDD have been published, and the kinetic model has again been able to simulate the results in a self-consistent fashion (107). Figure 15 illustrates these latest analyses using estradiol as an example.

A secondary aim of an effective model for TDD is to permit examination of experimentally inaccessible or poorly defined variables of the percutaneous absorption process. Two examples, in particular, may be cited: (a) the impact of cutaneous metabolism on the systemic availability of transdermally delivered drugs, and (b) the desirable properties required of putative penetration enhancers as a function of the physicochemical properties of the delivered drug.

The first case has been explored both for drug biotransformation by cutaneous enzymes within the viable epidermis (108) and for drug degradation on the skin surface by microorganisms (109). The former situation requires that the degree of effect be explored by assuming a range of metabolic transformation rate constants (108). These parameters, however, have not been quantified experimentally and the significance of the theoretical findings awaits, therefore, suitable accurate measurements of enzyme activity in skin. The latter situation has been addressed specifically for nitroglycerin making use of microbial degradation kinetics of the drug determined in culture (109). The simulations show that microorganisms on the skin surface elicit their maximal effect on drug delivered to the skin with first-order kinetics either from the contact adhesive of a transdermal delivery system or from a thinly spread film of topical ointment. The result for TDD is to delay the attainment of the target steady-state plasma concentration, an effect that can be circumvented by increasing the magnitude of the "loading" dose contained within the patch adhesive. Experimentally, in rhesus monkeys, a cutaneous "first-pass effect" of about 16–21% has been demonstrated for nitroglycerin (110). Given the sensitivity of nitroglycerin to metabolism, one might speculate that the magnitude of this effect reflects a maximum value. However,

Table 5 Pharmacokinetic and Physicochemical Parameters Utilized by the Kinetic Model (20,97,98,101,102) to Calculate the Predicted Curves in Figures 14 and 15 for Nitroglycerin, Clonidine, and Estradiol

	Nitroglycerin[a]	Clonidine[b]	Estradiol[c]
Molecular weight	227.1	230.1	272.4
log K	2.05	0.83	2.49
Half-life (hr)	0.04	8.5	0.05
V (L)	231	147	4.81
A (cm^2)	10	5	20
M (mg)	2	0.47	0.1
k^0 $(\mu g/cm^2/hr)$	36	1.6	0.21
k^I (hr^{-1})	1.3	1.3	1.3
k_r (hr^{-1})	10^{-4}	10^{-4}	10^{-4}
k_1 (hr^{-1})	0.15	0.15	0.14
k_2 (hr^{-1})	2.36	2.35	2.22
k_3 (hr^{-1})	53	3.2	222
k_4 (hr^{-1})	18.2	0.08	13.9

[a]Parameters from Ref. 102.
[b]Parameters from Ref. 101.
[c]Parameters from Ref. 107.

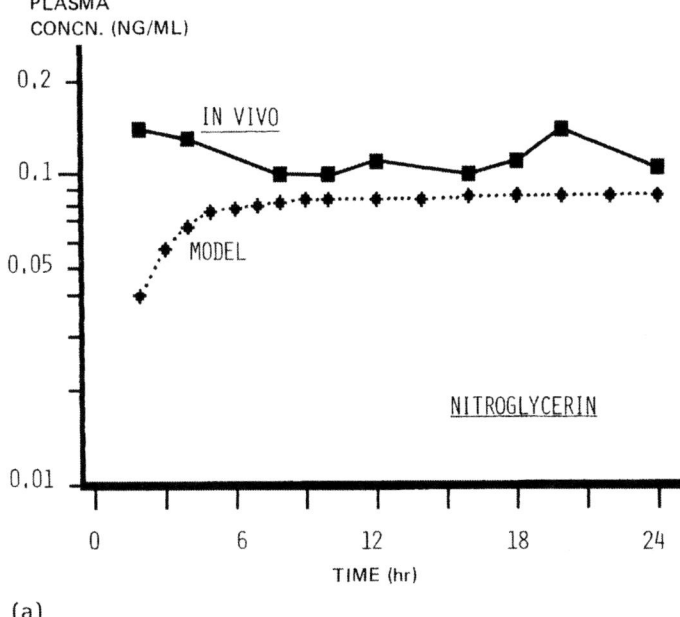

(a)

Figure 14 Comparison between theoretical predictions of the kinetic model (Fig. 12) (101,102) with in vivo plasma concentration versus time profiles for nitroglycerin and clonidine following transdermal delivery (9,11). The parameters used to calculate the simulated curves are given in Table 5. Time is measured in hours (a) and in days (b).

this hypothesis remains essentially untested, and the location of nitroglycerin metabolism (surface versus epidermal) is unknown. Considerably more work in this area is required, therefore, before the full significance of the model predictions can be assessed and acted upon.

The second case, the effect of penetration enhancers on TDD, has recently been examined by using the kinetic simulation to probe the action of "model" promoters as a function of the physicochemical properties of the penetrant (111). Two prospective enhancers, which act specifically in skin, have been considered: the first (PE1) increases the drug diffusion coefficient (D_S) across the stratum corneum by 10-fold; the second (PE2) increases D_S by the same amount but also reduces the effective stratum corneum/viable tissue partition coefficient of the drug by an order of magnitude from its

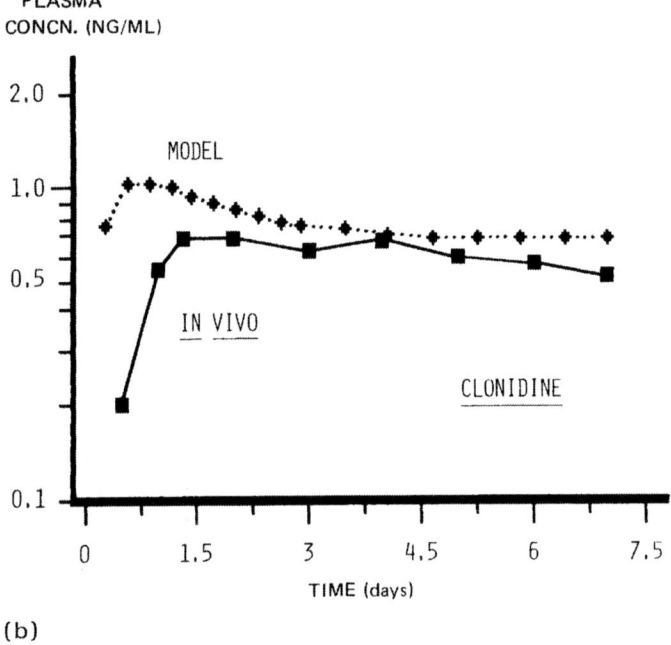

PLASMA
CONCN. (NG/ML)

(b)

Figure 14 (continued)

unperturbed value. Enhancer PE1 acts specifically to reduce the diffusional resistance of the stratum corneum, therefore, while PE2 demonstrates an additional, more subtle, role by which the lipophilic nature of the horny layer is somewhat masked. In terms of the model (Fig. 12), PE1 increases k_1 by 10-fold, PE2 again raises k_1 by a factor of 10 but also reduces k_3/k_2 by an order of magnitude.

Figure 16 shows that the action of these parameters is sensitive to the oil/water partitioning characteristics of the drug. We consider two drug molecules (D1 and D2) being delivered from a 10-cm^2 transdermal device that releases the active species with zero-order kinetics at 20 μg/cm^2/hr. The drugs have identical molecular weights (250), biological half-lives (0.5 hr), and volumes of distribution (100 L). They differ only in their respective octanol/water partition coefficient (K):

D1, log K = 1   D2, log K = 3

The simulations presented in Figure 16 show that PE1 is effective for the relatively hydrophilic drug D1 but is ineffectual in promoting

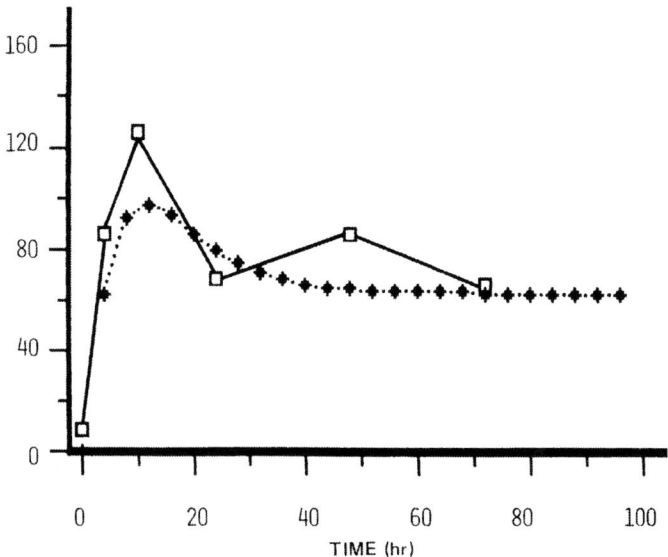

PLASMA
CONCN. (PG/ML)

Figure 15 Theoretical prediction (diamonds) of the plasma levels of estradiol as a function of time (107) following transdermal delivery compared to in vivo data (squares) (104). The parameters used to calculate the simulations are listed in Table 5.

penetration of the more lipophilic agent D2. The reverse differentiation is shown by PE2, which elicits minimal action on D1 but significantly enhances absorption of D2. It is apparent, therefore, that the desirable properties of a penetration enhancer may change depending on the physicochemical nature of the drug being delivered. For a relatively hydrophilic drug (log K ≤ 1–1.5), it is important for the enhancer to lower the diffusional resistance of the stratum corneum. For more hydrophobic compounds (log K ≤ 2), however, the enhancer must, in some way, promote the rate of stratum corneum to viable tissue partitioning. In this case, speeding the rate of stratum corneum diffusion is less important because transfer of drug *out* of the horny layer is the slowest step in the absorption process.

At the present time, the mechanisms of action of the various agents proposed as penetration enhancers are not well defined (27–29). The search for more effective promoters, therefore, lacks an obvious rationale. We suggest that theoretical investigations of the type discussed here may permit a more logical approach to the understanding

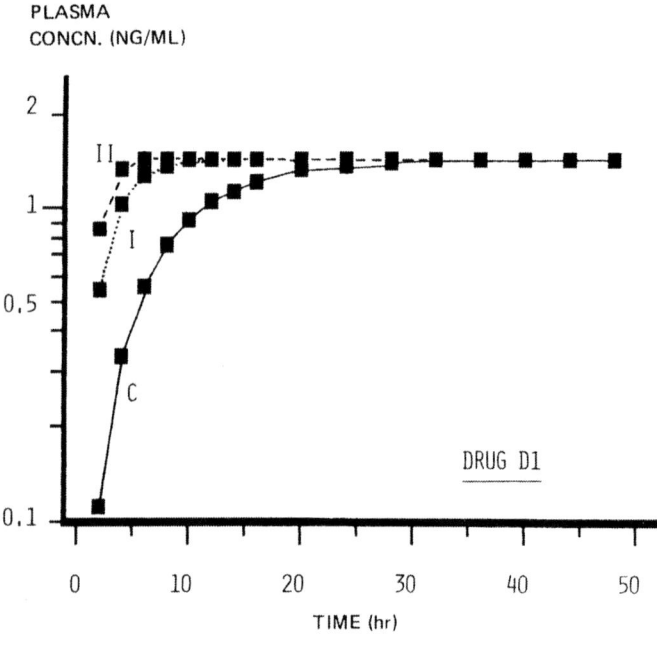

(a)

Figure 16 The predicted effects of two "model" percutaneous penetration enhancers (PE1 and PE2) on the plasma concentration versus
time profiles of two drugs (D1 and D2) delivered transdermally (111).
Curves C are the controls (no enhancer), curves I and II are those
resulting from transdermal delivery in the presence of PE1 and PE2,
respectively.

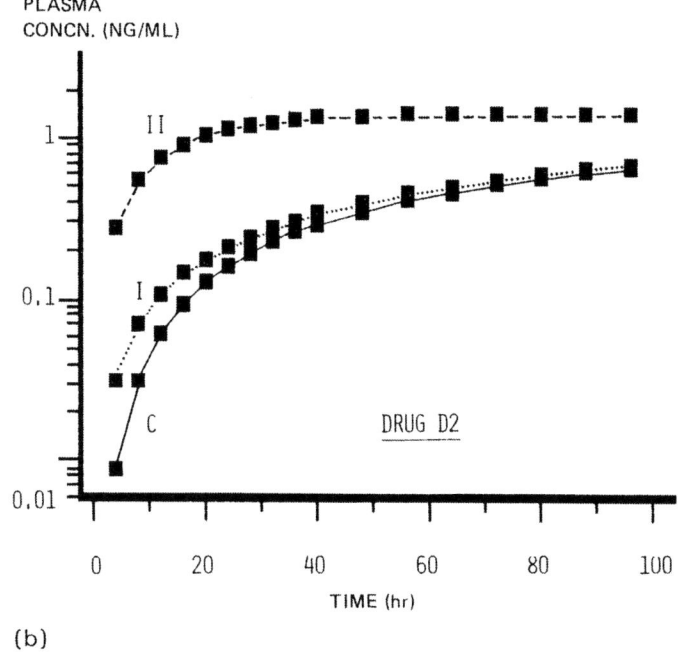

(b)

Figure 16   (continued)

and identification of compounds that can effectively and controllably facilitate percutaneous absorption.

V. SUMMARY

The in vivo evaluation of TDD represents a crucial stage in the development of a therapeutic device. Design of the appropriate test experiment and utilization of a relevant experimental system are of fundamental importance, therefore. The objective of this chapter has been to identify methodologies for assessing TDD in vivo and to elucidate the procedures that may prove most informative and indicative of potential success. There have been useful recent advances in the approaches to measure percutaneous absorption in vivo, and these procedures should be given careful attention when planning for TDD evaluation. The advantages and limitations of various animal models are now more clearly defined and, while there remains no "ideal" system, there is now no excuse for choosing a poorly representative species. Finally, our comprehension of the basic physicochemical and biological criteria, which determine the rate of drug passage across the skin, is becoming more sophisticated. We believe that in the foreseeable future it will be increasingly possible to define chemical structure/skin penetration relationships. Hence, we envisage the achievement of reliable predictions of TDD in vivo, from basic physical chemical and pharmacokinetic information.

ACKNOWLEDGMENTS

We acknowledge the advice of Drs. Howard I. Maibach and Ronald C. Wester. We thank Dr. J. M. Holland of the Upjohn Company, Kalamazoo, for Figure 4. Financial support was provided by National Institutes of Health grants GM-33395-02 and AG-04851, by a Special Emphasis Research Career Award to RHG from the National Institute of Occupational Safety and Health (K01-OH-00017-02) and by Vick International and Ciba-Geigy. Dr. Diana Villaflor provided invaluable assistance, and Andrea Mazel prepared a long manuscript with alacrity and care.

REFERENCES

1. S. K. Chandrasekaran, W. Bayne, and J. E. Shaw, Pharmacokinetics of drug permeation through human skin. *J. Pharm. Sci.*, 67: 1370–1374 (1978).

2. N. M. Price, L. G. Schmitt, J. McGuire, J. E. Shaw, and G. Trobough. Transdermal scopolamine in the treatment of motion sickness at sea. *Clin. Pharmacol. Ther.*, 29: 414–419 (1981).

3. S. K. Chandrasekaran, Controlled release of scopolamine for prophylaxis of motion sickness. *Drug. Dev. Ind. Pharm.*, 9: 627–646 (1983).

4. P. R. Imhof, T. Vuillemin, A. Gérardin, A. Racine, P. Müller, and F. Follath, Studies of the bioavailability of nitroglycerin from a transdermal therapeutic system (Nitroderm–TTS®). *Eur. J. Clin. Pharmacol.*, 27: 7–12 (1984).

5. P. Müller, P. R. Imhof, F. Burkart, L.-C. Chu, and A. Gérardin, Human pharmacological studies of a new transdermal system containing nitroglycerin. *Eur. Clin. Pharmacol.*, 22: 473–480 (1982).

6. P. R. Imhof, Anti-anginal therapy with transdermal nitroglycerin, in *Rate Control in Drug Therapy* (L. F. Prescott and W. S. Nimmo, eds.), Churchill-Livingstone, Edinburgh, 1985, pp. 201–214.

7. A. Karim, Transdermal absorption: A unique opportunity for constant delivery of nitroglycerin. *Drug. Dev. Ind. Pharm.*, *9*: 671-689 (1983).

8. A. Karim, Transdermal absorption of nitroglycerin from a microsealed drug delivery (MDD) system. *Angiology, 34*: 11-21 (1983).

9. W. R. Good, Transderm®-Nitro controlled delivery of nitroglycerin via the transdermal route. *Drug Dev. Ind. Pharm.*, *9*: 647-670 (1983).

10. M. Wolff, G. Cordes, and V. Luckow, In vitro and in vivo release of nitroglycerin from a new transdermal therapeutic system. *Pharm. Res.*, *2*: 23-29 (1985).

11. D. Arndts and K. Arndts, Pharmacokinetics and pharmacodynamics of transdermally administered clonidine. *Eur. J. Clin. Pharmacol.*, *26*: 79-85 (1984).

12. T. R. MacGregor, K. M. Matzek, J. J. Keirns, R. G. A. van Wayjen, A. van den Ende, and R. G. L. van Tol, Pharmacokinetics of transdermally delivered clonidine. *Clin. Pharmacol. Ther.*, *38*: 278-284 (1985).

13. A. A. H. Lawson, Clinical and pharmacological studies with transdermal clonidine, in *Rate Control in Drug Therapy* (L. F. Prescott and W. S. Nimmo, eds.), Churchill-Livingstone, Edinburgh, 1985, pp. 215-219.

14. L. R. Laufer, J. L. DeFazio, J. K. H. Lu, D. R. Meldrum, P. Eggena, M. P. Sambhi, J. M. Hershman, and H. L. Judd, Estrogen replacement therapy by transdermal estradiol administration. *Am. J. Obstet. Gynecol.*, *146*: 533-540 (1983).

15. L. B. Fisher, In vitro studies on the permeability of infant skin, in *Percutaneous Absorption* (R. L. Bronaugh and H. I. Maibach, eds.), Dekker, New York, 1983, pp. 213-222.

16. R. C. Wester and H. I. Maibach, Percutaneous absorption: Neonate compared to the adult, in *Environmental Factors in Human Growth and Development* (W. R. Hunt, M. K. Schmidt, and D. Worth, eds.), Cold Spring Harbor Press, Cold Spring Harbor, NY, 1982, pp. 3-15.

17. J. J. McCormack, E. K. Boisits, and L. B. Fisher, An in vitro comparison of the permeability of adult versus neonatal skin, in *Neonatal Skin: Structure and Function* (H. I. Maibach and E. K. Boisits, eds.), Dekker, New York, 1982, pp. 149-164.

18. V. A. Harpin and N. Rutter, Barrier properties of the newborn infant's skin. *J. Pediatr.*, *102*: 419-425 (1983).

19. D. R. Wilson and H. I. Maibach, An in vivo comparison of skin barrier functions, in *Neonatal Skin: Structure and Function* (H. I. Maibach and E. K. Boisits, eds.), Dekker, New York, 1982, pp. 101-110.

20. R. H. Guy and J. Hadgraft, Transdermal drug delivery: The ground rules are emerging. *Pharm. Int.*, *6*: 112–116 (1985).

21. J. E. Shaw and F. Theeuwes, Transdermal dosage forms, in *Rate Control in Drug Therapy* (L. F. Prescott and W. S. Nimmo, eds.), Churchill-Livingstone, Edinburgh, 1985, pp. 65–70.

22. P. K. Noonan and R. C. Wester, Cutaneous metabolism of xenobiotics, in *Percutaneous Absorption* (R. L. Bronaugh and H. I. Maibach, eds.), Dekker, New York, 1985, pp. 65–85.

23. D. A. W. Bucks, Skin structure and metabolism: Relevance to the design of cutaneous therapeutics. *Pharm. Res.*, *1*: 148–153 (1984).

24. P. K. Noonan and L. Z. Benet, Variable nitroglycerin metabolism to glyceryl-dinitrates as a function of the route of administration. *APhA, Acad. Pharmac. Sci.*, "*Abstracts,*" *14*(2): 251 (1984).

25. F. L. Brookes, W. B. Hugo, and S. P. Denyer, Transformation of betamethasone-17-valerate by skin microflora. *J. Pharm. Pharmacol.*, *34*: 61P (1982).

26. S. P. Denyer, W. B. Hugo, and M. O'Brien, Metabolism of glycerol trinitrate by skin staphylococci. *J. Pharm. Pharmacol.*, *36*: 61P (1984).

27. B. W. Barry, Optimizing percutaneous absorption, in *Percutaneous Absorption* (R. L. Bronaugh and H. I. Maibach, eds.), Dekker, New York, 1985, pp. 489–511.

28. E. R. Cooper, Vehicle effects on skin penetration, in *Percutaneous Absorption* (R. L. Bronaugh and H. I. Maibach, eds.), Dekker, New York, 1985, pp. 525–529.

29. C. L. Gummer, Vehicles as penetration enhancers, in *Percutaneous Absorption* (R. L. Bronaugh and H. I. Maibach, eds.), Dekker, New York, 1985, pp. 561–570.

30. C. Benezra, C. C. Sigman, L. R. Perry, C. T. Helmes, and H. I. Maibach, A systematic search for structure–activity relationships of skin contact sensitizers: Methodology. *J. Invest. Dermatol.*, *85*: 351–356 (1985).

31. R. C. Wester and H. I. Maibach, Animal models for percutaneous absorption, in *Models in Dermatology* (H. I. Maibach and N. J. Lowe, eds.), Vol. 2, Karger, Basel, 1985, pp. 159–169.

32. R. C. Wester and H. I. Maibach, In vivo animal models for percutaneous absorption, in *Percutaneous Absorption* (R. L. Bronaugh and H. I. Maibach, eds.), Dekker, New York, 1985, pp. 251–266.

33. K. E. Andersen, H. I. Maibach, and D. M. Anjo, The guinea pig: An animal model for human skin absorption of hydrocortisone, testosterone and benzoic acid. *Br. J. Dermatol.*, *102*: 447–453 (1980).

34. M. J. Bartek, J. A. La Budde, and H. I. Maibach, Skin permeability in vivo: Comparison in rat, rabbit, pig and man. *J. Invest. Dermatol.*, *58*: 114–123 (1972).

35. M. J. Bartek and J. A. La Budde, Percutaneous absorption in vitro, in *Animal Models in Dermatology* (H. I. Maibach, ed.), Churchill-Livingstone, New York, 1975, pp. 103–120.

36. R. L. Bronaugh, R. F. Stewart, and E. R. Congdon, Methods for in vitro percutaneous absorption studies. II. Animal models for human skin. *Toxicol. Appl. Pharmacol.*, *62*: 481–488 (1982).

37. N. Hunziker, R. J. Feldmann, and H. I. Maibach, Animal models of percutaneous absorption: Comparison in Mexican hairless dogs and man. *Dermatologica*, *156*: 79–88 (1978).

38. F. N. Marzulli, D. W. C. Brown, and H. I. Maibach, Techniques for studying skin penetration. *Toxicol. Appl. Pharmacol.*, *Suppl. 3*: 79–83 (1969).

39. A. H. McGreesh, Percutaneous toxicity. *Toxicol. Appl. Pharmacol.*, *Suppl. 2*: 20–26 (1969).

40. R. T. Tregear, *Physical Functions of Skin*, Academic Press, New York, 1966.

41. R. J. Feldmann and H. I. Maibach, Regional variation in percutaneous penetration of [^{14}C]cortisone in man. *J. Invest. Dermatol.*, *48*: 181–183 (1967).

42. R. J. Feldmann and H. I. Maibach, Percutaneous penetration of steroids in man. *J. Invest. Dermatol.*, *52*: 89–94 (1969).

43. R. J. Feldmann and H. I. Maibach, Absorption of some organic compounds through the skin in man. *J. Invest. Dermatol.*, *54*: 399–404 (1969).

44. H. I. Maibach and R. J. Feldmann, Effect of applied concentration on percutaneous absorption in man. *J. Invest. Dermatol.*, *52*: 381–386 (1969).

45. H. I. Maibach, R. J. Feldmann, T. H. Milby, and W. F. Serat, Regional variation in percutaneous penetration in man. *Arch. Environ. Health*, *23*: 208–211 (1971).

46. R. J. Feldmann and H. I. Maibach, Percutaneous penetration of some pesticides and herbicides in man. *Toxicol. Appl. Pharmacol.*, *28*: 120–132 (1974).

47. P. Campbell, T. Watanabe, and S. K. Chandrasekaran, Comparison of in vitro skin permeability of scopolamine in rat, rabbit and man. *Fed. Proc. (Fed. Am. Soc. Exp. Biol.)*, *35*: 639 (1976).

48. M. Walker, P. H. Dugard, and R. C. Scott, In vitro percutaneous absorption studies: A comparison of human and laboratory species. *Hum. Toxicol.*, *2*: 561 (1983).

49. R. C. Wester and H. I. Maibach, Percutaneous absorption in the rhesus monkey compared to man. *Toxicol. Appl. Pharmacol.*, *32*: 394–398 (1975).

50. R. C. Wester and H. I. Maibach, Rhesus monkey as an animal model for percutaneous absorption, in *Animal Models in Dermatology* (H. I. Maibach, ed.), Churchill-Livingstone, New York, 1975, pp. 133-137.

51. R. C. Wester and H. I. Maibach, Relationship of topical dose and percutaneous absorption in rhesus monkey and man. *J. Invest. Dermatol.*, *67*: 518-520 (1976).

52. R. C. Wester and H. I. Maibach, Percutaneous absorption in man and animal: A perspective, in *Cutaneous Toxicity* (V. Drill and P. Lazar, eds.), Academic Press, New York, 1977, pp. 111-126.

53. R. C. Wester and P. K. Noonan, Topical bioavailability of a potential antiacne agent (SC-23110) as determined by cumulative excretion and areas under plasma concentration-time curves. *J. Invest. Dermatol.*, *70*: 92-94 (1978).

54. R. C. Wester and P. K. Noonan, Relevance of animal models for percutaneous absorption. *Int. J. Pharm.*, *7*: 99-110 (1980).

55. R. C. Wester, P. K. Noonan, M. P. Cole, and H. I. Maibach, Percutaneous absorption of testosterone in the newborn rhesus monkey: Comparison to the adult. *Pediatr. Res.*, *11*: 737-739 (1977).

56. R. C. Wester, P. K. Noonan, and H. I. Maibach, Frequency of application on percutaneous absorption of hydrocortisone. *Arch. Dermatol.*, *113*: 620-622 (1977).

57. R. C. Wester, P. K. Noonan, and H. I. Maibach, Recent advances in percutaneous absorption using the rhesus monkey model. *J. Soc. Cosmet. Chem.*, *30*: 297-307 (1979).

58. R. C. Wester, P. K. Noonan, and H. I. Maibach, Variations in percutaneous absorption of testosterone in the rhesus monkey due to anatomic site of application and frequency of application. *Arch. Dermatol. Res.*, *267*: 229-235 (1980).

59. R. C. Wester, P. K. Noonan, and H. I. Maibach, Percutaneous absorption of hydrocortisone increases with long-term administration: In vivo studies in the rhesus monkey. *Arch. Dermatol.*, *116*: 186-188 (1980).

60. R. C. Wester and H. I. Maibach, Cutaneous pharmacokinetics: 10 steps to percutaneous absorption. *Drug Metab. Rev.*, *14*: 169-205 (1983).

61. R. L. Bronaugh and H. I. Maibach, Percutaneous absorption of nitroaromatic compounds: In vivo and in vitro studies in the human and monkey. *J. Invest. Dermatol.*, *84*: 180-183 (1985).

62. H. I. Maibach and L. J. Wolfram, Percutaneous penetration of hair dyes. *J. Soc. Cosmet. Chem.*, *32*: 223-229 (1981).

63. L. J. Wolfram, Hair dye penetration in monkey and man, in *Percutaneous Absorption* (R. L. Bronaugh and H. I. Maibach, eds.), Dekker, New York, 1985, pp. 409–422.

64. W. G. Reifenrath, E. M. Chellquist, E. A. Shipwash, and W. W. Jederberg, Evaluation of animal models for predicting skin penetration in man. *Fund. Appl. Toxicol.*, *4*: S224–S230 (1984).

65. W. G. Reifenrath, E. M. Chellquist, E. A. Shipwash, W. W. Jederberg, and G. G. Krueger, Percutaneous penetration in the hairless dog, weanling pig, and grafted athymic nude mouse: Evaluation of models for predicting skin penetration in man. *Br. J. Dermatol.*, *111* (Suppl. 27): 123–135 (1984).

66. A. M. Kligman, A biological brief on percutaneous absorption. *Drug Dev. Ind. Pharm.*, *9*: 521–560 (1983).

67. R. H. Guy, A. H. Guy, H. I. Maibach, and V. P. Shah, The bioavailability of dermatological and other topically administered drugs. *Pharm. Res.*, *3* (1986).

68. A. Rougier, D. Dupuis, C. Lotte, R. Roguet, and H. Schaefer, In vivo correlation between stratum corneum reservoir function and percutaneous absorption. *J. Invest. Dermatol.*, *81*: 275–278 (1983).

69. D. Dupuis, A. Rougier, R. Roguet, C. Lotte, and G. Kalopissis, In vivo relationship between horny layer reservoir effect and percutaneous absorption in human and rat. *J. Invest. Dermatol.*, *82*: 353–356 (1984).

70. A. Rougier, D. Dupuis, C. Lotte, and R. Roguet, The measurement of the stratum corneum reservoir. A predictive method for in vivo percutaneous absorption studies: Influence of application time. *J. Invest. Dermatol.*, *84*: 66–68 (1985).

71. R. C. Wester, H. I. Maibach, D. A. W. Bucks, and R. H. Guy, Malathion percutaneous absorption after repeated administration to man. *Toxicol. Appl. Pharmacol.*, *68*: 116–119 (1983).

72. B. A. Gilchrest, *Skin and Aging Processes*, CRC Press, Boca Raton, FL, 1984.

73. E. Christophers and A. M. Kligman, Percutaneous absorption in aged skin, in *Advances in Biology of Skin*, Vol. VI, *Aging* (W. Montagna, ed.), Pergamon Press, New York, 1964, pp. 163–175.

74. H. Tagami, Functional characteristics of aged skin. *Acta Dermatol. (Kyoto)*, *66*: 19–21 (1971).

75. A. M. Kligman, Perspectives and problems in cutaneous gerontology. *J. Invest. Dermatol.*, *73*: 39–46 (1979).

76. R. R. Kohn, Age variation in rat skin permeability. *Proc. Soc. Exp. Biol. Med.*, *131*: 521–522 (1969).

77. R. H. Guy, E. Tur, S. Bjerke, and H. I. Maibach, Are there age and racial differences to methyl nicotinate-induced vasodilatation in human skin? *J. Am. Acad. Dermatol.*, *12*: 1001–1006 (1985).

78. K. V. Roskos, R. H. Guy, and H. I. Maibach, Percutaneous absorption in the aged, in *Dermatologic Clinics, Skin Aging* (B. A. Gilchrest, ed.), Saunders, Philadelphia, Vol. 4, (1986).

79. S. E. Friberg, D. W. Osborne, and T. L. Tombridge, X-Ray diffraction study of human stratum corneum. *J. Soc. Cosmet. Chem.*

80. S. E. Friberg and D. W. Osborne, Interaction of a model skin surface lipid with a glyceridacid. *J. Am. Oil. Chem. Soc.*

81. S. E. Friberg and D. W. Osborne, Small angle X-ray diffraction patterns of stratum corneum and a model structure for its lipids. *J. Dispersion Sci. Technol.*

82. M. Gibaldi and D. Perrier, *Pharmacokinetics*, 2nd ed., Dekker, New York, 1982.

83. B. W. Barry, *Dermatological Formulations: Percutaneous Absorption*, Dekker, New York, 1983.

84. H. Schaefer, A. Zesch, and G. Stüttgen, *Skin Permeability*, Springer Verlag, Berlin, 1982.

85. W. J. Albery and J. Hadgraft, Percutaneous absorption: Theoretical description. *J. Pharm. Pharmacol.*, *31*: 129–139 (1979).

86. W. J. Albery and J. Hadgraft, Percutaneous absorption: In vivo experiments. *J. Pharm. Pharmacol.*, *31*: 140–147 (1979).

87. J. Hadgraft, The epidermal reservoir: A theoretical approach. *Int. J. Pharm.*, *2*: 177–194 (1979).

88. J. Hadgraft, Theoretical aspects of metabolism in the epidermis. *Int. J. Pharm.*, *4*: 229–239 (1980).

89. R. H. Guy and J. Hadgraft, A theoretical description relating skin penetration to the thickness of the applied medicament. *Int. J. Pharm.*, *6*: 321–332 (1980).

90. R. H. Guy and J. Hadgraft, Percutaneous absorption with saturable metabolism. *Int. J. Pharm.*, *11*: 187–197 (1982).

91. R. H. Guy and J. Hadgraft, Physicochemical interpretation of the pharmacokinetics of percutaneous absorption. *J. Pharmacokinet. Biopharm.*, *11*: 189–203 (1983).

92. W. J. Albery, R. H. Guy, and J. Hadgraft, Percutaneous absorption: Transport in the dermis. *Int. J. Pharm.*, *15*: 125–148 (1983).

93. R. H. Guy, J. Hadgraft, and H. I. Maibach, A pharmacokinetic model for percutaneous absorption. *Int. J. Pharm.*, *11*: 119–129 (1982).

94. R. H. Guy, J. Hadgraft, and H. I. Maibach, Percutaneous absorption: Multidose pharmacokinetics. *Int. J. Pharm.*, *17*: 23–28 (1983).

95. R. H. Guy and J. Hadgraft, Percutaneous absorption kinetics of topically applied agents liable to surface loss. *J. Soc. Cosmet. Chem.*, *35*: 103–113 (1984).

96. R. H. Guy and J. Hadgraft, Prediction of drug disposition kinetics in skin and plasma following topical administration. *J. Pharm. Sci.*, *73*: 883–887 (1984).

97. R. H. Guy, J. Hadgraft, and H. I. Maibach, Percutaneous absorption in man: A kinetic approach. *Toxicol. Appl. Pharmacol.*, *78*: 123–129 (1985).

98. R. H. Guy and J. Hadgraft, The prediction of plasma levels of drugs following transdermal application. *J. Control. Rel.*, *1*: 177–182 (1985).

99. R. H. Guy and J. Hadgraft, Transdermal drug delivery: A simplified pharmacokinetic approach. *Int. J. Pharm.*, *24*: 267–274 (1985).

100. N. Evans, R. H. Guy, J. Hadgraft, G. D. Parr, and N. Rutter, Transdermal drug delivery to neonates. *Int. J. Pharm.*, *24*: 259–265 (1985).

101. R. H. Guy and J. Hadgraft, Pharmacokinetic interpretation of the plasma levels of clonidine following transdermal delivery. *J. Pharm. Sci.*, *74*: 1016–1018 (1985).

102. R. H. Guy and J. Hadgraft, Kinetic analysis of transdermal nitroglycerin delivery. *Pharm. Res.*, *2*: 206–211 (1985).

103. C. Hansch and A. J. Leo, *Substituent Constants for Correlation Analysis in Chemistry and Biology*, Wiley-Interscience, New York, 1979.

104. L. Schenkel, J. Balestra, L. Schmitt, and J. Shaw, Transdermal estrogen substitution in the menopause, in *Rate Control in Drug Therapy* (L. F. Prescott and W. S. Nimmo, eds.), Churchill-Livingstone, Edinburgh, 1985, pp. 294–303.

105. C. Muir and R. Metcalfe, A comparison of plasma levels of hyoscine after oral and transdermal administration. *J. Pharm. Biomed. Anal.*, *1*: 363–367 (1983).

106. P. H. Vlasses, L. G. T. Ribeiro, H. H. Rotmensch, J. V. Bondi, A. E. Loper, M. Hichens, M. C. Dunlay, and R. K. Ferguson, Initial evaluation of transdermal timolol: Serum concentrations and β-blockade. *J. Cardiovasc. Pharmacol.*, *7*: 245–250 (1985).

107. R. H. Guy and J. Hadgraft, Interpretation and prediction of the kinetics of transdermal drug delivery: Hyoscine, oestradiol and timolol. *Int. J. Pharm.* (1986).

108. R. H. Guy and J. Hadgraft, Pharmacokinetics of percutaneous absorption with concurrent metabolism. *Int. J. Pharm.*, *20*: 43–51 (1984).

109. S. P. Denyer, R. H. Guy, J. Hadgraft, and W. B. Hugo, The microbial degradation of topically applied drugs. *Int. J. Pharm.*, *26*: 89–97 (1985).

110. R. C. Wester, P. K. Noonan, S. Smeach, and L. Kosobud, Pharmacokinetics and bioavailability of intravenous and topical nitroglycerin in the rhesus monkey. Estimate of percutaneous first-pass metabolism. *J. Pharm. Sci.*, *72*: 745–748 (1983).
111. R. H. Guy and J. Hadgraft, The effect of penetration enhancers on the kinetics of percutaneous absorption. *J. Control. Rel.*, in press (1987).

CLINICAL ASSESSMENTS OF TRANSDERMAL THERAPEUTIC SYSTEMS

9

Transdermal Delivery of Nitroglycerin I

NATHANIEL REICHEK / *Hospital of the University of Pennsylvania, Philadelphia, Pennsylvania*

I. INTRODUCTION

Chronic angina pectoris, characterized by chest discomfort with physical exertion or emotional stress, is by far the most common chronic, recurrent symptom of coronary artery disease. Consequently, a large number of pharmacological and mechanical treatments for this disorder have been developed, including organic nitrates, calcium channel blockers, beta blockers, coronary bypass surgery, and coronary angioplasty. Of these therapeutic modalities, the nitrates are by far the oldest, the most widely used, and perhaps, the most commonly misunderstood.

While the nitrates have been used for treatment of angina for more than 100 years (1), many important aspects of their mechanism of action, pharmacokinetics, and pharmacodynamics remain incompletely understood. Furthermore, recent developments in clinical research in the field have challenged long-held practices and beliefs. Thus, despite the antiquity of the nitrates as a therapeutic class, it would be fair to say that, at this writing, the field is in turmoil. Much of the controversy and many of the important lessons currently being learned have been precipitated by the development and widespread clinical use of nitroglycerin-releasing transdermal devices. These devices, introduced to the marketplace only a few years ago, now account for more than $130 million in annual sales and roughly one-third million patient years of treatment per year in the United States alone. Despite this, fundamental questions have been raised about the efficacy of these devices and, indeed, the assumptions about nitroglycerin pharmacology on which their design has been based. In this chapter, we will review the history of transdermal delivery of nitroglycerin, problems in the assessment of antianginal effects of nitrates, and the current state of information on nitroglycerin ointment and nitroglycerin patches. We will also consider the studies presently in progress, as well as potential new developments that may further modify our approach to nitrates as a class.

II. HISTORY OF TRANSDERMAL NITROGLYCERIN

Cutaneous absorption of nitroglycerin was first reported by Albers in 1864, but was not used therapeutically (2). By the end of the century, nitroglycerin had become an essential commodity for mining and for war. Because of the extreme explosive hazard it engendered, work with nitroglycerin was virtually all manual, by small groups of workers dispersed in small wooden structures (3). Workers in these facilities soon learned that initiation into the environment was accompanied by severe headaches, which waned over a few days. However, if a worker was absent from the environment for a day or two, recrudescence of severe headaches was associated with reintroduction into the plant. Workers rapidly learned that tolerance to nitroglycerin-induced headache could be sustained by application of small amounts of nitroglycerin to clothes or a hatband. Thus, the phenomenon of transdermal absorption of nitroglycerin was discovered. Furthermore, sufficient absorption could produce not only tolerance to nitrate headache, but a syndrome of apparent dependence, characterized by cardiac ischemia, infarction, or death during periods of withdrawal (3). Angiographic documentation of this phenomenon was finally obtained in the 1970s (4).

Interest in the therapeutic applications of transdermal nitroglycerin did not begin until the 1940s. Initial trials for the treatment of intermittent claudication, due to peripheral vascular disease, with topical application of nitroglycerin to the affected extremity proved unrewarding. Yet, it was serendipitously discovered that patients with both claudication and angina pectoris experienced subjective improvement in exertional angina if treated with a 2% nitroglycerin ointment (5). A brief period of enthusiasm for the preparation ensued. However, during the 1960s, skepticism about the efficacy of all long-acting nitrates mounted and nitroglycerin ointment fell into disuse.

As part of a series of studies on the antianginal effects of nitroglycerin and its congeners, the first controlled, randomized, blinded study of nitroglycerin ointment against placebo was performed in

1971-1972 at the then National Heart Institute and published in 1974 (6). Surprisingly, striking effects were observed, which were confirmed by other groups and led to a rapid and widespread recrudescence of clinical use of nitroglycerin ointment. Since, at the time, no other "long-acting" nitrate had been shown to have similarly demonstrable antianginal effects, mainly because of improper study designs, interest in nitroglycerin ointment was at a peak in the mid-1970s.

Not surprisingly, the messiness, inconvenience, and imprecision in the application of ointment formulation promptly led a number of pharmaceutical companies to seek the development of better methods for transdermal administration of nitroglycerin that would be tidy, convenient, accurate, and hopefully, longer lasting. Transdermal nitroglycerin delivery devices were thus developed. When regulatory approval was sought in the United States, nitroglycerin patches were treated as new formulations of an old medication, nitroglycerin ointment. Since the efficacy of nitroglycerin ointment was not under challenge, regulatory approval of nitroglycerin patches for marketing evidently was based largely on bioavailability data, principally the blood nitroglycerin levels, which were shown to be comparable to those resulting from the topical application of 0.5 in. of 2% nitroglycerin ointment (roughly 6.25 mg) for 6 hr (7). Since such plasma levels were sustained for at least 24 hr, the claim on once-a-day medication was viewed as acceptable.

Unfortunately, there was reason to suspect that such bioavailability data would not be sufficient to assure efficacy. First, as will be discussed further below, there were no data to demonstrate that the selected reference standard (0.5 in. of 2% nitroglycerin ointment at 6 hr) was clinically effective. Second, measurement of nitroglycerin in plasma is a difficult assay, mainly because of the short biological half-life of nitroglycerin ($t_{1/2} < 5$ min) and the very low concentrations that must be detected (8). Third, the relationship between plasma nitroglycerin levels and antianginal effects has not been well characterized. Finally, whereas plasma nitroglycerin levels following sublingual administration are as high as 3 ng/ml, the plasma levels produced by the patches and their reference standard were only on the order of 0.5 ng/ml (7). When appropriately designed, blinded, controlled, clinical efficacy trials from experienced investigators began to report disappointing results, it became clear that our understanding of the clinical pharmacology of nitroglycerin was less satisfactory than many had supposed.

III. PROBLEMS IN ASSESSMENT OF LONG-ACTING NITRATES FOR ANGINA PROPHYLAXIS

Before considering existing data with respect to the clinical efficacy of transdermal nitroglycerin, it is essential to review the complexities that beset such studies. First, the dose-response relationship for nitrates varies widely among individuals (9). Thus, one cannot assume that a given dose administered or a given plasma concentration achieved will have a predictable biological effect. Second, in a given individual, there may not be a constant dose-response relationship over time (10). Third, nitroglycerin has multiple biological effects in a given individual, which could have a different time courses and dose-response relationships. Thus, in patients with angina, a single dose of nitroglycerin could also produce systemic venodilation, systemic arterial dilation, coronary vasodilation, lowering of blood pressure, lowering of ventricular filling pressures, and/or improvement of exercise tolerance. However, one cannot predict any one response simply based on information from another.

As a result of all the factors discussed above, it is essential to evaluate nitrates by using a relevant bioassay, namely occurrence of angina in the patients with coronary artery disease. This might be achieved by a simple diary count of angina prevalence on treatment with active drug versus placebo in a crossover design.

Unfortunately, diary studies have, in general, proved to be relatively unreliable. Therefore, studies based on provocative testing, using treadmill or bicycle exercise, have become the accepted standard. Variables that can be measured include exercise time to the onset of angina, exercise time to the onset of the level of angina at which the patient customarily stops exercise voluntarily (often termed "moderately severe angina"), heart rate and blood pressure responses to each level of exercise, the product of heart rate and systolic pressure (so-called double product, a useful indirect index of myocardial oxygen demand), and electrocardiographic ST-segment changes during exercise. Designs may include either active/placebo crossover studies or parallel active- and placebo-treated groups. The crossover design has greater statistical power for a given number of subjects, provided no effects resulted from either treatment sequence or training are observed.

The dose-response problem can be addressed in a variety of ways. A particularly convenient one is to pretitrate each subject to doses that have matched physiological effects (e.g., blood pressure reduction or heart rate increase) in each subject (11). Alternatively, maximal tolerated doses may be administered to each patient. More rigorously, one may evaluate each of a series of doses in all subjects in a multiple crossover design or treat parallel groups with a range of doses and placebo. To date, all widely accepted studies on the antianginal effects of nitrates follow one of these designs in either a single-dose acute study or a multiple-dose chronic study. Despite the subjective nature of the principal endpoint, anginal chest pain, a high degree of reproducibility can be achieved (Fig. 1) (12), particularly if a placebo lead-in pretreatment is performed prior to

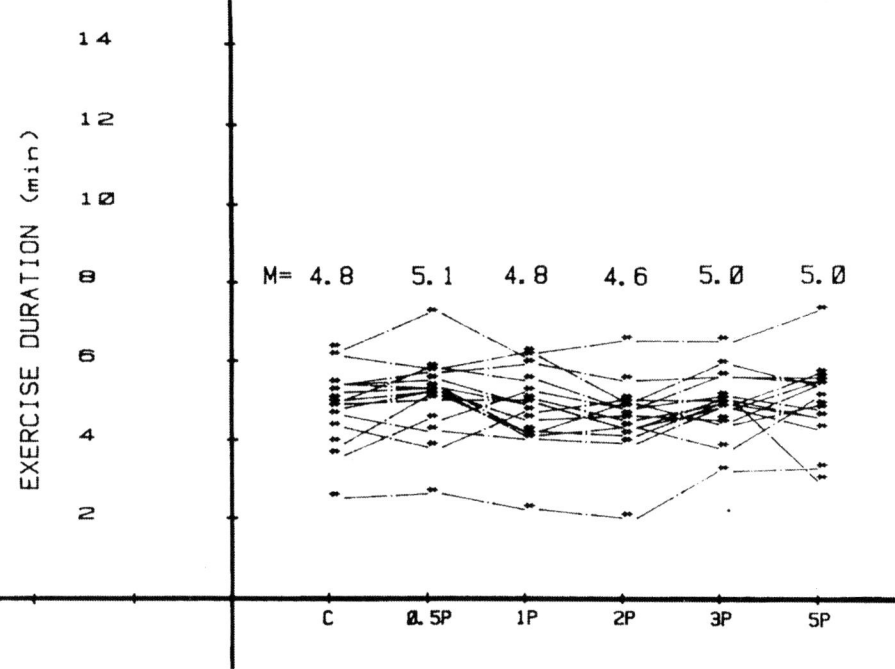

Figure 1 Exercise duration in anginal patients before (C) and after treatment with placebo formulation (P) for 0.5–5 hours. No placebo effect was evident. Exercise duration varied somewhat in each patient from one time period to another, but all the mean values were very similar. (From Ref. 12. Reprinted with permission from N. Reichek and *European Journal of Clinical Pharmacology*.)

the beginning of study to wash out the placebo effect. Performance of such studies is complex, time-consuming, costly, and often limited by the availability of suitable patients. Nonetheless, no reasonable alternative exists at present.

IV. ANTIANGINAL EFFECT OF NITROGLYCERIN OINTMENT

Antianginal effect of 2% nitroglycerin ointment was first described clinically by Davis and co-workers in 1954 (5). However, the first controlled trial was not published until 1974 (6). This study was based on the methods developed by Goldstein and associates (11)

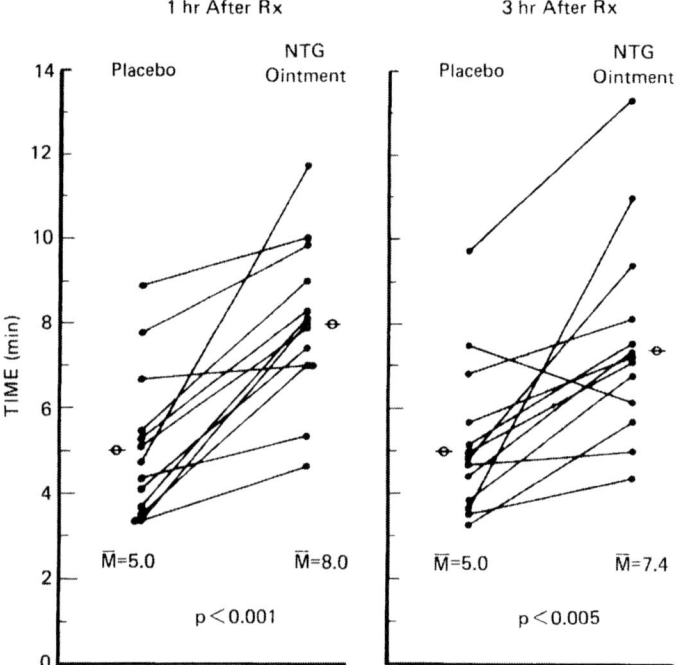

Figure 2   Comparison of the duration of exercise before the onset of angina (vertical axis) between treatment with placebo (left of each panel) and with nitroglycerin ointment (right of each panel). Data points from the same patient are connected. Mean values (the circled bars and the number beneath each column) demonstrate that a significant increase in exercise capacity is present 1 hr after nitroglycerin ointment (left panel), which persists essentially undiminished 2 hr later (right panel). (From Ref. 6. Reprinted with permission from N. Reichek and the American Heart Association.)

and Redwood et al. (13), using a randomized, blinded crossover design, comparing active drug to placebo at serial intervals after acute administration.   Provocative testing was performed using individualized bicycle ergometer progressive exercise tests, with 20-W increments every 3 min.   Each study was so designed that, in the absence of any test antianginal agent, angina occurred within 3–6 min of exercise.   Furthermore, nitroglycerin ointment doses were pretitrated to produce a fall in systolic blood pressure of at least 10 mmHg or a pulse increase of at least 10 beats per minute in each subject.   The ointment used contained an estimated 12.5 mg of nitroglycerin per inch, and the mean applied dose was 5 mg (or, 0.4 in.) (6). This dose was observed to produce a significant increase in exercise tolerance (Fig. 2) at 1 and 3 hr after administration as compared to placebo medication. No difference in effects was observed at the two time points tested. Furthermore, the increase in the duration of exercise time was noted to be similar to that produced by sublingually administered nitroglycerin in each subject.

A small number of patients were studied again after 3-month administration of nitroglycerin ointment at the intervals of every 6 hr. A dose of placebo was substituted in this group of patients for a dose of active nitroglycerin ointment in each subject and the results were then compared to those continuously administered with a routine dose. Again, the active ointment was found to be associated with greater exercise tolerance than the placebo and no significant reduction in the effects was noted as compared to the results obtained from the acute studies (Fig. 2). The study was performed using an application area of 225 cm^2 with an occlusive dressing. Subsequent studies of acute treatment confirmed these results (14, 15). A recent study further demonstrated that with larger doses (2 in. or 25 mg), the increase in the exercise tolerance can persist for up to 8 hr following the acute medication (16). However, no adequate body of data has been generated to this day on the effects of nitroglycerin ointment after chronic administration.

The lack of such data is of considerable importance, since a number of studies have suggested that chronic administration of oral isosorbide dinitrate to achieve a continuous high blood level of nitrate results in a dramatic attenuation of the antianginal effect (17). There is no reason to assume that cutaneous nitroglycerin will behave differently. Recent preliminary reports further suggest that the attenuation of antianginal effects of oral nitrates can be avoided by providing a prolonged daily nitrate-free period, during which plasma levels are dramatically diminished (18).

V. ANTIANGINAL EFFECT OF NITROGLYCERIN PATCHES

Initial encouraging results on the clinical efficacy of nitroglycerin patches, which were originally reported abroad (19), coupled with the plasma concentration data that had led to regulatory approval for marketing of the patches in United States have generated considerable enthusiasm for the new preparations. Unfortunately, subsequent studies by investigators in both North America and the United Kingdom were quite discouraging (20-23).

Our own laboratory set out to apply the same methods that had been used to demonstrate the acute efficacy of nitroglycerin ointment (20). Using the study design described above, we determined that

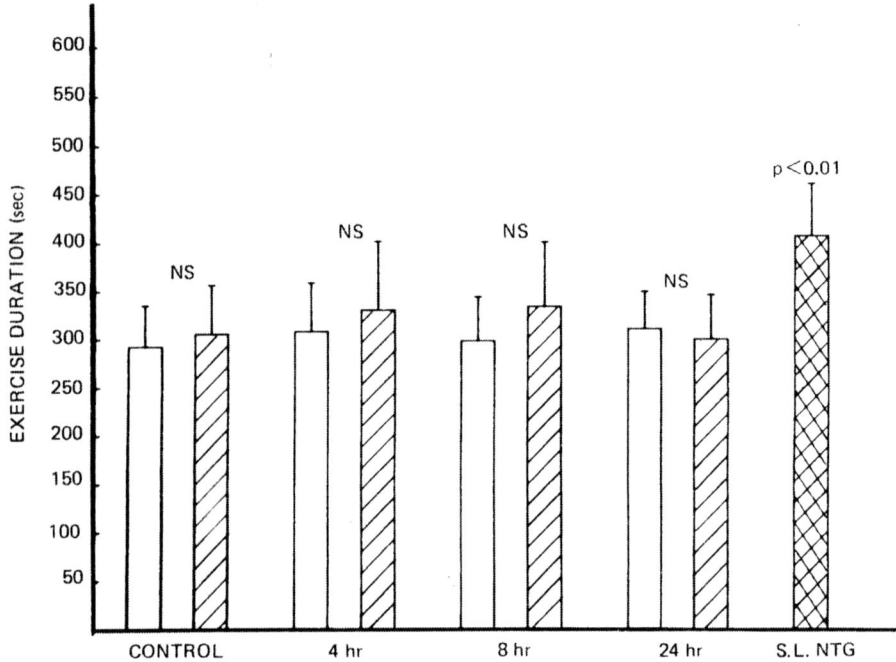

Figure 3   The duration of exercise to the onset of angina measured before (as the control) and at 4, 8, and 24 hr after the application of either placebo patches (clear bars) or nitroglycerin-releasing patches (cross-hatched bars). Sublingual nitroglycerin (SL.NTG) was also administered, as a positive control, to the same group of patients. Cross bars indicate standard deviations. There is a trend to increase the length of exercise time at 4 and 8 hr after administration but not at 24 hr. This trend was not statistically significant. On the other hand, sublingual nitroglycerin produced a highly significant increase. (From Ref. 20. Reprinted with permission from N. Reichek and *The American Journal of Cardiology*.)

the mean dose required to produce a detectable alteration in blood
pressure or heart rate was 1.9 of the "5-mg" patches. However,
it rapidly became apparent, in the first studies with six patients,
that no demonstrable effects on exercise tolerance could be detected (Fig. 3). These results were particularly striking because
all other nitrates, including the sublingual and oral isosorbide dinitrate, nitroglycerin ointment, and buccal nitroglycerin tablet studied
in identical fashion produced effects that were comparable to those
of sublingual nitroglycerin, suing comparably selected doses (24).
The reason for the dissociation between the hemodynamic effects at

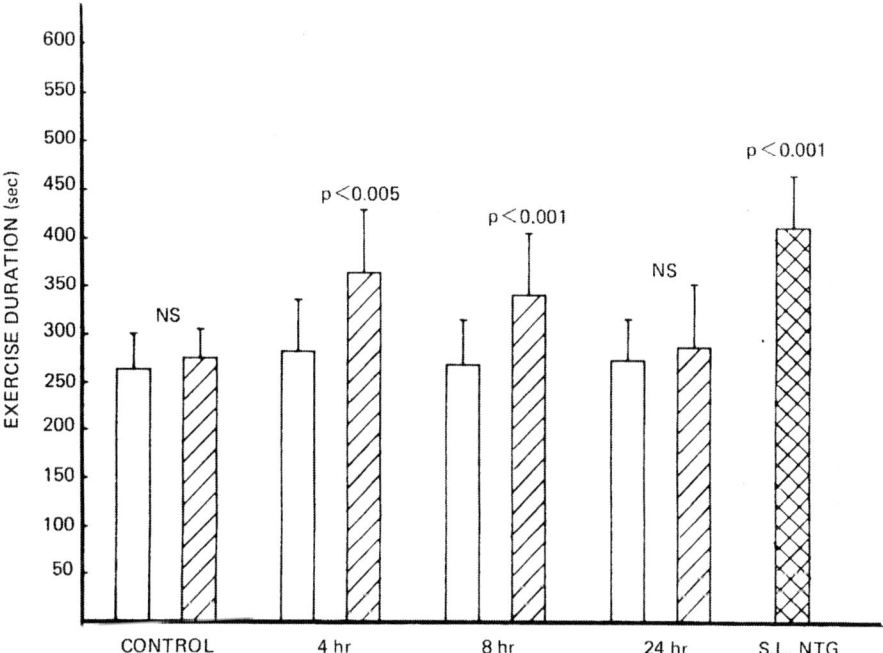

Figure 4   The duration of exercise to the onset of angina measured
before and at 4, 8, and 24 hr after the application of placebo patches
or the maximal dose of nitroglycerin-releasing patches. Sublingual
nitroglycerin was also evaluated as a positive control. A significant
increase in exercise duration was observed with nitroglycerin patches
at 4 and 8 hr. At 24 hr, however, exercise duration was similar to
that with placebo patches. Sublingual nitroglycerin was noted to
produce a more substantial increase in exercise time than the active
patches. (From Ref. 20. Reprinted with permission from N. Reichek
and *The American Journal of Cardiology.*)

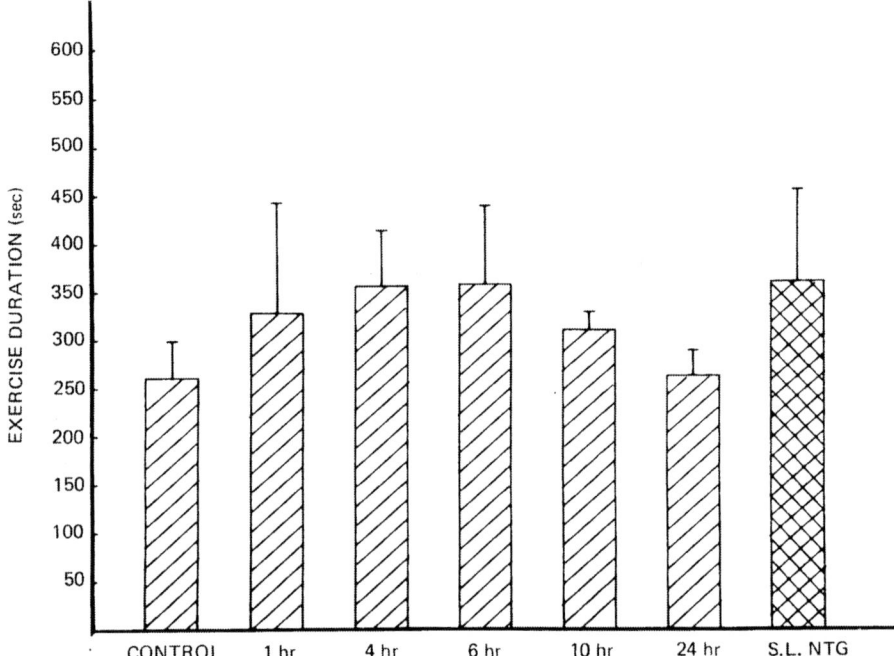

Figure 5   The duration of exercise to the onset of angina measured before and at 1, 4, 6, 10, and 24 hr after the application of the maximal dose of a second type of nitroglycerin patch. Sublingual nitroglycerin was also evaluated as a positve control. The results indicated a significant increase in the exercise duration at 1, 4, 6, and 10 hr after administration, but not at 24 hr. (From Ref. 20. Reprinted with permission from N. Reichek and *The American Journal of Cardiology*.)

rest and the antianginal effects during exercise remained obscure. Subsequent studies by a number of other groups also confirmed the lack of antianginal effects for the low-dose nitroglycerin patches (22,23).

To determine whether antianginal effects could be achieved and sustained using nitroglycerin patches with a larger dose, we performed another study using the maximal patch dose tolerated during acute titration. The maximal tolerated dose was defined as the dose that produced either a systolic blood pressure of 90 mmHg in normotensive subjects, a systolic pressure of 110 mmHg in hypertensive subjects, or a dose just smaller than the dose that produced symptomatic orthostatic hypotension. In eight subjects, the dose required was found to be that which released 25 mg of

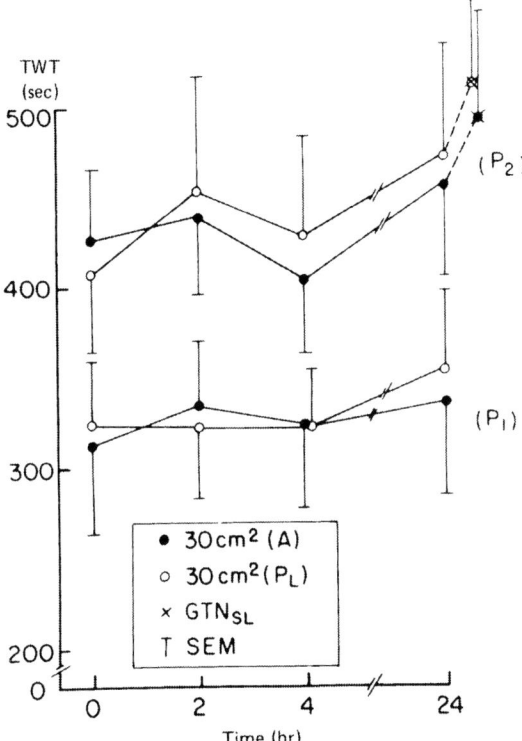

Figure 6 Treadmill walking time (TWT) required to trigger the development of angina (P_1) and of moderate angina (P_2) measured before (0) and at 2, 4, and 24 hr after the application of 30 cm^2 of active (A) and placebo (P_L) nitroglycerin (GTN) patches during sustained therapy. There was no difference in the duration of TWT between active and placebo therapy. On the other hand, sublingual (SL) nitroglycerin was observed to produce a significant prolongation of TWT to P_2 in the same group of anginal patients. (From Ref. 21. Reprinted with permission from *The American Journal of Cardiology* and the authors.)

nitroglycerin in 24 hr or 5 units of the $10\text{-}cm^2$ patches. This dose produced a significant increase in the exercise tolerance at both 4 and 8 hr after administration, but not at 24 hr (Fig. 4).

Analogous studies with another type of nitroglycerin-releasing patch produced similar results: no increase in exercise tolerance at 24 hr (Fig. 5). These results on acute first-dose testing were subsequently confirmed by Parker and Fung (21). The same investigators further demonstrated that after 2 weeks of continuous administration, there was no difference in exercise tolerance between active nitroglycerin patches and placebo (Fig. 6).

In summary, existing evidence indicates that "low-dose" nitroglycerin patches, which deliver nitroglycerin at roughly double the daily dose most commonly prescribed clinically, are completely ineffective for the prophylaxis of exertional angina. On the other hand, the maximal acutely tolerated doses can produce an effective antianginal effect, which lasts for 4–10 hr but disappears completely within 24 hr. Furthermore, available data suggest that chronic administration of "high-dose" nitroglycerin patches becomes essentially ineffective within 2 weeks.

VI. ATTENUATION OF ANTIANGINAL EFFECTS OF OTHER NITRATES

Other types of antianginal medication, including other nitrates, have not been evaluated as extensively as nitroglycerin patches with respect to their efficacy after 24-hr continuous administration. This is hardly surprising in that no other nitrate has sought to claim continuous 24-hr efficacy from a single dose. Nonetheless, the available evidence suggests that attenuation of antianginal effects within 24 hr is a property of all continuously administered "high-dose" nitrates, as is a marked attenuation of the antianginal effects during a chronic administration.

With respect to oral nitrates, no 24-hr studies have been published. However, Thadani and co-workers demonstrated that during the acute administration of oral isosorbide dinitrate in doses ranging from 15 to 120 mg, a clear dose–response curve was demonstrated, with the higher doses producing a larger, more sustained increase in the exercise tolerance (17). In contrast, the dose–response curve was found to be washed out after 2 weeks of continuous administration, and all isosorbide dinitrate doses yielded an antianginal effect with magnitude and duration comparable to those produced by a 15-mg dose (Fig. 7).

Preliminary studies indicate that when maximal tolerated doses of nitroglycerin patches and buccal nitroglycerin tablets are administered for 24 hr, attenuation of the antianginal effects occurs

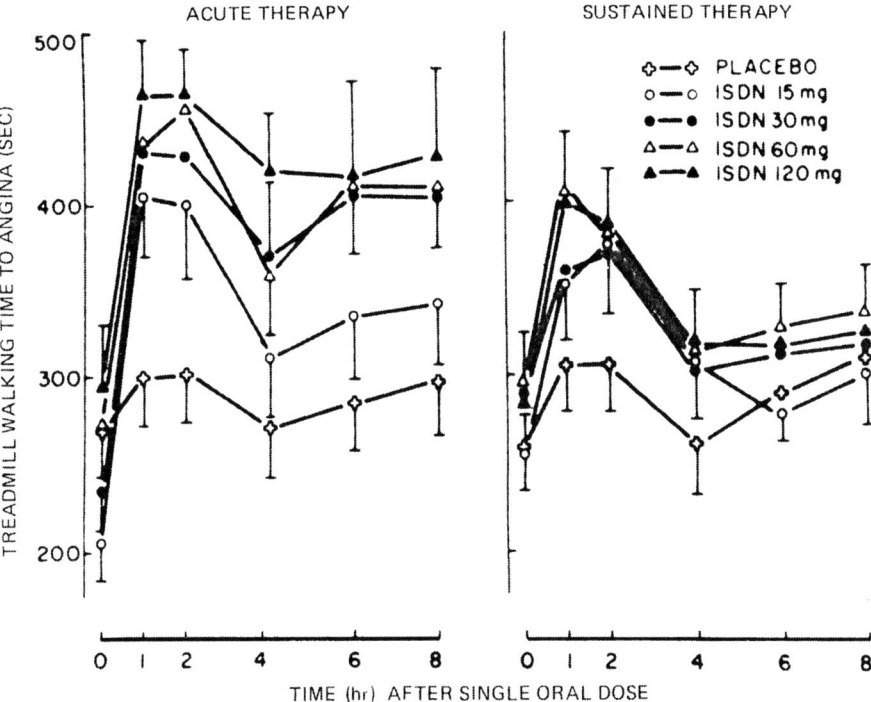

Figure 7 The dose–response relationship for treadmill walking time (TWT) after various doses of oral isosorbide dinitrate (ISDN) during acute (short-term) therapy (left panel) and after chronic (long-term) treatment (right panel). Little change was seen for the 15-mg dose; but for higher dose levels (30–210 mg), the magnitude and the duration of TWT were markedly reduced. (From Ref. 17. Reprinted with permission from the American Heart Association and the authors.)

with both preparations; even though the attenuation is more marked and occurs earlier with the patches (25,26). Recent preliminary data with intravenous nitroglycerin (10) also indicated that infusion of maximal tolerated doses also results in a marked attenuation of the antianginal effects at 24 hr (Table 1).

Thus, it can be concluded that attenuation of the antianginal effects is a common property of all high-dose continuously administered nitrates. Conversely, recent preliminary reports suggest that with oral nitrates, provision of a daily nitrate-free interval or even a low-plasma-level period, which lasts 12–14 hr, can effectively eliminate the attenuation phenomenon (18).

Table 1   Mean Exercise Duration After Intravenous Nitroglycerin[a]

	Mean exercise duration (sec)				
	C	1 hr	4 hr	8 hr	24 hr	SL[b]
IV NTG	278	449*	409*	381**	325	384
Placebo	268	286	257	253	282	426*

[a]Mean exercise duration in six subjects measured before (C) and at 1, 4, 8, and 24 hr after intravenous (IV) administration of maximal tolerated nitroglycerin (NTG) dose. Plasma NTG was unchanged over the time course of experiment (mean = 5.3 ± 1.2 ng/ml).
[b]Response to sublingual (SL) NTG at 24.5 hr. NTG prolongs the exercise duration at 1, 4, and 8 hr but not at 24 hr. SL NTG response is diminished after IV NTG.
*$p < 0.01$ and **$p < 0.05$ versus placebo.
Source: From Ref. 25; reprinted with permission from the American Heart Association and the authors.

VII. STUDIES IN PROGRESS

Existing data on the nitroglycerin patches and, indeed, on all long-acting nitrates, have raised many important questions. Specifically, the mechanism underlying the development of nitrate tolerance requires further elucidation. Since the attenuation of nitrate effects has often been observed to occur within less than 24 hr during continuous exposure to nitroglycerin, it is reasonable to explore the possibility of utilizing an interrupted pattern of nitrate administration, with a prolonged daily nitrate-free interval. Preliminary data with both oral and transdermal nitrates suggest that this approach may prevent the occurrence of nitrate "tolerance." Additionally, since the patients with angina treated chronically with nitrates generally have their symptoms only with physical activity, it may be quite feasible to protect them from symptoms effectively with an interrupted administration plan, designed to give protection during daytime hours. Many studies currently under way aim to explore this hypothesis.

Furthermore, it has been argued that existing data on nitroglycerin patches have not fully explored the issue of overcoming the "tolerance" resulting from the long-term continuous administration of nitroglycerin. The argument goes that it may be possible to administer to patients a dose far larger than has yet been tested by gradual upward titration. Studies reported to data have used only the maximal tolerated doses during an acute titration procedure. In consequence, a large multicenter trial is now in progress to compare the effects of high doses, using multiple nitroglycerin patches and placebo, in a double-blind, parallel group design, using chronic upward titration to reach each dose level. In all, 480 subjects may be so tested. It is the opinion of the author that the results will not differ significantly from those already reported.

VIII. FUTURE DIRECTIONS

A novel approach that holds the potential for pharmacological prevention of nitrate "tolerance" has recently emerged from studies done by Horowitz and his associates (27,28). These investigators noted that the cellular mechanism behind the action of nitroglycerin appears to be the formation of nitrosothiols by the combination of NO_2 with a sulfhydryl donor, which results in the activation of cyclic GMP, leading to the relaxation of smooth muscle. They further noted that the availability of sulfhydryl groups might play a rate-limiting role in nitrate effect. Consequently, Horowitz and co-workers examined the effects of concomitant administration of N-acetylcysteine (NAC) with nitroglycerin, both in man and in experimental animal models, and observed a marked potentiation of nitroglycerin effect by the coadministration of NAC. This observation of potentiation was recently confirmed in man by other investigators (29). It is tempting to speculate that chronic administration of a sulfhydryl donor might prevent the development of nitrate tolerance during long-term continuous medication with nitrates. Vigorous exploration of this possibility is anticipated in the next several years.

IX. CONCLUSIONS

In summary, despite its familiarity, nitroglycerin remains a perplexing pharmacological agent. It is extremely well suited to transdermal delivery, but the prolonged administration of nitroglycerin by this route appears to be self-defeating due to the rapid development of a tolerancelike phenomenon. It is clear that transdermal nitroglycerin patches deliver the drug effectively and would be likely to be effective for up to 10-12 hr, if used intermittently and removed after 12 hr. It remains to be seen whether the use of higher nitroglycerin doses or the coadministration of a thiol donor will possibly avoid the development of nitrate tolerance during the long-term, continuous administration of nitroglycerin by transdermal rate-controlled drug delivery.

ACKNOWLEDGMENTS

The author is indebted to Mrs. Mary Johnson for her very able assistance in preparation of this chapter and to Cheryl Priest, R.N., Thelma Chandler, R.N., Kathleen Bogin, R.N., Martin St. John Sutton, FRCP, David Zimrin, M.D., Pamela Douglas, M.D., and Barbara Berko, M.D., for their contributions to the performance of studies described in this chapter.

REFERENCES

1. T. L. Brunton, On the use of nitrate of amyl in angina pectoris. *Lancet, 2*: 97 (1867).
2. W. B. Fye, Nitroglycerin: A homeopathic remedy. *Circulation, 73*: 21–29 (1986).
3. P. Carmichael and J. Leben, Sudden death in explosives workers. *Arch. Environ. Health (Chicago), 7*: 424 (1963).
4. R. L. Lange, M. S. Reid, D. D. Tresch, M. H. Keelan, V. M. Bernhard, and G. Coolidge, Nonathermomatous ischemic heart disease following withdrawal from chronic industrial nitroglycerin exposure. *Circulation, 46*: 666 (1972).
5. T. A. Davis and B. H. Wiesel, The treatment of angina pectoris with a nitroglycerin ointment. *Am. J. Med. Sci., 230*: 259 (1955).
6. N. Reichek, R. E. Goldstein, D. R. Redwood, and S. E. Epstein, Sustained effects of nitroglycerin ointment in patients with angina pectoris. *Circulation, 50*: 348–356 (1974).
7. Data on file, Ciba-Geigy Pharmaceuticals Co., Searle Pharmaceuticals Inc., and Key Pharmaceuticals, Inc.
8. H. L. Fung, Pharmacokinetics of nitroglycerin and long-acting nitrates. *Am. J. Med., 72*: 13–19 (1983).
9. R. E. Goldstein and S. E. Epstein, Nitrates in the prophylactic treatment of angina pectoris. *Circulation, 48*: 917 (1973).
10. D. Zimrin, N. Reichek, K. Bogin, S. Cameron, P. Douglas, and H. L. Fung, Anti-anginal effects of IV nitroglycerin. *Circulation, 72*(III): 460 (1985).
11. R. E. Goldstein, D. R. Rosing, D. R. Redwood, G. D. Beiser, and S. E. Epstein, Clinical and circulatory effects of isosorbide dinitrate. *Circulation, 43*: 629 (1971).
12. N. Reichek, C. Priest, M. Kienzle, J. P. Kleaveland, S. Bolton, and M. St. John Sutton, Angina prophylaxis with buccal nitroglycerin: A rapid onset long-acting nitrate. *Adv. Pharmacother., 1*: 1 (1982).
13. D. R. Redwood, D. R. Rosing, R. E. Goldstein, G. D. Beiser, and S. E. Epstein, Importance of the design of an exercise

protocol in the evaluation of patients with angina pectoris. *Circulation, 43:* 618 (1971).

14. J. O. Parker, R. J. Augustine, J. R. Burton, R. O. West, and P. W. Armstrong, Effect of nitroglycerin ointment on the clinical and hemodynamic response to exercise. *Am. J. Cardiol.,* 38: 162–166 (1976).

15. M. E. Davidov and W. J. Mroczek, The effect of nitroglycerin ointment on the exercise capacity in patients with angina pectoris. *Angiology, 27:* 205–211 (1976).

16. G. Nyberg and V. Panfilov, Effect of nitroglycerin ointment (Nitrong) on exercise tolerance and several circulatory parameters in patients with angina pectoris. *Eur. J. Clin. Pharmacol.,* 24: 733–739 (1983).

17. U. Thadani, H. L. Fung, A. C. Darke, and J. O. Parker, Oral isosorbide dinitrate in angina pectoris. Comparison of duration of action and dose–response relationship during acute and sustained therapy. *Am. J. Cardiol., 49:* 411–417 (1982).

18. S. Silber, K. Theisen, and H. Jahrmarker, Circumvention of nitrate tolerance combined with maximal effects for 12 hours. *Circulation, 72:* III–431 (1985).

19. R. H. Thompson, The clinical use of transdermal delivery devices with nitroglycerin. *Angiology, 34:* 23–31 (1983).

20. N. Reichek, C. Priest, D. Zimrin, T. Chandler, S. Bolton, W. Laskey, and M. St. John Sutton, Antianginal effects of nitroglycerin patches. *Am. J. Cardiol., 54:* 1–7 (1984).

21. J. D. Parker and H. L. Fung, Transdermal nitroglycerin in angina pectoris. *Am. J. Cardiol., 54:* 471–476 (1984).

22. P. A. Crean, P. Ribeiro, F. Crea, G. J. Davies, D. Ratcliffe, and A. Maseri, Failure of transdermal nitroglycerin to improve chronic stable angina: A randomized placebo-controlled, double-blind crossover trial. *Am. Heart J., 108:* 1494–1500 (1985).

23. M. Sullivan, M. Savvides, N. Abouantoun, E. B. Madsen, and V. Froelicher, Failure of transdermal nitroglycerin to improve exercise capacity in patients with angina pectoris. *J. Am. Coll. Cardiol., 5:* 1220–1223 (1985).

24. N. Reichek, Long-acting nitrates: Relative utility of nitroglycerin patches. *Am. J. Med., 76(6A):* 63 (1984).

25. N. Reichek, C. Priest, D. Zimrin, T. Chandler, N. Berger, P. Douglas, and M. St. John Sutton, Antianginal effect of nitroglycerin over 24 hours: Role of the method of administration. *Circulation, 70:* II–190 (1984).

26. J. D. Horowitz, E. M. Antman, B. H. Lorell, W. H. Barry, and T. W. Smith, Potentiation of the cardiovascular effects of nitroglycerin by N-acetylcysteine. *Circulation, 68:* 1247–1253 (1983).

27. J. Torresi, J. D. Horowitz, and G. H. Dusting, Prevention and reversal of tolerance to nitroglycerine with N-acetylcysteine. *J. Cardiovasc. Pharmacol.*, 7: 777–783 (1985).

28. M. D. Winniford, P. L. Kennedy, P. J. Wells, and L. D. Hillis, Potentiation of nitroglycerin-induced coronary dilatation by N-acetylcysteine. *Circulation*, 73: 138–142 (1986).

10

Transdermal Delivery of Nitroglycerin II

DŽENANA E. REZAKOVIĆ / University Hospital and University of
Zagreb, Zagreb, Yugoslavia

I. INTRODUCTION

Nitroglycerin has been the most important drug in the treatment of
angina pectoris for more than a century. Sublingual administration
provides rapid relief of anginal attacks, but the duration of action
is short, in the range of 15–30 min. Thus there have been many
efforts to design delivery systems that would prolong the duration
of nitrate action. Finally, in 1982, nitroglycerin became available in
a transdermal formulation known as the nitroglycerin patch. This
formulation provides transdermal nitroglycerin absorption directly
to venous circulation at a constant rate, bypassing the gastrointestinal tract and the extensive enterohepatic clearance and resulting
in a steady plasma concentration over 24 h. It was assumed that
the application of a single patch would provide continuous nitroglycerin delivery and constant plasma concentrations, affording sustained antianginal efficacy day and night. Nitroglycerin patches were
accepted immediately and widely by physicians and patients alike as
a comfortable and simple form of therapy.

However, some authors very soon raised serious doubts about
the duration of action and the clinical efficacy of nitroglycerin
patches, based on several trials in which 24-h antianginal efficacy
was not demonstrated, and they anticipated the need for more studies

to assess objectively the place of this formulation in the treatment of angina pectoris (1,2). Investigators have accumulated enough documentation to separate the facts from the fancies about the efficacy of nitroglycerin patches in angina pectoris and congestive heart failure. The aim of this chapter is to give a critical review of all articles and abstracts about the clinical performance of nitroglycerin patches and, founded on all these results, to define objectively the efficacy, the duration of action, and the role of transdermal nitroglycerin among other nitrate formulations in the treatment of the patients with angina pectoris and congestive heart failure.

II. CLINICAL TRIALS OF NITROGLYCERIN PATCHES IN CORONARY ARTERY DISEASE

This section summarizes the results of all acute and chronic clinical trials of nitroglycerin patches in coronary artery disease (stable angina pectoris, unstable angina pectoris, and variant angina pectoris). All trials in which clinical and hemodynamic variables were monitored for 24 h after patch application are included as acute studies (Table 1). Trials that evaluated the efficacy of therapy with nitroglycerin patches over 2 days up to 12 months are treated as semichronic and chronic studies (Tables 2 and 3). An effort is made to present in a standardized way all available and indispensable data from each study; this approach makes available for evaluation and comparison the same criteria with respect to trials resulting in differing reports of clinical efficacy. The original literature data are presented in the greatest possible detail in Tables 1, 2, and 3.

Each study is described with several standardized data. The reference is cited, together with the number of trials if more than one trial was presented in the publication. The name of the nitroglycerin patch preparation is given. The dose of nitroglycerin released from the patch per 24 h after a fixed-dose, sliding scale of doses or after a titrated dose is listed for each item, as well as concurrent antianginal or other cardiac therapy and the total number of patients included in the trial. Comparison with another antianginal agent in the same or a parallel group of patients is also noted. The trials are analyzed according to their design characteristics: placebo control, double-blind fashion, crossover, and randomization.

Since the exercise test was applied as a diagnostic method in most of the trials, the maximum exercise time and maximum ST-segment depression are used as criteria for the assessment of clinical efficacy, calculated as the percentage of increase or decrease versus placebo or control (washout) value. The results of ST-depression at the comparable exercise time, used by German authors to mean the time achieved in all exercise tests in the trial, are sometimes also cited. All studies are qualified arbitrarily as "positive" or "negative" according to the statistical significance of nitroglycerin patch effects on these variables of the exercise test.

Acute and chronic clinical trials were carried out to assess the duration of action over 24 h after single or long-term nitroglycerin patch application. Since the time periods of investigation were very different in the studies cited, the results are noted as early (1–12 h) and late (13–24 h) efficacy, which could be assigned as positive and negative, as previously explained (see Tables 1, 2, and 3).

The term "not studied," used when an early (1–12 h) assessment was planned without data in the later period, is introduced to give better insight into the duration of action after acute, single nitroglycerin patch application (Table 1.1). Information about acute and subsequent chronic investigation of the same group of patients is also given (Tables 1, 2, and 3).

A. Acute Clinical Trials in Coronary Artery Disease

Acute clinical trials of nitroglycerin patch are described as early-positive and late-not studied efficacy (Table 1.1), early-positive and late-negative efficacy (Table 1.2), early-positive and late-positive efficacy (Table 1.3), and early-negative and late-negative efficacy (Table 1.4).

The data for placebo or control (washout) values of the exercise time and ST-segment depression are also added for better insight into the original patients' values.

1. Acute Clinical Trials: Early-Positive/ Late-Not Studied Efficacy (Table 1.1)

1. In Hollenberg and Go (3) (article), 10 patients with stable angina pectoris on a sliding scale of nitroglycerin doses (2.5, 5.0, 7.5, and 10.0 mg per 24 h) were studied in a placebo-controlled single-blind design. The fall in resting systolic blood pressure and the rise in heart rate occurred with each dose of patch. The treadmill exercise score (TES), a computerized analysis of ST-segment changes during exercise, was improved by 31% and the time required for 1 mm ST-segment depression was improved by 33% at 4 and 7 h after patch application. Variables improved more (by 82 and 55%) with sublingual nitroglycerin (0.4–0.8 mg) than with nitroglycerin

Table 1.1. Acute Clinical Studies of Transdermal Nitroglycerin in Angina Pectoris (Early and Late Efficacy)

Author	Prepa-ration	Dose mg/24 hours	Other the-rapy	Pats. No.	Placebo control	Double-blind	Cross-over	Placebo*/control** exercise time/min	Placebo*/control** ST depression/mm	NTG-exercise time % of increase vs. P* / C** Early(h)	Late(h)	NTG-ST depression % of decrease vs. P*/ C** Early(h)	Late(h)	Chronic study	Other results
Table 1.1 :								POS	POS (NOT STUDIED)	POS (NOT STUDIED)		POS (NOT STUDIED)			
1. Hollenberg[3] Nitro-dur		2.5	-a	10	X	X Sgl. 0 bl.				4 – 7 h		4 – 7 h			° Treadmill exercise score
		5.0	-									°-33% (TES)		X	33% increase in time
		7.5						7.9**	°-17.6** (TES)	10%		-29%			to ST (-1,0 mm)
		10.0										-31%			depressions
												-31%			
2. Kennedy[4] Deponit		5	No	48	0	0 0	0	°501**	-1.6**	2 h 6%		2 h - 17% m - 22% c		X	° Working capacity (Watt x min)
3. Reiniger[5]₁ Deponit		5	No	6	0	0 0	0	-	-	-		2,5 h - 59%** - 63% - 77% - 82%		0	
		10													
		20													
		30													

248

								1 – 5 h	1 – 5 h	
4. Zeiher[6]	Trans-derm	5	HH DIG	12	X X O	R	-	°1.25 0.70mm**	°°20.9 11.6mm**	° Increase of exercise time (min)
	2 % NTG ointment	10 mg		12		C				°° Decrease of the sum of ST depressions
	2 % NTG ointment	30 mg		20						
								2 h		
5. Bassan[7]	Trans-derm		HH	10	X Sgl. bl.	4.13**	-	56 %	-	° Dose titration
		5–60								
	ISN	10–40 mg				C				
								1 – 3 h		
6. Nyberg[8]	Trans-derm		HH	10	O O X	R °76**	-	°23% 16%	-	° Work load (Watt/min) at the onset of AP
		10	CAA			C		°°50% 45%		°° Maximum work load
	NTG SL tbl 0.5 mg									
	NTG buccal 2.5 mg									
								4 h		
7. Colombo[9]	Trans-derm		No	9	X X X	R 6.8*	-	23 %	-	° Maximum work load (Watt/min)
		10				C		° 18%		
	ISN SR	20 mg								
								5 h	5 h	
8. Goldstein[10]	Trans-derm		No	20	O X	R -	-	°Significant increase	°Significant increase	° Time to the onset of AP and ST depressions, same efficacy as ISN SR 20 mg
		10				C				
	ISN SR	2×20 mg								

patch. A very weak dose-response relationship was demonstrated. Acute investigation was followed by chronic study after 28 days of patch therapy (Table 2, item 58) (3).

2. In Kenedy (4) (article), an open study, 48 patients with stable angina pectoris showed improvement by 6% of working capacity and by 17% of ST depression at maximum and 22% at comparable exercise time 2 h after the application of nitroglycerin patch (5 mg per 24 h). Acute study was followed by chronic investigation after 6 weeks and 3 and 6 months of long-term therapy (Table 2, item 65).

3. In Reiniger et al. (5) (article), an open study, six patients with stable angina pectoris achieved a reduction of 59, 63, 77, and 82% in ST-segment depression on a sliding scale (5, 10, 20, and 30 mg per 24 h) of nitroglycerin delivered, 2.5 h after patch application. Dose-response relationships were significant.

4. In Zeiher et al. (6) (article), 44 patients were investigated in a placebo-controlled double-blind randomized manner comparing three nitrate formulations. The 12 patients on nitroglycerin patch (5 mg per 24 h; 25 mg per 10 cm^2) showed improvement in maximum exercise time and a decrease in the sum of exercise-induced ST-segment depression 1 and 5 h after patch application. The 12 patients on 10 mg of 2% nitroglycerin ointment (40 cm^2) achieved an increase in maximum work load (watt/minute) and a reduction in the sum of ST-segment depression at 1 h but not at 4 h after application. The remaining 20 patients on 30 mg of 2% nitroglycerin ointment (40 cm^2) demonstrated in the same variables an improvement at 1 h but only in maximum work load at 6 h. This study shows that transdermal nitrate delivery and the duration of action depend not only on the nitroglycerin doses and the surface of administration but also on the mode of topical application.

5. In Bassan (7) (abstract), 10 men with stable angina pectoris were investigated in a placebo-controlled single-blind and comparison study between nitroglycerin patches in the dose range from 5 to 60 mg per 24 h and isosorbide dinitrate from 10 to 40 mg. The initial work load was individualized so that the starting level chosen provoked angina during 3-6 min. The patients showed a similar increase in the exercise time 2 h after nitroglycerin patch and 1 h after isosorbide dinitrate administration. The 9 patients with positive efficacy received different doses of nitroglycerin in patches: 1-5, 1-10, 1-15, 2-20, 2-30, 1-50, and 1-60 mg per 24 h.

6. In Nyberg (8) (abstract) the efficacy of single dose of a sublingual nitroglycerin tablet (0.5 mg), a buccal nitroglycerin tablet (2.5 mg), and nitroglycerin patch (10 mg per 24 h) was investigated in an open, randomized crossover trial in 10 patients with stable angina pectoris. Sublingual and buccal nitroglycerin had equal effect on ischemia and chest pain intensity during the exercise test within 5 min of application. The nitroglycerin patch and buccal

nitroglycerin increased the maximum exercise work load (by 50 and 45%, 56 and 51%) and the level of work load to the onset of angina pectoris (by 25 and 16%, 34 and 24%) approximately the same extent at 1 and 3 h after administration.

7. In Colombo et al. (9) (article), the nitroglycerin patch (10 mg per 24 h) was investigated in nine patients with stable angina pectoris in a placebo-controlled double-blind, randomized crossover trial and in comparison with isosorbide dinitrate (20 mg, slow release). Both nitrates lowered lying and standing systolic blood pressure and increased the duration of exercise time (NTG patch, 23%; ISDN, 29%) and maximum work load (NTG patch and ISDN, 18%) to a similar extent 4 h after dosing.

8. In Goldstein et al. (10) (abstract), 20 patients with stable angina pectoris were investigated in a double-blind, randomized crossover design comparing nitroglycerin patch (10 µg/24 h) with isosorbide dinitrate (20 mg slow release). Both nitrates increased the maximum exercise work load and the time to onset of anginal attacks and decreased ST-segment depression to the same extent at 5 h after topical application or oral intake.

2. *Acute Clinical Trials: Early-Positive / Late-Negative Efficacy* (Table 1.2)

9. Müller$_1$ (11) (article; see also items 36, 44, 60, 74, and 82), in an open trial, nine patients with stable angina pectoris (with ST-segment depression between 1.0 and 2.0 mm at 100 W/min work load) showed a reduction in ST-segment depression at 1 h but not 24 h after the application of a nitroglycerin patch (5 mg per 24 h), but they did not demonstrate any change in the working capacity (watt × minute) at either period. The study was continued by the chronic investigation over 2 months of patch therapy (Table 2, item 60).

10. In Parker$_1$ and Fung (12) (article; see also items 18, 43, and 93), a placebo-controlled, double-blind design, 11 patients with stable angina pectoris showed improved exercise time 2 and 4 h (11 and 9%, 11 and 16%, 11 and 13%) but not 24 h after application, with nitroglycerin patches on a sliding dose scale (5, 10, and 15 mg per 24 h). The control value of exercise time (exercise test was carried out before patch application) was not constant; it improved by 20% during the trial, complicating the interpretation of therapeutic effects. The acute phase of the investigation was followed by semichronic investigation after 7–14 days of nitroglycerin patch administration (Table 3, item 93).

11. In James et al. (13) (article), 12 patients with stable angina pectoris were studied in a placebo-controlled, double-blind, randomized crossover manner after nitroglycerin patch (5 mg per 24 h) application. The time to the onset of angina pectoris and ST-segment

Table 1.2. Acute Clinical Studies of Transdermal Nitroglycerin in Angina Pectoris (Early and Late Efficacy)

Table 1.2. :

Author	Prepa-ration	Dose mg/24 hours	Other the-rapy	Pats. No.	Placebo control	Double-blind	Cross-over	Placebo*/control** exercise time/min	Placebo*/control** ST depres-sion/mm	NTG-exercise time % of increase vs. P*/C** Early (h) POS	Late (h) NEG	NTG-ST depression % of decrease vs. P*/C** Early (h) POS	Late (h) NEG	Chronic study	Other results
9. Müller[11]	Depotit	5	No	9	O	O	O	°750**	-1.9**	1 / °NS	24 h / NS	1 / -46%	24 h / -23%(NS)c	X	°Working capacity (Watt x min)
10. Parker[12]	Nitro-dur	5	BB	11	O	O Sgl.bl. O		°5.8**	–	2 / 11% ; 4 / 9%	24 h / 6%(NS)**	2 / – ; 4 / –	24 h / –	X	°21% increase in control value
		10	1 pts.		X	X		6.7**	–	11% ; 16%	1%(NS)*	– ; –	–	(during study)	
		15		(10)	X	X		7.0**	–	11% ; 13%	6%(NS)*	– ; –	–		
11. James[13]	Trans-derm	5	BB 9 pts.	12	X	X	X	8.1*	-1.8*	3 / 6%	24 h / -1%(NS)	3 / -39%	24 h / -6%(NS)	O	
12. Sellier[14]	Nitro-dur	5	–	9	X	X R	X	–	–	4 / 20%	28 h / NS	4 / –	28 h / –	O	
13. Thadani[15]	Trans-derm	°5	–	(14)	X	X R	X	5.4**	–	4 / 41%	24 h / 10%(NS)	4 / –	24 h / –	O	°Dose titration
		10		7				°°3.9*	–	°°62%	7%(NS)	–	–		°°Time to the onset of AP
		20		5, 2											
14. Reifart[16]	Depotit	5	No	12	X	X R	X	–	–	2 - 6 / –	24 h / –	2 - 6 / °45% ; 16%	24 h / NS**	O	°Sum of ST depressions
		10			X	C		–	–	–	–	55% ; 31%	NS		
	ISDN	10mg													
15. Gohlke-Barwolf[17]	Depotit	10	No	12	X	X R	X	7.2* / °44%*	-0.20*	2 / 20% ; °55%	8 h / 7% (NS) ; 32% (NS)	2 / -38%	8 h / -24%c(NS)	O	°Working capacity (Watt x min)

16.	Mertens[18]	Deponit		-	12	X X X			2.5 / 12 - 24 h	2.5 / 12 - 24 h		° Working capacity
			10			R	°256*	°°-3.0*	°59% NS	-48% NS^{c}		(Watt x min)
		Trans-derm	10			C	-	-	38% NS	-28% NS	0	°° Sum of
		Nitro-disc	10				-	-	50% NS	-45% NS		ST depressions No difference between the patches.
17.	Lönne[19]	Deponit		No	14	X X X			2 4 10 / 24h	2 4 10 / 24h		
			10			R	-	-2.3**	- - - -	-45% -40% -20% -14%^{c} NS	0	
18.	Parker[12] 2	Nitro-		No	6	X X X			2 - 4 / 24h	2 - 4 / 24h		
		dur	15			R	5,3**	-	34% 41% 8%(NS)	- - -		
			30				5,6**	-	44% 43% 16%(NS)	- - -	0	
19.	Reiniger[20]	Trans-		-	-	X X X			2.5 8 14 / 24h	2.5 8 14 / 24h	X	° Time to the onset
		derm	15			R	-	-	°132% 39% 34% NS	-64% -37% -20% NS -10%** NS		of ST-1,0 mm
20.	Reichek[21] 1	Nitro-disc		BBL	8	X X X			4 8 / 24h	4 8 / 24h		° Dose titration
		NTG SL	°25 0.34 mg	CAA		R	°°4,7*	-1.25*	°°30% 26% 4%(NS)	-20% NS NS	0	°° Time to the onset of AP
21.	Reichek[21] 2	Trans-		BBL	5	X X X			1 4 6 10 24	1 4 6 10 24		° Dose titration
		derm	°22	CAA		R	°°4,2**	-	°°31% 40% 33% 17% 2%°°°	- -	0	°° Time to the onset of AP °°° No statistics
22.	Reichek[22]	Nitra-		—	5	X X 0			1 6 10 / 24	- -		
		disc	19.2			R	4,4**	-	34% 36% 21% 0%(NS)	- -	0	
		NTG buccal	6x2.8 mg									
		NTG SL	0.38 mg			C				- -		
23.	Reiniger[5] 2	Deponit	30	-	10	X X X	°230 *	-1.75 *	2.5 8 24 / °143% 49% NS	2.5 8 24 / -89% -30% NS	X	° Working capacity (Watt x min)
						R	m494*		57% 35% NS			to the onset of ST - 1.0 mm, m-maximal w. capacity

depression of 1.0 mm and maximum exercise time were prolonged at 3 h but not 24, 48, 72 h after patch administration.

12. In Sellier et al. (14) (abstract), the efficacy of nitroglycerin patches (5 and 10 mg per 24 h) was assessed in nine patients with stable angina pectoris in a placebo-controlled, double-blind, randomized crossover design. At 4 h, exercise time was improved with the 5-mg patch by 20%, but there was no change at 28 h. However, the 10-mg patch (Table 1.3) improved exercise time (25 and 22%) and total work (48 and 41%) after 4 and 28 h. The dose-response relationship was significant.

13. In Thadani et al. (15) (abstract), the nitroglycerin patch was investigated in 14 patients with stable angina pectoris in a placebo-controlled, double-blind, randomized crossover study. An equipotent dose was identified by dose titration: 7 patients received 5 mg per 24 h, 5 patients 10 mg per 24 h and 2 patients 20 mg per 24 h. Nitroglycerin patches increased exercise time at 4 h (41%) but not at 24 h.

14. In Reifart and Bussmann (16) (article), 12 patients with stable angina pectoris were investigated in a placebo-controlled, double-blind, randomized crossover and comparison study of nitroglycerin patches (5 and 10 mg per 24 h) and isosorbide dinitrate (10 mg). The nitroglycerin patches decreased the sum of exercise-induced ST-segment depression (5 mg, 45%; 10 mg, 55%) at 90 min as well as isosorbide dinitrate (57%). At 6 h, nitroglycerin patches exhibited a decrease in the same variable (5 mg, 16%; 10 mg, 31%), and at 24 h the changes were no longer significant. The nitroglycerin patch dose-response relationship is significant.

15. In Gohlke-Bärwolf et al (17) (article), the nitroglycerin patch (10 mg per 24 h) was investigated in a placebo-controlled, double-blind, randomized crossover study in 12 patients with stable angina pectoris. They showed an improvement in exercise time (20%), working capacity (55%), and ST-segment depression (38%) at 2 h after patch application, but at 8 h the changes were no longer significant (7, 32, and 24%).

16. In Mertens et al. (18) (article), three patch preparations releasing 10 mg per 24 h of nitroglycerin were studied in a placebo-controlled, double-blind, randomized crossover design. At 2.5 h, nitroglycerin patches improved the working capacity and the sum of ST-segment depressions (Deponit, 59 and 48%; Transderm, 38 and 28%; Nitrodisc, 50 and 45%). After 12 and 24 h there were no more changes with either of the patches. Differences between the patches could not be proved. All three systems lead to an increase in heart rate and to a reduction in the systolic blood pressure at rest and during exercise.

17. In Lönne and Chvatik (19) (article), the nitroglycerin patch (10 mg per 24 h) was studied in 14 patients with stable angina

pectoris in a placebo-controlled, double-blind, randomized crossover design. A decrease in exercise-induced ST-segment depression was demonstrated at 2, 4, and 10 h (45, 40, and 20%) but there was no significant change (14%) 24 h after application. No significant changes in the blood pressure were found.

18. In Parker$_2$ and Fung (12) (article; see also items 10, 43, and 93), six patients with stable angina pectoris were investigated in a placebo-controlled, double-blind, randomized crossover fashion on sliding scale of nitroglycerin patch doses (15, 30, and 45 mg per 24 h). Maximum exercise time was prolonged for all three doses at 2 and 4 h, but at 24 h only the 45 mg per 24 h patch (Table 1.3) demonstrated a significant increase (15 mg, 34%; 41 and 8% NS; 30 mg, 44%, 43 and 16% NS; 45 mg, 44%, 43 and 16%).

19. In Reiniger et al. (20) (abstract), the data for a number of patients are missing. The nitroglycerin patch (15 mg per 24 h), studied in a placebo-controlled, double-blind, randomized crossover design, demonstrated an improvement in the time to the onset of angina pectoris (132, 39, and 34%) at 2.5, 8, and 14 h and in exercise-induced ST-segment depression (64 and 37) only at 2.5, and 8 h, while at 14 h ST segment change was not significant (20% NS). At 24 h chan0es in the variables were no longer significant. The patch was continued on days 2 and 3 with repeated exercise tests, in a semichronic study (Table 3, item 94).

20. In Reichek$_1$ et al. (21) (article; see also items 21 and 47), eight patients with stable angina pectoris were studied with an individualized initial exercise work load in which angina pectoris was elicited between 3 and 6 min of exercise in the absence of nitrate therapy in a placebo-controlled, double-blind, randomized crossover design. Patients received the maximum tolerated nitroglycerin patch dose (mean dose 25 mg per 24 h) identified by dose titration that demonstrated an improvement in the exercise time to the onset of angina pectoris at 4 and 8 h (30 and 26%) and a decrease in ST-segment depression at 4 h (20%) but not at 8 h. There were no significant changes at 24 h. Sublingual nitroglycerin (0.34 mg) affected significantly more the time to the onset of angina pectoris (50%) than the nitroglycerin patch.

21. In Reichek$_2$ et al. (21) (article; see also items 20 and 47), five patients with stable angina pectoris were studied by the same protocol as in the previous trial (item 20) but with a different patch preparation and a maximum nitroglycerin dose of 22 mg per 24 h to determine the influence of patch design on the results. The time to the onset of angina pectoris showed a change in 1, 4, 6, 10, and 24 h of 31, 40, 33, 17, and 2%, but no statistical analysis was carried out.

22. In Reichek et al. (22) (abstract), six patients with stable angina pectoris were investigated in a placebo-controlled, double-blind,

randomized crossover and comparison study between the maximum tolerated nitroglycerin patch dose of 19.2 mg per 24 h and long-acting transmucosal nitroglycerin tablets (mean dose, 2.8 mg, administered at 4–5 h). The nitroglycerin patches demonstrated an improvement in the exercise time at 1, 4, 6, and 10 h but not at 24 h; transmucosal nitroglycerin was effective in all periods from 1 to 24 h.

23. In Reiniger$_2$ et al. (5) (article; see also item 96), the nitro-glycerin patch (30 mg per 24 h) was investigated in 10 patients with stable angina pectoris in a placebo-controlled, double-blind, randomized crossover study. An increase in the exercise capacity to the onset of 1.0 mm ST-segment depression (143 and 49%) and a decrease in ST-segment depression (89 and 30%) were demonstrated at 2.5, and 8 h, but at 24 h there were no significant effects on either parameter. No changes in blood pressure were found. In 7 of these patients, testing was again performed after repeated application on day 2 (Table 3, item 96).

3. *Acute Clinical Trials: Early-Positive/ Late-Positive Efficacy* (Table 1.3)

24. In Naafs et al. (23) (article), 10 patients with stable angina pectoris were studied in a placebo-controlled, double-blind, randomized crossover study after single application of a nitroglycerin patch (5 mg per 24 h). The patients demonstrated an improvement in the maximum exercise time (16%), in the time to the onset of angina pectoris (29%), and in ST-segment depression (16%) at 12–16 h. There were no significant changes in either heart rate or blood pressure.

25. In Müller (24) (article), 20 patients with stable angina pectoris were studied in a placebo-controlled, double-blind randomized protocol after nitroglycerin patch (5 mg per 24 h) administration. Patients showed a reduction in ST-segment depression at the maximum (28 and 30%) and comparable (28 and 32%) exercise test at 1 and 24 h but without significant change in the working capacity. The study was continued with nitroglycerin patch therapy for 17 days (Table 2, item 56).

26. In Weisbort et al. (25) (article), 12 patients with stable angina pectoris were investigated in a double-blind, randomized crossover and comparison study between the nitroglycerin patch (5 mg per 24 h) and nitroglycerin capsules (slow release, 2.5 mg twice a day). The nitroglycerin patch did not affect the working capacity (watt × minute) at 1 and 24 h but decreased ST-segment depression during maximum and comparable exercise test (58 and 82%) at 24 h without a significant change at 1 h (36 and 59% NS). The nitroglycerin capsules did not show any significant effect on the exercise test values. The study was continued with chronic

patch treatment, and exercise testing was repeated after 14 days and 3 months (Table 2, item 61).

27. In Hey (26) (article), an open randomized and comparison study between two nitroglycerin patch preparations (5 mg per 24 h; Deponit and Transderm) was carried out in 48 patients with stable angina pectoris. Deponit demonstrated an improvement in the working capacity (19 and 16%) and ST-segment depression (38 and 28%), and Transderm a decrease in ST-segment depression (33 and 31%) at 2 and 24 h. Resting systolic blood pressure was decreased only 24 h after dosing. No significant difference in the efficacy was found between two patch preparations. The study was followed by semichronic investigation with continuous patch therapy for 14 days (Table 2, item 49).

28. In Krepp (27) (abstract), a placebo-controlled, double-blind randomized trial, the nitroglycerin patch (5 mg per 24 h) was investigated in 20 (18 statistically analyzed) patients with stable angina pectoris. An improvement in the maximum work load (watt/ minute) (15 and 24%) and ST-segment depression (33 and 36%) was shown at 2 and 24 h.

29. In Rezakovic et al. (28) (article), the nitroglycerin patch (5 mg per 24 h) was studied in a placebo-controlled single-blind protocol in 24 patients with stable angina pectoris. The study confirmed an improvement in the maximum exercise time (21 and 15%), the time to the onset of angina pectoris (49 and 36%), the time to the onset of ST-segment depression of 1.0 mm (56 and 46%), and the reduction in ST-segment depression (23 and 18%) at 5 and 24 h. Resting systolic blood pressure was lowered only at 5 h. The trial was continued during 3 months of chronic treatment (Table 2, item 62).

30. In Georgopoulos et al. (29) (article), in a placebo-controlled, single-blind protocol, the nitroglycerin patch (5 mg per 24 h) was tested in 11 patients with stable angina pectoris. A reduction in the sum of ST-segment depression (47, 44, and 48%) was assessed at 2, 8, and 24 h.

31. In Thompson (30) (abstract), 20 patients with stable angina pectoris were tested in a placebo-controlled, double-blind, randomized crossover protocol after single nitroglycerin patch (5 mg per 24 h) application. An improvement in the exercise time to the onset of angina pectoris and ST-segment depression of 2.0 mm (38 and 44%) was confirmed at 2 and 26 h after patch administration.

32. In Sabin and Görlitz (31) (abstract), a placebo-controlled, double-blind comparison study was performed of nitroglycerin patches in 5 and 10 mg per 24 h doses in 10 patients (total, 20) with stable angina pectoris. Both doses of the nitroglycerin patch affected a similar reduction in ST-segment depression at the comparable exercise test (5 mg, 40 and 33%; 10 mg, 54 and 41%) at 2 and 24 h.

Table 1.3. Acute Clinical Studies of Transdermal Nitroglycerin in Angina Pectoris (Early and Late Efficacy)

Author	Prepa-ration	Dose mg/24 hours	Other the-rapy	Pats. No.	Placebo control	Double-blind	Cross-over	Placebo*/control** exercise time/min	Placebo*/control** ST depres-sion/mm	NTG-exercise time % of increase vs. P* / C** Early (h)	Late (h)	NTG-ST depression % of decrease vs. P* / C** Early (h)	Late (h)	Chronic study	Other results
										POS	POS	POS	POS		
Table 1.3. :															
24. Naafs[23]	Trans-derm	5	No	10	X	X	X / R	6.2* 4.4*	-2.2*		16 h 16% °29%		16 h -16%	0	° Time to the onset of AP
25. Müller[24]	Deposit	5	No	20	X	X / R	O	°750**	-3.9**	1	24 h NS	°NS	24 h -30%m -32%c	X	° Working capacity (Watt x min)
26. Weisbort[25]	Deposit NTG SR 2x 2,5 mg	5	No	12	O	X / R	X / C	°452**	-1.4**	1 °NS	24 h NS	-36%(NS) -59%(NS)	24 h -58%m -8%c	X	° Working capacity (Watt x min)
27. Hey[26]	Deposit Trans-derm	5 5	No	24 24	O	O / R	O / C	°651** °480	-2.1** -2.3	2 °19% NS	24 h 16% NS	2 -8% -33%	24 h -29%c -31%c	X	° Working capacity (Watt x min)
28. Krepp[27]	Deposit	5	No	18 (20)	X	X / R	X	°85 **	-4.5**	2 °15%	24 h 24%	2 -33%	24 h -36%c	0	° Maximum work load (Watt /min)
29. Pezakovic[28]	Deposit	5	No	24	X Sgl. bl.	O		5.6*	-2.72*	5 21% °49% °°56%	24 h 15% 30% 46%	5 -3%	24 h -18%	X	° Time to the onset of AP °° Time to ST depression - 1.0 mm

#	Reference	Drug	n		n				2	8	24 h	2	8	24 h	Notes	
30.	Georgopoulos[29]	Trans-derm	5	–	11	X Sgl. 0	–	-7.5*	–	–	–	°-17%	-44%	-48%	°Sum of ST depressions. Only 3 pts developed AP during exercise	0
31.	Thompson[30]	Nitro-disc	5	No	20	X X X / R	12.1*	–	26%	– – – – – >	44%	2	–	26 h –	°Time to AP and ST depressions -2.0 mm	0
32.	Sabin[31]	Deponit	5 / 10	No	20 / 10 / 10	X X O	°78* / °75*	-2.1* / -2.2*	NS / °20%	NS	NS	-40% / -54%		-33°C / -41°C 24 h	°Maximum work load (Watt/min)	X
33.	Cerri[32]	Trans-derm	5 / 10	No	20	X X X / R	6.7**	–	28% / 30%	22% / 22%	24 h	3	–	24 h –	No difference between 5 and 10 mg patches.	0
34.	Fazio[33]	Trans-derm	10	–	10	X O X / R	–	–	°64%	20 h			–	20 h –	°Work capacity (Watt/min). Improved myocardial perfusion during Th Th-201 stress scintigraphy P < 0.001*	0
35.	Pucci[34]	Nitro-dur	10	EEL / 1 pts Verapamil / 1 pts	10	O O X / R	°132*	–	°64%	45%	21 h	3	–	21 h –	°Total work during exercise (kgm)	0
		ISDN LA 3x 80 mg				C										

Table 1.3 (continued)

Table 1.3. (cont.)

Author	Prepa-ration	Dose mg/24 hours	Other the-rapy	Pats. No.	Placebo control	Double-blind	Cross-over	Placebo*/control** exercise time/min	Placebo*/control** ST depression/min	NTG-exercise time % of increase vs. P*/O** Early (h)	POS	Late (h)	POS	NTG-ST depression % of decrease vs. P*/O** Early (h)	POS	Late (h)	POS	Chronic study	Other results
36. Müller[11] 2	Deponit	10	No	10	O	O	O	°750**	-3.4**	1	°NS	24 h	NS	1	-46%	24 h	-46%^c	X	° Working capacity (Watt x min)
37. Krepp[35]	Deponit	10	No	18 (20)	X	O	O	°333*	-2.5*	2	°48%	24 h	33%	2	-15%(NS) -36%	24 h	-20%^m -37%^c	X	° Working capacity (Watt x min)
38. Wagner[36]	Deponit	10	No	20	X Sgl. bl.		O	°220*	-2.3*	4	°30%	24 h	51%	4	-34%	24 h	-35%^c	X	° Working capacity (Watt x min)
39. Scardi[37]	Trans-derm	10 20	No	15	X	X R	X	5.3*	-	4	53% 58%	24 h	37% 39%	4	-	24 h	-	O	22-16% /10 mg 20-18% /20 mg increase of maximum work load (Watt / min)
40. Heepe[38]	Deponit	10	BL 29	40	X	X R	X	-	-2.0*	8	-	24 h	-	8	-51% -51%	24 h	-36%^m -36%^c	X	
41. Schiavoni[39]	Nitro-dur	10	No	12	O	O	O	6.0**	-2.1**	6	29%	24 h -	28%	6	-66%	24 28 h	-76% -23%	O	
42. Sellier[14]	Nitro-dur	10	-	9	X	X R	X	-	-	4	25% °48%	28 h	22% 41%	4	-	28 h	-	O	° Total work load (Watt / min)
43. Parker[12] 2	Nitro-dur	45mg	-	6	X	X R	X	5.6*	-	2	44% 43%	24 h	16%	2	-	24 h	-	O	° Total work load (Watt / min)

The trial was continued with exercise testing after 28 days of continuous therapy with nitroglycerin patches (Table 2, item 59).

33. In Cerri et al. (32) (article), the effectiveness of the nitroglycerin patches in 5 and 10 mg per 24 h doses was assessed in a placebo-controlled, double-blind, randomized crossover protocol in 20 patients with stable angina pectoris. Both nitroglycerin patches showed a similar improvement in the maximum exercise time (5 mg, 28 and 22%; 10 mg, 30 and 22%) at 3 and 24 h but the fall in blood pressure and increase in the resting heart rate were significantly more changed by the 10-mg patch. The fall in blood pressure was more pronounced after 3 h than after 24 h.

34. In Fazio et al. (33) (abstract), the nitroglycerin patch (10 mg per 24 h) was investigated in a placebo controlled and randomized protocol, in 10 patients with stable angina pectoris and showed an increase in the working capacity (watt × minute) by 64% at 20 h, with improved myocardial perfusion in thallium-201 stress scintigraphy.

35. In Pucci et al. (34) (article), an open randomized, crossover comparison trial was carried out between the nitroglycerin patch (10 mg per 24 h) and oral long-acting isosorbide dinitrate (20 mg every 8 h) in 10 patients with stable angina pectoris. Both nitrate formulations had a similar positive effect on improvement in the exercise total work (kilogram meter) at 3 and 21 h of treatment, for the nitroglycerin patch by 64 and 45% and for isosorbide dinitrate by 39 and 40%. Resting systolic blood pressure was only lowered 3 h after the nitroglycerin patch.

36. In Müller$_2$ (11) (article; see also items 9, 44, 60, 74, and 82), ten patients with stable angina pectoris (with ST-segment depression of more than 2.0 mm at a 100 watt/minute work load) demonstrated in an open trial a reduction in ST-segment depression during a comparable exercise test at 1 and 24 h (46 and 42%), but there was no significant change in the working capacity (watt × minute). The study was continued by chronic investigation during 2 months of patch therapy (Table 2, item 74).

37. In Krepp (35) (article), the nitroglycerin patch (10 mg per 24 h) was tested in a placebo-controlled and open study in 20 patients (18 patients statistically analyzed) with stable angina pectoris. An improvement was demonstrated in the maximum exercise time (48 and 33%) and ST-segment depression at the comparable exercise test (36 and 37%) at 2 and 24 h. The exercise testing was repeated after 7 days of nitroglycerin treatment (Table 2, item 68).

38. In Wagner (36) (article), in a placebo-controlled single-blind study, the nitroglycerin patch (10 mg per 24 h) was tested in 20 patients with stable angina pectoris. An improvement in the working capacity (30 and 51%) and in ST-segment depression at the comparable exercise test (34 and 35%) was found at 4 and 24 h after patch

administration. No change in blood pressure was found. The acute
study was followed by repeated nitroglycerin patch treatment for 21
days (Table 2, item 73).

39. In Scardi et al. (37) (article), a placebo-controlled, double-
blind, randomized crossover study, the efficacy of the nitroglycerin
patches in two doses (10 and 20 mg per 24 h) was assessed in 15
patients with stable angina pectoris. Both nitroglycerin patches
induced at 4 and 24 h an increase in the maximum exercise time
(10 mg, 53 and 37%; 20 mg, 58 and 38%), the maximum work load
(watt/minute) (10 mg, 22 and 16%; 20 mg, 20 and 18%) and the time
to the onset of ST-segment depression (10 mg, 70 and 55%; 20 mg,
55 and 44%). At 4 h after dosing, an increase in heart rate and a
decrease in supine and upright systolic blood pressure was also shown.
No difference was found in efficacy between two doses of nitroglycerin
patch.

40. In Heepe (38) (article), the efficacy of a 10 mg per 24 h
nitroglycerin patch was assessed in a placebo-controlled, double-
blind, randomized crossover trial in 40 patients with stable angina
pectoris. A reduction in ST-segment depression in the maximum
exercise test (51 and 36%) was demonstrated at 8 and 24 h after
dosing. No significant change in blood pressure was found. The
trial was continued by chronic 12-month therapy (Table 2, item 75).

41. In Schiavoni et al. (39) (article), the nitroglycerin patch
(10 mg per 24 h) was investigated in an open study of 12 patients
with stable angina pectoris. An improvement was seen in the exercise time (29 and 28%) and in the maximum work load (watt/minute)
(41 and 39%) at 6 and 24 h; the reduction in ST-segment depression
was assessed at 6, 24, and 28 h (66, 76, and 23%), as was the fall
in resting systolic blood pressure.

42. In Sellier et al. (14) (abstract), the nitroglycerin patches
in two doses (5 and 10 mg per 24 h) were studied, and it was concluded that only the 10-mg patch showed an improvement at 4 and
28 h after application in maximum exercise time (25 and 22%) and in
the total work load (watt/minute) (48 and 41%) (see Table 1.2,
item 12).

43. In Parker3 and Fung (12) (article; see also items 10, 18,
and 93), six patients were investigated with different doses of the
nitroglycerin patch (15, 30, and 45 mg per 24 h). Maximum exercise
time over 24 h was increased only with 45 mg per 24 h patch at 2, 4,
and 24 h postdosing by 44, 43, and 16% (see Table 1.2, item 18).

4. Acute Clinical Trials: Early-Negative /
Late-Negative Efficacy (Table 1.4)

44. In Müller3 (11) (article; see also items 9, 36, 60, 74, and
82), 11 patients with stable angina pectoris (with ST-segment
depression of 1.0 mm at 100 watt/minute work load) showed in

Table 1.4. Acute Clinical Studies of Transdermal Nitroglycerin in Angina Pectoris (Early and Late Efficacy)

Table 1.4. :

Author	Prepa-ration	Dose mg/24 hours	Other the-rapy	Pats. No.	Placebo control. / Double-blind / Cross-over	Placebo*/control** exercise time/min	Placebo*/control** ST depre-ssion/mm	NTG-exercise time % of increase vs. P*/C** Early(h)	Late (h)	NTG-ST depression % of decrease vs. P*/C** Early (h)	Late (h)	Chronic study	Other results
44. Müller[11], 3	Deponit	2.5	No	11	O O O	°750**	-1.0**	NEG / 1 °NS	NEG / 24 h NS	NEG / 1 NS	NEG / 24 h NS	X	° Working capacity (Watt x min)
45. O'Hara[40], 1	Trans-derm	5 10	–	18	O O O	-	-	NEG / 1 - 8 h NS	NEG / 8 h NS	NEG / 1 - 8 h NS	NEG / 8 h NS	X	
46. Kohli[41]	Trans-derm	5 10 20	–	20	X X X R	-	-		22 h NS		22 h NS	O	° NS for all doses
47. Reichek[21], 3	Nitro-disc / NTG SL	°9.4 / 0.36 mg	BBL CAA	7	X X X R	°°4,9	-	4 8 °°NS	24 h NS	4 8 -	24 h NS	O	° Dose titration °° Time to AP

POS/NEG-positive/negative efficacy; BBL - beta-blockers; DIG - digitalis; CAA - calcium antagonist blockers; Sgl.bl. - single blind; X - presented data

a - no data
O - not planned
R - randomized study
C - comparison study
c - comparable exercise test
m - maximum attained exercise test

263

an open trial no changes in the exercise test over 25 h of therapy with the nitroglycerin patch (2.5 mg per 24 h). (See items 9 and 36).

45. In O'Hara$_1$ et al. (40) (abstract; see also items 86, 87, and 92), 18 patients were randomized to a 5 or 10 mg per 24 h nitroglycerin patch and demonstrated no therapeutic effect on the exercise variable at 1 h or at 7–8 h after single patch application. The study was followed by testing at the end of 14 days therapy with nitroglycerin patches (Table 3, item 87).

46. In Kohli et al. (41) (abstract), a placebo-controlled, double-blind, randomized crossover trial, 20 patients with stable angina pectoris were assessed with a sliding scale of nitroglycerin patch doses of 5, 10, and 20 mg per 24 h. Exercise testing at 22 h after patch application showed no significant changes at any dose.

47. In Reichek$_3$ et al. (21) (article; see also items 20 and 21), 7 patients, as a part of a 14-patient group (see items 20 and 21), were assessed in a placebo-controlled, double-blind, randomized crossover trial with the nitroglycerin patch in the mean titrated dose of 9.4 mg per 24 h. During exercise testing with an individualized work load, no improvement was demonstrated at 4, 8, and 24 h. However, the exercise time was improved significantly by 3 min after sublingual nitroglycerin (0.36 mg).

B. Semichronic and Chronic Clinical Trials in Coronary Artery Disease

Semichronic and chronic clinical trials of nitroglycerin patch are divided in two tables into studies showing positive chronic efficacy (Table 2) and those showing negative efficacy (Table 3). The tables are constructed the same way as those for the acute trials. Data for the duration of semichronic or chronic nitroglycerin patch therapy are added. Data about the angina pectoris episodes and sublingual nitroglycerin consumption are presented, both expressed as a number per week or per day before (control or placebo value) and during patch therapy and calculated as a percentage versus control or placebo value. The results of the acute study are presented with the duration of action whenever an acute trial preceded the chronic investigation.

1. Semichronic and Chronic Clinical Trials: Positive Efficacy (Table 2)

48. In Schneider et al. (42) (article), nitroglycerin patches on a sliding dose scale (2.5, 5, and 10 mg per 24 h) were investigated in a placebo-controlled, single-blind, randomized crossover trial over 1 week in 12 patients with stable angina pectoris. The 2.5-mg patch did not elicit any reduction in ST-segment depression (Table 3).

The 5- and 10-mg patches prolonged the time to onset of angina pectoris at 3 and 24 h (5 mg, 20 and 20%; 10 mg, 44 and 27%) and reduced the sum of ST-segment depression only at 3 h (5 mg, 23%; 10 mg, 44%) with a decrease in the number of angina pectoris episodes (33 and 72%) and sublingual nitroglycerin consumption (29 and 59%). Arterial blood pressure was decreased only with the 10-mg patch after 3 h. The dose-response relationship was significant.

49. In Hey (26) (article), an acute study with two preparations of nitroglycerin patch (5 mg per 24 h) had been positive over 2–24 h (see item 27). Chronic trial was continued in an open protocol for 14 days in 48 patients. An improvement was found at 2 h in the working capacity (5 mg, 18%; 10 mg, 37%) and in ST-segment depression (5 mg, 43%; 10 mg, 44%) with a decrease in the number of angina episodes (75 and 60%) and sublingual nitroglycerin consumption (77 and 65%). Chronic trial showed that all effects of acute nitroglycerin patch administration on the exercise test were sustained and even slightly improved for both preparations after 14 days' therapy. The resting systolic blood pressure was lowered in both the acute and chronic phase.

50. In Rezaković (43) (article), 40 patients with stable angina pectoris were investigated with 5 mg per 24 h nitroglycerin patch over 14 days in a placebo-controlled, double-blind, randomized crossover protocol. An improvement was found during exercise testing at 5 h, in the exercise time (13%), in the time to the onset of ST-segment depression of 1.0 mm (48%), and in the ST-segment depression at maximum exercise time (32%) and 3 min after the test (24%). The resting systolic blood pressure showed a fall. The number of angina episodes (33%) and the nitroglycerin consumption (37%) also decreased.

51. In Kapor et al. (44) (article), 30 patients with stable angina pectoris were tested with a 5 mg per 24 h nitroglycerin patch over 14 days in a placebo-controlled, double-blind, randomized crossover design. The exercise time improved for 35% at 48 h after patch application. Angina pectoris episodes and nitroglycerin consumption also decreased by 60 and 67%.

52. In Löllgen et al. (45) (article), an open, randomized, crossover comparison study, the nitroglycerin patch (5 mg per 24 h) and isosorbide mononitrate (2 × 30 mg/day) were investigated over 14 days in 13 patients with stable angina pectoris. Both nitrates showed a similar decrease in the sum of ST-segment depression (5 mg patch, 39%; 60 mg isosorbide mononitrate, 42%) after 14 days of therapy. The time of testing was not indicated. Angina pectoris episodes also diminished for the 5-mg patch by 57% and for isosorbide mononitrate by 30%.

53. In Georgopoulos et al. (46) (article), 13 patients with angina pectoris were assessed in a placebo-controlled, double-blind, randomized crossover trial with a nitroglycerin patch (5 mg per 24 h) over 14 days. A decrease in the sum of ST-segment depression (51%) was

Table 2 Semichronic and Chronic Clinical Studies with Positive Efficacy in Angina Pectoris

Author	Preparation	Dose mg/24 hours	Other therapy	Pats. No.	Placebo control	Double-blind	Cross-over	Duration	NTG exercise time % of increase vs. placebo*/ control** Early(h)	Late (h)
48. Schneider [42]	Nitrodur	5 10		No	12	X	Sgl. bl. R	X	7 days	3 °20% 44%	24 h 20% 27%
49. Hey [26]	Deponit	5		No	24	0	0 R	0	14 days	2 h °18%**	
	Trans derm	5			24		C			°37%	
50. Rezaković [43]	Deponit	5		No	40	X	X R	X	14 days	5 h 13%* °48%*	
51. Kapor [44]	Trans derm	5		–	30	X	X R	X	14 days	48 h 35%*	
52. Löllgen [45]	Trans derm IS-5-MN	5 3x20 mg	BBL CAA	13	0	0 R C	X	14 days	–	
53. Georgopoulos [46]	Trans derm	5		No	13	X	X R	X	14 days	–	
54. Wester [47]	Trans derm Nifedipine	5 2x20 mg		No	12	0	0 R C	0	14 days	2 h °37%** °37%	
55. Imhof [48]	Trans derm ISDN R	5 2x40 mg		No	10	X	X R C	X	14 days	3 – 4 h 36%* 34%*	
56. Müller [24]	Deponit	5		No	20	X	X R	0	17 days	1 °NS	24 h NS

NTG ST depression % of decrease vs. placebo*/ control** Early (h)	Late (h)	Angina episodes No. / week/ day P*/C** NTG	SL NTG consumption No. / week/ day P*/C** NTG	Acute study	Other results
3	24 h				° Time to AP
°°-23%	NS*	9.3* / 6.2/-33%	9,8*/ 7.0/-29%^{W}	0	°°Sum of ST depression
-44%	NS	2.6/-72%	4.0/-59%		in exercise
2 h				POS	° Working capacity
-43%** c		13,5**/ 3.4/-75%	10.4**/2.4/-77%^{W}	2-	(Watt x min)
-44% c		8,7**/3.5/-60%	10.3**/3.6/-65%	24 h	
5 h					° Time to ST - 1,0 mm
-32%*		12.4*/ 8.2/ -33%	8.7*/ 5.5/ -37%^{W}	0	°°ST depressions
°°-24%*					3 min after test
18 h					
-		10*/ 4/-60%	9*/ 3/ -67%^{W}	0	
-					
°-39%***		5.1**/2.2/-57%^{W}		0	° Sum of ST depressions
°-42%**		3.6/-30%^{W}			
-					
°-51%*		-67%*	-63%*	0	° Sum of ST depressions
2 h					° Working capacity
-35%**		0.57**/0.29/-49%	°°0.45**/0.23/-49%^{d}		(Watt x min)
-45%		0.24/-58%	0.21/-53%	0	°°NTG SL mg
3 - 4 h					
NS		19.4*/4.3/-78%	19.1*/3.9/-80%^{W}	0	
NS		6.4/-67%	6.2/-68%		
1	24 h			POS	° Working capacity
-35%	-35%** c	1.7*/ 0.6/-75%	1.8*/ 0.3/-82%^{d}	1-	(Watt x min)
-35%	-36% m			24 h	

Table 2 (continued)

Author	Preparation	Dose mg/24 hours	Other therapy	Pats. No.	Placebo control	Double-blind	Cross-over	Duration	NTG exercise time % of increase vs.placebo*/control** Early (h)	Late (h)
57. Martines[49]	Trans-derm	5 10	No	24	X	X	X R	21 days	3 33%* 59%#	°14% °35%
58. Hollenberg[3]	Nitro-dur	5	–	5	X	0	0	28 days	4 – 7 h –	
59. Sabin[31]	Deponit	5 10	No	20 10 10	X	X	0	28 days	2 h °NS 20%	
60. Müller[11]	Deponit	5	No	9	0	0	0	2 months	– °44%**	
61. Weisbort[25]	Deponit	5	No	12	0	X	X R	14 days	1 NS	24 h NS
					0	0	0	3 months		
	NTG SR(2x2.5mg)					C			NS	NS
62. Rezaković[28]	Deponit	5	No	24	X Sgl. bl.	0	3 months	5 30% °86%	24 h 22%# 71%
63. Georgopoulos[29]	Trans-derm	5	No	13	X Sgl. bl.	0	5,6 months	– –	
64. Höhfeld[50]	Deponit	5	No	21	X	0	0	2 months 4 months 6 months	4 °18%** °°33%	5 h
65. Kenedy[4]	Deponit	5	No	48 41 29 15	0	0	0	6 weeks 3 months 6 months	2 h °20%** 37% 27%	

NTG depression % of decrease vs. placebo*/ control**		Angina episodes		SL NTG consumption		Acute study	Other results
Early (h)	Late (h)	No./week/ day P*/C** NTG		No./ week/ day P*/C** NTG			
3 h							5mg/10mg effects
–		8.3*/ –67%		–61%[W]		0	P < 0,01
–		–87%		–90%			° Maximal work load (Watt/min)
–						POS 4-7 h	°Time to ST - 1,0 mm ·Fall of control values
°25%**		–		–			
2 h						POS 2-24 h	•Maximum work load (Watt/min)
–14%[m]	–40%°*	–		–			
–20%	–50%						
–						POS 1 h	° Working capacity (Watt x min)
–40%°**		13.2**/3.7/-72%		13.8**/2.8/-80%[W]			
1	24 h						
–48%(NS)	–42%°**	–		–		POS 1-24 h	
–68%	–50%°(NS)						
–42%	–18% (NS)						
–77%	–41% (NS)						
NS	NS						
5	24 h	–		–		POS 5-24 h	° Time to ST - 1,0 mm °°ST depression 3 min after test
–31%	–24%*						
°°–35%	–27%						
–							° Sum of ST depressions
°–40%**		26.6**/2.5/– 80%[W]		–		0	
4	– 5h						° Maximum load (Watt/min)
–46%°**		–		–		0	°°Working capacity (Wat x min)
–60%							
–57%							
2 h						POS 2 h	° Working capacity (Watt x min)
–52%°**		7.8**/1.8/-77%		6.9/1.6/-77%[W]			
–67%							
–50%							

Table 2   (continued)

	Preparation	Dose mg/24 hours	Other therapy	Pats. No	Placebo control	Double-blind	Cross-over	Duration	NTG exercise time % of increase vs.placebo*/control** Early (h)	Late (h)
66. Rezaković[51]	Deponit	5	No	24	X Sgl. bl.	0		6 month 12 months	5 21%* 22%	24 h 14%*
67. Shell[52]	-	°10.4	BBL	8	0	0	0	2-3 days		
68. Krepp[35]	Deponit	10	No	18	X	0	0	7 days	2 °59%	24 h 43%*
69. Greco[53]	Deponit	10	No	19	X	X R	X	7 days	$\frac{3}{30\%}$	24 h 16%*
70. Agabiti-Rosei[54]	Trans-derm	10	-	35	X	X	X	7 days	4 h 21%* °36%	
71. Midtbø	Trans-derm	10	-	10	X	X R	X	7 days	22 °38%* °°80%	26 h
72. Giani[56]	Trans-derm Metoprolol SR	10 200 mg	No	12	X	X R C	X	14 days	24 h 30%* °34%	
73. Wagner[36]	Deponit	10	No	20	X Sgl. bl.	0		21 days	4 °62%	24 h 40%**
74. Müller[11] 2	Deponit	10	No	10	0	0	0	2 months	- °45%** (NS)	
75. Heepe[38]	Deponit	10	BBL (29)	40	0	0	0	12 months	8 -	24 h -

NTG depression % of decrease vs.placebo[*]/ control[**]		Angina episodes No./ week/ day P[*]/C[**] NTG	SL NTG consumption No. / week/ day P[*]/C[**] NTG	Acute study	Other results
Early (h)	Late (h)				
5 -37%[*] -34%	24 h -27%[**]	-	-	0	
[oo]5,8[**]/0,9/-85% [oo]110[**]/21/ -81%	24 h	-	-	0	[o] Dose titration [oo] Number of ishemic ST episodes and [ooo]time during Holter ECG (min)
2 -16% -44%	24 h -8%(NS)[m*] -27%[c]	1.06[*]/0.34/-68%	1.2[*]/0.34/-72%[d]	PCS 2-24 h	[o] Working capacity (Watt x min)
3 NS -67%	24 h NS[m*] -42%[c]	3.9[*]/2.7/-31%	3.9[*]/2.6/-34%[W]	0	
	4 h	3.9[*]/1.9/-51%	2.5[*]1.4/-21%[W]	0	[o] Time to ST - 1,0 mm
22 [o]-42%[*]	26 h	-	-	0	[o] No statistical analysis [oo]Working capacity (Watt x min) P < 0,01
	24 h -	-	-	0	[o] Total work (Kpm)
4 - 31%	24 h -23% (NS)	16.5[**]/8.7/-47%	17.8[**]/8.7/-51%[W]	PCS 4-24 h	[o] Working capacity (Watt x min)
- -52%[c**]		11.7[**]/3.6/-69%	15.1[**]/2.4/-84%[W]	PCS 1-24 h	[o] Working capacity (Watt x min)
8 47% 47%	24 h 35%[m*] 36%[c*]	5.3[**]/3.8/-28%[W]	-	PCS 8-24 h	

Table 2 (continued)

Author	Preparation	Dose mg/24 hours	Other therapy	Pats. No	Placebo control	Double-blind	Cross-over	Duration	NTG exercise time % of increase vs. placebo*/control** Early (h)	Late (h)
76. Thompson[57]	Nitra-disc	° 10-20	No	8	X	X	X	3 days / 12 days	2 / 30 / °°39%	26 h / 25%** / 44%
					R					
77. Salerno[58]	Trans-derm	10 20	-	9	X	0	X	2 days	-	
					R					
78. Lin[59]	Nitro-dur	°22,5	BBL Nitr. CAA °10		0	0	X	2-8 days		
	NTG i.v.°84 mg/min		C							
79. Dickstein[60]1	Trans-derm	10-30 10 20 30	BBL 18 29 CAA 22 24 3 Nitr.9 2		X	X	X	28 days	-	
80. Mahapatra[61]	Trans-derm	10 15-20	BBL 21 43 CAA 6		0	0	0	5 months	-	

W - per week

d - per day

found, as well as a lower number of angina episodes (65%) and lower nitroglycerin consumption (63%). Systolic and diastolic blood pressures at rest were also lowered with this therapy. The time of testing was not indicated.

54. In Wester and Mouselimis (47) (article), the nitroglycerin patch (5 mg per 24 h) was investigated in an open randomized comparison with Nifedipin (2 × 20 mg) in 12 patients with stable angina pectoris. Testing was carried out 14 days after continuous therapy, 2 h after drug administration. The investigation by M-mode echocardiography showed a decrease with both medicaments of left ventricular end-systolic diameter and, with only the nitroglycerin patch, a decrease in left ventricular end-diastolic diameter. Mean arterial blood pressure fell with both drugs, but the fall was more pronounced with Nifedipine. A similar improvement in the exercise test was demonstrated in the working capacity (watt × minute) (5 mg patch

NTG depression % of decrease vs. placebo*/ control** Early (h) Late(h)		Angina episodes No./week/day P*/C** NTG	SL NTG consumption No./week/day P*/C** NTG	Acute study	Other results
		--	-63%**	0	° Dose titration °° Time to ST - 1,5 mm and AP
°23**	24 h ‾‾‾‾‾‾ -54%* -56%*	-	-	0	° Number of ischemic ST episodes
No pain in 10 patients No pain in 10 patients	24 h ‾‾‾‾‾			0	° Patients with unstable angina pectoris °° Dose titration
——		2.5* 1.4/-44%	3.6* 2.3/-36%^{d}	0	
-		11** 5/ -55%^{W} 3/ -73%	-	0	

and Nifedipine by 37%) and in ST-segment depression (5 mg patch, 35%; Nifedipine, 45%), as well as in the number of angina episodes (49 and 58%) and the nitroglycerin consumption (49 and 53%).

55. In Imhoff et al. (48) (article), the nitroglycerin patch (5 mg per 24 h) was assessed in a placebo-controlled, double-blind, randomized crossover comparison with slow-release isosorbide dinitrate (2 × 40 mg) in 10 patients with stable angina pectoris, 14 days after sustained therapy and 3–4 h after drug administration. Similar improvement in the prolongation of exercise time (patch, 36%; ISDN, 34%) was found for both drugs, without significant change in ST-segment depression but with a decrease in the angina episodes (patch, 78%; ISDN, 67%) and in the nitroglycerin consumption (patch, 80%; ISDN, 68%). Systolic blood pressure was lowered with both treatments, the nitroglycerin patch being slightly more active than ISDN. However, the nitroglycerin patch was shown to be superior to ISDN

in the reduction of nitroglycerin consumption and ST-segment depression immediately after the exercise test.

56. In Müller (24) (article), the acute study with a nitroglycerin patch (5 mg per 24 h) was carried out and showed a positive effect on the exercise tolerance from 1 to 24 h. The chronic trial was continued in 20 patients with nitroglycerin patch (5 mg per 24 h) therapy over 17 days, with testing at 1 and 24 h post-dosing. There was no improvement in the working capacity (watt × minute), but there was a reduction in ST-segment depression with the comparable (35 and 35%) and maximum exercise test (35 and 36%), with a decrease in angina episodes (75%) and nitroglycerin consumption (82%). The positive acute effects were completely sustained during 17 days of therapy.

57. In Martines (49) (article), nitroglycerin patches in two doses (5 and 10 mg per 24 h) were investigated, in a placebo-controlled, double-blind, randomized, crossover study, in 24 patients with stable angina pectoris, for 21 days of sustained therapy. The nitroglycerin patches improved the exercise time (5 mg, 33%; 10 mg, 59%) and the maximum work load (watt/minute) (5 mg, 14%; 10 mg, 35%) at 3 h after patch application. The number of angina episodes (5 mg, 67%; 10 mg, 87%) and nitroglycerin consumption (5 mg, 61%; 10 mg, 90%) were also reduced. No differences in resting heart rate and arterial blood pressure were found with either patch. The dose-response relationship was significant.

58. In Hollenberg and Go (3) (article), acute study showed improvement in exercise-induced ischemic changes at 4-7 h with doses from 2.5 to 10 mg per 24 h (see item 1). The chronic trial was continued with five patients treated with a 5 mg per 24 h nitroglycerin patch over 28 days. Improvement in the time to the onset of ST-segment depression and the treadmill exercise score seems to be the same as in the acute study, although no statistical analysis is shown. A decrease and an increase appeared in control baseline values during 4 weeks of therapy, which complicated the analysis of results. Response to sublingual nitroglycerin was also preserved, and it seemed greater than the nitroglycerin patch effects. A fall in resting and erect systolic blood pressure was seen, but it was much smaller than in the acute trial.

59. In Sabin and Görlitz (31) (article), acute study with the 5 and 10 mg per 24 h nitroglycerin patch showed positive effects on the exercise test at 2 and 24 h. (See item 32.) The chronic trial was continued in 20 patients over 28 days. The testing was carried out at 2 h post-dosing. The positive effects found in the acute study were completely sustained; the maximum work load (watt/minute) was improved by 20% with the 10 mg per 24 h nitroglycerin patch, and ST-segment depression was reduced during the comparable exercise test with both doses (5 mg, 40%; 10 mg, 50%).

60. In Müller (11) (article; see also items 9, 36, 44, 74, and 82), acute trial with the 5 mg per 24 h nitroglycerin patch showed a reduction in ST-segment depression at 1 h but not at 24 h (see item 9). Chronic investigation in nine patients 2 months after continuous therapy with the 5-mg patch demonstrated an improvement not only in ST-segment depression during the comparable exercise test (40%) but also an increase in the working capacity by 44%, which was not demonstrated in the acute test. A reduction in angina episodes (72%) and in nitroglycerin consumption (80%) was also demonstrated.

61. In Weisbort et al. (25) (article), acute comparison between the nitroglycerin patch (5 mg per 24 h) and the sustained-released nitroglycerin capsules (2.5 mg twice a day) showed nitroglycerin patch efficacy over 24 h and no changes in the exercise test with the nitroglycerin capsules (see item 26). A double-blind, randomized crossover trial lasting 14 days in 12 patients revealed that the nitroglycerin patch induced a reduction of 42% in ST-segment depression during the maximum exercise test at 24 h postdosing; there were no significant changes with nitroglycerin capsule therapy. An open study with a 5 mg per 24 h nitroglycerin patch was continued over 3 months of therapy. It showed sustained reduction of ST-segment depression during the maximum (42%) and comparable exercise test (77%) at 1 h but no reduction 24 h after patch application.

62. In Rezaković et al. (28) (article), acute study with the 5 mg per 24 h nitroglycerin patch was previously carried out and demonstrated a positive effect on the exercise test over 24 h (see item 29). A partly placebo-controlled single-blind trial in 24 patients was continued during 3 months of chronic therapy with the 5-mg patch. It demonstrated sustained improvement of exercise test at 5 and 24 h, in the maximum exercise time (30 and 22%), in the time to onset of ST-segment depression (86 and 71%), in ST-segment depression (31 and 24%), and ST depression 3 min after the test (35 and 27%).

63. In Georgopoulos et al. (29) (article), a placebo-controlled single-blind study, the nitroglycerin patch (5 mg per 24 h) was assessed in 13 patients with stable angina pectoris over 5.6 months of continuous therapy. A reduction in the sum of ST-segment depression (40%) at 24 h and in the angina episodes (80%) was found at the end of treatment. The resting systolic blood pressure, as well as the exercise systolic and diastolic blood pressures, was significantly lowered.

64. In Höhfeld (50) (article), a partly placebo-controlled open trial was carried out in 21 patients with stable angina pectoris during 6 months' therapy with the 5 mg per 24 h nitroglycerin patch. A reduction in ST-segment depression was found at 4–5 h at the end of 2, 4, and 6 months of therapy (46, 60, and 57%). Improvement in the maximum work load (watt/minute) and the working

capacity (watt × minute) was shown at the end of 6 months' therapy (18 and 33%).

65. In Kenedy (4) (article), acute testing of the nitroglycerin patch (5 mg per 24 h) showed a positive effect on exercise tolerance 2 h after application. An open trial was continued for 6 months in 48 patients. Improvement was demonstrated in the exercise test after 6 weeks, 3 months, and 6 months of therapy, in the working capacity (watt × minute) (20, 37, and 27%), and in ST-segment depression (52, 67, and 50%) at 2 h after dosing. The number of angina episodes and the nitroglycerin consumption were reduced by 77% each at the end of 6 weeks of therapy.

66. In Rezaković (51) (article), the nitroglycerin patch (5 mg per 24 h) was investigated in a partly placebo-controlled single-blind study in 24 patients with stable angina pectoris during 12 months of continuous treatment. The testing was carried out at 5 h after dosing at the end of 3, 6, and 9 months and at 5 and 24 h at 12 months. An improvement in the exercise time (22 and 14%) and in ST-segment depression (34 and 27%) was sustained during 12 months of therapy at 5 and 24 h after patch application.

67. In Shell (52) (article), an open trial was carried out on eight patients with stable angina pectoris to assess the effects of the nitroglycerin patch on the number, duration, and magnitude of ischemic events registered by 24-h ECG monitoring. The dosage of nitroglycerin patch was titrated until the number of symptomatic events were abolished, ranging from 5 to 20 mg (mean, 10.4 mg per 24 h) nitroglycerin patch. The total number and the duration of ischemic events decreased by 85 and 81%, as did the ischemia-magnitude integral.

68. In Krepp (35) (article), acute trial with the 10 mg per 24 h nitroglycerin patch showed improvement in the working capacity and in ST-segment depression from 2 to 24 h after dosing. (See item 37). The study was continued in 18 patients over 7 days in an open and partly placebo-controlled (4 days) protocol. It demonstrated a sustained improvement of the working capacity (watt × minute) (59 and 43%) and in ST-segment depression during the comparable exercise test (44 and 27%) at 2 and 24 h. The number of angina episodes and the sublingual nitroglycerin consumption were also reduced by 68 and 72% during the 7 days of therapy.

69. In Greco (53) (abstract), the nitroglycerin patch (10 mg per 24 h) was studied in a placebo-controlled, double-blind, randomized crossover protocol in 19 patients with stable angina pectoris during 7 days of continuous therapy and at 3 and 24 h after dosing. Improvement in the exercise time (30 and 16%) and in ST-segment depression (67 and 42%) was found, as well as a decrease in the number of angina pectoris episodes (31%) and in sublingual nitroglycerin consumption (34%).

70. In Agabiti-Rosei et al. (54) (abstract), a placebo-controlled, double-blind crossover trial, the nitroglycerin patch (10 mg per 24 h) was investigated in 35 patients with stable angina pectoris after 7 days of therapy and 4 h after the patch application. Improvement was found in the exercise time (21%) and in the time to the onset of ST-segment depression of 1.0 mm (36%), as well as a reduced number of angina episodes (51%) and reduced sublingual nitroglycerin consumption (21%).

71. In Midtbo (55) (article), a placebo-controlled, double-blind, randomized crossover trial, the nitroglycerin patch (10 mg per 24 h) was investigated in 10 patients with stable angina pectoris at the end of 7 days' therapy and at 22–26 h after dosing. The exercise time (38%) and ST-segment depression (42%) seemed to improve compared with placebo values, although the exercise test values were not statistically analyzed, except that the working capacity was significantly better than placebo values by 80%.

72. In Giani et al. (56) (abstract), a placebo-controlled, double-blind, randomized crossover comparison was carried out between the nitroglycerin patch (10 mg per 24 h) and metoprolol (200 mg slow release) in 12 patients with stable angina pectoris during 14 days of therapy and at 24 h postdosing. Both treatments improved the exercise time (10-mg patch, 30%; metoprolol, 40%) and the total work (kilopondmeter) (10-mg patch, 34%; metoprolol, 50%) and the combination has greater effect (48 and 66%). There are no data about statistical significance.

73. In Wagner (36) (article), acute study with the 10 mg per 24 h nitroglycerin patch demonstrated a positive effect on the exercise test 4 and 24 h after patch application (see item 38). A partly placebo-controlled single-blind trial was continued in 20 patients with testing on day 21 at 4 and 24 h after dosing. The improvement in the working capacity (watt × minute) (62 and 40%) at 4 and 24 h and in ST-segment depression (31%) at 4 h was sustained at the end of 21 days' therapy, with a reduced number of angina episodes (47%) and reduced nitroglycerin consumption (51%). Blood arterial pressure and heart rate showed no changes.

74. In Müller$_2$ (11) (article; see also items 9, 36, 44, 60, and 82), acute study with the 10 mg per 24 h nitroglycerin patch showed improvement in ST-segment depression over 24 h but not in the working capacity. (See item 36.) An open trial in 20 patients was continued for 2 months and demonstrated improvement not only in ST-segment depression (52%) during the comparable exercise test but also an increase in the working capacity (45%), with a reduction in the number of angina episodes (69%) and in sublingual nitroglycerin consumption (84%).

75. In Heepe (38) (article), acute study with the 10 mg per 24 h nitroglycerin patch demonstrated improvement in ST-segment

depression during the maximum and comparable exercise test at 8 and 24 h after patch application. (See item 40.) A chronic, open trial was continued in 40 patients with testing after 1, 3, 6, and 12 months of therapy at 8 and 24 h after dosing. It showed a sustained improvement in ST-segment depression during the maximum (47 and 35%) and comparable (47 and 36%) exercise test at 8 and 24 h during the 12 months of therapy and a reduction in the number of angina episodes (28%).

76. In Thompson (57) (article), the nitroglycerin patch in the titrated dose (from 10 to 20 mg per 24 h) was assessed in a placebo-controlled, double-blind, randomized crossover study in eight patients (five patients received 10 mg per 24 h) with stable angina pectoris in two periods of 3 and 12 days. Improvement in the exercise time (30 and 25%) and in the time to the onset of ST-segment depression of 1.5 mm and a reduction in the number of angina pectoris episodes (38 and 44%) were found at 2 and 26 h after dosing, along with a reduction in sublingual nitroglycerin consumption (63%).

77. In Salerno et al. (58) (abstract), the nitroglycerin patch in two doses (10 and 20 mg per 24 h) was assessed in nine patients with vasospastic angina at rest in a placebo-controlled, randomized crossover protocol lasting 48 h. Follow-up for the ischemic episodes was carried out by 24-h Holter ECG recording. The number of ischemic episodes was reduced with the 10-mg patch by 54% and with the 20-mg patch by 56% over 24 h of ECG monitoring.

78. In Lin and Flaherty (59) (article), the efficacy of nitroglycerin patch in 10 patients with unstable angina pectoris was assessed in a crossover and comparison study with nitroglycerin infusion. Intravenous and transdermal nitroglycerin was administered in equipotent doses, inducing a 10% reduction in mean arterial pressure (IV NTG in the range 10–200 μg/min; mean, 84 ± 74 μg/min; transdermal NTG in the range 5–40 mg per 24 h; mean, 22.5 ± 10 mg per 24 h). After the initial hemodynamic endpoint was reached by nitroglycerin infusion 9 patients were free of chest pain episodes; after an additional nitroglycerin dose all 10 patients were free of pain. After the equipotent transdermal nitroglycerin dosage and an additional 10 mg per 24 h nitroglycerin patch, 8 patients were free of chest pain. All 10 patients were without pain during further stay in the coronary care unit. Of the 10 patients, 7 had no further chest pains at rest during their hospitalization and were changed to oral antianginal treatment without the nitroglycerin patch. Another 2 patients needed permanent transdermal nitroglycerin in the same dosage; they had recurrent chest pains with discontinuation or reduction in treatment. The remaining patient underwent cardiovascular surgery. This study showed that intravenous nitroglycerin could be followed by transdermal nitroglycerin in unstable angina, maintaining anti-ischemic effects even during long-term treatment.

79. In Dickstein[1] and Knutsen (60) (article; see also item 88), a placebo-controlled, double-blind, multiple crossover study, the nitroglycerin patch (10-30 mg per 24 h) was investigated in 29 patients with stable angina pectoris (24 patients, 10 mg; 3 patients, 20 mg; 2 patients, 30 mg) in 2-day periods over 28 days. Reduction in the number of angina episodes (44%) and in sublingual nitroglycerin consumption (36%) was demonstrated.

80. In Mahapatra et al. (61) (abstract), 43 patients with stable angina pectoris were investigated using doses of nitroglycerin patches titrated on the basis of the frequency of the angina pectoris (10 mg, 33 patients; 15 mg, 22 patients; 20 mg per 24 h, 7 patients) during follow-up for 5 months. The treatment with the 10 mg per 24 h nitroglycerin patch reduced angina episodes by 55% and the 15-20 mg per 24 h patch by 73% over the period of the patch therapy.

2. Semichronic and Chronic Clinical Trials:
   Negative Efficacy (Table 3)

81. In Schneider et al. (42) (article), the testing of the 2.5-mg nitroglycerin patch was carried out as part of study of 12 patients on a sliding scale of nitroglycerin patch doses, from 2.5 to 10 mg per 24 h (see item 48). Although the 5 and 10 mg per 24 h patches demonstrated positive efficacy during the exercise test, the 2.5 mg per 24 h showed only slight improvement in the time to onset of angina pectoris (13 and 15%) at 3 and 24 h after dosing. There was no reduction in ST-segment depression, the number of angina episodes, or nitroglycerin consumption.

82. In Müller[3] (11) (article; see also items 9, 36, 44, 60, and 74), acute study with the 2.5-mg per 24 h nitroglycerin patch showed no efficacy over 24 h (see item 44). A chronic, open study was continued in 11 patients. No change in the exercise testing was shown, but an important reduction in the number of angina episodes (72%) and sublingual nitroglycerin consumption (75%) was found during 2 months of nitroglycerin patch therapy.

83. In Crean et al. (62) (article; see also item 95), the nitroglycerin patch (5 mg per 24 h) was assessed in a placebo-controlled, double-blind, randomized multiple crossover trial in 10 patients with stable angina pectoris during four 1-week periods. No significant changes either in the exercise testing 2 and 4 h after dosing or in the number of angina episodes and nitroglycerin consumption were demonstrated after 7 days' patch therapy. During 96-h continuous ECG monitoring, a reduction in ST-segment depression (35%) was found, but this finding was not statistically significant.

84. In Subramanian et al. (63) (article), the nitroglycerin patch (5 mg per 24 h) was assessed in a placebo-controlled, double-blind, randomized crossover study in 18 patients with stable angina pectoris.

Table 3   Semichronic and Chronic Clinical Studies with Negative Efficacy in Angina Pectoris

Author	Preparation	Dose mg/24 hours	Other therapy	Pats. No.	Placebo control	Double-blind	Cross-over	Duration	NTG exercise time % of increase vs. placebo*/ control** Early (h)	Late (h)
81. Schneider[42]	Nitro-dur	2.5		No.	12	X	Sgl. bl.	X	7 days	3 °13%	24 h 15%
82. Müller[11/3]	Deponit	2.5		No	11	0	0	0	2 months	1 NS	24 h NS
83. Crean[62]	Trans-derm	5		No	10 (11)	X	X	X R	7 days	2 NS	4h NS
84. Subramanian[63]	Trans-derm	5		-	18	X	X	X R	14 days	20 NS	22h NS
85. Petersen[64]	Trans-derm	5	BBL CA	27	X	X	X	14 days	-	
86. O'Hara[40/2]	Trans-derm	5		-	18	X	X	X R	14 days	21 NS	23 h NS
87. O'Hara[40/1]	Trans-derm	5 10		-	18	0	0	0 R	14 days	1 NS	8h NS
88. Dickstein[60/2]	Trans-derm	5	BBL CAA LANitrate DIG.	27	X	X	X R	28 days	-	
89. Sullivan[65]	Trans-derm	10	BBL 8 Nifedipine 1	16	X	X	X R	3 days	1 NS	24h NS
90. Jackson[66/1]	Trans-derm	10		-	10	X	X	X R	7 days	24 h NS	
91. Jackson[66/2]	Trans-derm	20		-	20	X	X	X R	7 days	24 h NS	

NTG depression % of decrease vs. placebo*/ control**		Angina episodes No./ week/ day P*/C** NTG	SL NTG consumption No./ week/ day P*/C** NTG	Acute study	Other results
Early (h)	Late (h)				
3	24 h				° Time to the
NS	NS	9.3*/ 8.0/ NS	9.8*/ 10/ NS^W	0	onset of angina pectoris
1	24 h			Neg.	
NS	NS	7.4**/ 2.1/ -72%	6.5**/16/-75%^{W}	1-24 h	
2	4h				35% fewer minutes of ST depressions per 96 hours of continuous ECG monitoring (NS)
NS	NS	9*/ 10/ NS	13*/ 14/ NS^W	0	
20	22 h				
NS	NS	-	-	0	
-		14.4*/19.4/ NS	15.3*/19.3/ NS^W	0	
21	23 h				
-		-	-	0	
1	8 h			Neg.	
-		-	-	1-8	
-		1.2*/1.0/ NS	2.0*/1.7/ NS^d	0	
1	24 h				
NS	NS	-	-	0	
	24 h				
	NS	-	-	0	
	24 h				
	NS	-	-	0	

Table 3   (continued)

Author	Prepa-ration	Dose mg/24 hours	Other the-rapy	Pats. No.	Placebo control	Double-blind	Cross-over	Duration	NTG exercise time % of increase vs. placebo*/ control'** Early (h)	Late(h)
92. O`Hara[40] [3]	Trans-derm	10	-	12	X R	X	X	14 days	21 NS	23 h NS
93. Parker[12] [1]	Nitro-dur NTG SL	10-15 0,6	No	11	X R	X	X	7 - 14 days	during 24 h NS 16%	
94. Reiniger[20]	Trans-derm	15	-	-	X R	X	X	2 days	- -	
95. Crean[62]	Trans-derm	°15-20	No (9)	2 7	0	0	0	6 - 8 days	4 h NS	
96. Reiniger[5] [2]	Deponit	30	No	7	X R	X	X	2 days	2.5 h °37% NS	

No positive effect could be demonstrated on exercise testing at 20–22 h after dosing at the end of 14 days' nitroglycerin patch therapy.

85. In Petersen et al. (64) (abstract), the nitroglycerin patch (5 mg per 24 h) was investigated in a placebo-controlled, double-blind crossover study in 27 patients with stable angina pectoris during 14 days. No improvement was found in the number of angina episodes or in sublingual nitroglycerin consumption.

86. In O'Hara₂ et al. (40) (abstract; see also items 45, 87, and 92), a placebo-controlled, double-blind, randomized crossover trial, the nitroglycerin patch (5 mg per 24 h) was studied in 18 patients with stable angina pectoris. No changes in the exercise testing could be shown at 21–23 h postdosing after 14 days of patch therapy.

87. In O'Hara₁ et al. (40) (abstract; see also items 45, 86, and 92), acute study was carried out with two doses of the nitroglycerin patch (5 and 10 mg per 24 h) and demonstrated no changes in the exercise testing at 1–8 h after dosing (see item 45). A chronic open and randomized trial was continued in 18 patients. This demonstrated no positive efficacy at 1–8 h postdosing after 14 days of patch therapy.

88. In Dickstein₂ and Knutsen (60) (article; see also item 79), the nitroglycerin patch (5 mg per 24 h) was assessed in a placebo-controlled, double-blind, randomized multiple crossover study with 2-day periods over 28 days in 27 patients with stable angina pectoris.

NTG depression % of decrease vs. placebo*/ control** Early(h) Late (h)	Angina episodes No./week/day P*/C** NTG	SL NTG consumption No./week/day P*/C** NTG	Acute study	Other results
21 23 h				
-	-	-	0	
during 24 h			Pos	
NS	-	-	2-4h	
-	-	-		
2.5 h			Pos	
-17% NS	-	-	2.5-8h - 14 h	
4 h				° Dose
NS	-	-	0	titration
2.5 h			Pos	°Working capacity (Watt X min)
-17% NS	-	-	2.5-8h	to onset of ST - 1.0 mm

No reduction was demonstrated in the number of angina episodes or in sublingual nitroglycerin consumption.

89. In Sullivan et al. (65) (article), the nitroglycerin patch (10 mg per 24 h) was tested in a placebo-controlled, double-blind, randomized crossover trial of 16 patients with stable angina pectoris. No effect was demonstrated during exercise testing at 1 and 24 h postdosing after 3 days' patch therapy.

90. In Jackson et al. (66) (abstract), the nitroglycerin patch (10 mg per 24 h) was investigated in a placebo-controlled, double-blind, randomized crossover trial in 10 patients with stable angina pectoris. No effect was seen on exercise testing at 24 h after dosing at the end of 7 days' patch therapy.

91. In Jackson$_2$ et al. (66) (abstract), the nitroglycerin patch (20 mg per 24 h) was studied using the same design as with the 10-mg patch (see item 90), but in 20 patients with stable angina pectoris. No efficacy was seen at 24 h after 7 days of patch therapy.

92. In O'Hara$_3$ et al. (40) (abstract; see also items 45, 86, and 87), the nitroglycerin patch (10 mg per 24 h) was investigated in a placebo-controlled, double-blind, randomized crossover trial in 12 patients with stable angina pectoris. No efficacy was shown during exercise testing at 21-23 h postdosing at the end of 14 days' patch therapy.

93. In Parker[4] and Fung (12) (article; see also items 10, 18, and 43), acute trial with 5-15 mg per 24 h patch doses demonstrated improvement in the exercise time at 2 and 4 h but not at 24 h postdosing. (See item 10.) A chronic study was continued in a placebo-controlled, double-blind, randomized crossover protocol in 11 patients (10 patients, 15-mg patch; 1 patient, 10-mg patch). No improvement was found at 2, 4, and 24 h postdosing after 7-14 days of patch therapy.

94. In Reiniger et al. (20) (abstract), acute study with the 15 mg per 24 h nitroglycerin patch was carried out and demonstrated an effect on exercise testing at 2.5, 8, and 14 h postdosing (see item 19). The investigation was continued. The day 2 application showed an insignificant improvement in ST-segment depression (17%) at 2.5 h. After a 10-h therapy-free interval and the third patch application, the improvement in ST-segment depression (15%) and in the exercise capacity to the onset of ST-segment depression of 1.0 mm (21%) at 2.5 h postdosing was lower than during acute testing.

95. In Crean et al. (62) (article), the first study on 10 patients (see item 83) was continued to test the efficacy of incremental doses of the nitroglycerin patch. In an open trial, nine patients were investigated with 15-20 mg per 24 h nitroglycerin patch (15 mg, two patients; 20 mg, seven patients). No change was demonstrated in the exercise test at 4 h postdosing at the end of 6-8 days' patch therapy.

96. In Reiniger[2] et al. (5) (article), acute study with the 30 mg per 24 h nitroglycerin patch showed a positive anti-ischemic effect during the exercise test at 2.5 and 8 h but not 24 h postdosing (see item 23); day 2 application did not elicit any significant improvement in ST-segment depression (17% NS) at 2.5 h after dosing.

III. HEMODYNAMIC TRIALS OF NITROGLYCERIN PATCHES

Published studies about the hemodynamic efficacy of nitroglycerin patches during acute, semichronic, or chronic investigation are presented here. Data for the trials are shown in the standardized way in Table 4.

Hemodynamic monitoring was carried out by catheterization of the right heart. The most important parameters for the evaluation of cardiac function, the pulmonary capillary pressure, mean pulmonary artery pressure, cardiac output or cardiac index, and systemic vascular resistance, are presented as a baseline-control value and as a calculated percentage of the nitroglycerin patch-induced changes versus the control value. The time of hemodynamic investigation and the duration of the study are also noted, as well as the following data: name of the author, name of patch preparation, administered

dose per 24 h (from 5 to 120 mg per 24 h), number of patients, and
the patient diagnosis (coronary artery disease, acute or chronic
heart failure, and pulmonary hypertension).

97. In Noseda and Pfister (67) (article), the hemodynamic
efficacy of the nitroglycerin patch (5 mg per 24 h) after a single
application was investigated in 10 patients with chronic heart failure
due to coronary artery disease in a placebo-controlled, single-blind
crossover manner. All patients were in NYHA class IV, stabilized
on digitalis and diuretics. They showed a decrease in elevated
(23 mm Hg) pulmonary capillary pressure (16, 33, and 38%) and an
increase in the cardiac output (5, 12, and 16%) at 1, 4, and 8 h
after dosing.

98. In Sharpe and Coxon (68) (article), 16 patients with severe
chronic heart failure (4 patients, NYHA class IV; 11 patients, class
III; 2 patients, class II) taking digoxin (12 patients), oral furosemide,
and spironolactone (16 and 8 patients) were assessed in two acute
and one chronic investigation. In an open trial after a single application of the nitroglycerin patch (5 and 10 mg per 24 h), 8 patients
were investigated. No significant change was found in blood pressure or heart rate. A significant decrease in elevated (29 mm Hg)
pulmonary capillary pressure (41%) and in mean pulmonary artery
pressure (30%) was observed from 1 to 24 h after the 5 mg per 24 h
nitroglycerin patch. However, a decrease in the systemic vascular
resistance (28%) and an increase in the cardiac index (35%) were
assessed only at 4 h after dosing. There was a rise in the pulmonary
capillary pressure nearly to control values (27 mm Hg) following the
removal of the 5-mg patch, with a repeated decrease in the pulmonary
capillary pressure (41%) and mean pulmonary artery pressure (30%)
during 8 h of monitoring with the 10 mg per 24 h nitroglycerin
patch, without any change in afterload parameters.

The 8 patients were given in an open, random study either the
nitroglycerin patch (5 mg per 24 h) or oral and topical nitrates on
consecutive days. The only parameter affected was the pulmonary
capillary pressure, with a decrease of 18% at 4 h after the nitroglycerin patch (5 mg per 24 h), of 27% after 1 h of oral isosorbide
dinitrate (20 mg), and of 16% after 1 h of nitroglycerin ointment
(1 inch).

The 10 patients who responded to the 5 mg per 24 h nitroglycerin
patch in the acute trial continued to receive the same therapy and
were re-evaluated after 3 months. They showed that acute changes
in hemodynamic parameters 4 h after dosing were sustained, although
attenuated, during 3 months; a reduction in pulmonary capillary pressure, from 32 to 12%, and systemic vascular resistance, from 19 to
15%. There was an increase in cardiac index, from 17 to 12%.

These studies showed that 10 mg per 24 h nitroglycerin patch
had the same effect on the preload as the 5 mg per 24 h patch and

Table 4   Hemodynamic Studies

Author	Prepa-ration	Dose mg/24 hours	Other the-rapy	Pats. No.	Diag-nosis	PCP (mm Hg)		
97. Noseda [67]	Trans-derm	5	DIG. DIUR.	10	CHR HF	1 $^c23/-16\%$	4 -33%	8h -38%
98. Sharpe [68]	Trans-derm	5 10	DIG. (16) DIUR.	8	CHR HF	1 $^c29/\ -41\%$ -41% ------>	8 ------->	24h ----->
		5		10	Acute 3 months	4h $^c_25/\ -32\%$ $^c_26/\ -12\%$		
99. Lempereur [69]	Trans-derm	5- 10	-	8	CHR HF	2-10 $^c24/\ -51\%$ ------->		24h
100. Bergbauer [70]	Depo-nit	5 10	No	20 10 10	CAD	2h $^c_12/$ $^c_13/$	-30% -39%	
101. Osterspey [72]	Trans-derm	5 10 20	No	24 8 8 8	CAD			
102. Wiechmann [73]	Trans-derm	10	No	30	CAD			
103. Vogt [74]	Depo-nit	10	No	10	CAD ACHF	2-16 $^c24/\ -25\%$		24h NS
104. Yasky [75]	Trans-derm	10	DIG. DIUR.	10	CHR HF	2 $^c27/\ -17\%$		24h -31%
105. Daum [76]	Depo-nit	10	No	10	PULM. HYPER. After 4 weeks	2 6 10 14 24h $^c_9/-45\%-67\%-67\%-56\%-33\%$ $^c_6/-50\%-33\%$		
106. Reale [77]	Trans-derm	10 20	No	8	CAD	4 NS NS		24h

MPAP (mm Hg)			SVR dynes s cm^{-5}		CO* / CI** L/min L/min/m^2	

| | | | | | 1 4 8h |
| | | | | | $^c4.2^*/$ 5% 12% 16% |

2 8 24h			$^c2050/$ -28%	24h NS	4 24h $^c1.76^{**}/$ 35% NS
$^c40/$ -30% ------->------>					
-30%------->			NS		NS

| | | | 4h | | 4h |
| | | | $^c1962/$ -19% | $^c2349/$ -15% | $^c1.87^{**}/$ 17%
$^c1.74^{**}/$ 12% |

| | | | | | 2 - 24h |
| | | | | | NS |

2h					2h
$^c20/$ -22% -13%^{E}					$^c3.5^{**}$ / NS -15%^{E}
$^c21/$ -30% -25%^{E}					$^c3.9^{**}$ /-19% NS^E

2h					
$^c17/$ -18% -13%^{E}					
16/ -22% -21%^{E}					
16/ -26% -39%^{E}					

2 24 h	2	24h	2 24h
$^c16/$ -27% -32%	NS	NS	NS NS
-21%^{E} -26%^{E}	NS^E	NS^E	NS^E NS^E

| 2-12 24 h | | | 2 24h |
| $^c32/$ -21% NS | | | NS NS |

| 2 24 h | 2 | 24h | 2 24h |
| $^c39/$ -19% -27% | -11% | -32% | 2.0**/15% 30% |

2 6 10 14 24 h			2 6 10 14 24h
$^c30/$-20%-30%-30%-27%-13%			$^c4.5^*/14\%$ 22% 10% NS NS
$^c27/$-22%-19%			$^c4.9/$NS

4 24 h			4 24h
NS			NS
NS			NS

Table 4 (continued)

Author	Preparation	Dose mg/24 hours	Other therapy	Pats. No.	Diagnosis	PCP (mm Hg)				
107. Packer[78]	Trans-derm	°10-40	-	11	CHR HF		1			24h
						c_{27}/ -23%				-15%
108. Taylor[79]	Trans-derm		-	48	AMI		1.5			4h
		10			8/8+ AC HF+	-		c_{23}/ -9% +		
		20			8/8+	-		22/ -23% +		
		40			8/8+	c_{11}/ -27%		21/ -23% +		
109. Olivari[80]	Nitro-dur	5-10		9	N		1-6			24h
		15-20	DIG	9	CHR HF	c_{23}/ -22%				NS
110. Verma[81]	Trans-derm	20	-	8	AC HF	c_{21}/	1,5 h	- 24%		
	ISDN iv	50-200 mg/kg/h		8	AMI	c_{25}/		- 24%		
111. Rajfer[82]	Nitro-disc		No	9	CHR HF	c_{24}/ -25%	0.5-6			24h -17%
		15-40		(6)						
	i.v.NTG	156 µg/min								
112. Elkayam[83]	Trans-derm	30-60	-	10	CHR HF		2 8 12			24h
						c_{30}/NS NS 20% 20%				
113. Jordan[84]	Trans-derm	60	DIG	15 (8)	CHR HF		2 4 12			24h
						c_{22}/-23% -36% -18% NS				
114. Elkayam[85]	Trans-derm	90	DIG	10	CHR HF		2 6 10 16			24h
						c_{27}/-30 NS - - - - NS				
115. Roth[86]	Trans-derm	120	-	11	CHR HF		2 4 6			24h
						1 day c_{26}/-35% -39% -39% -27%				
						2 days -16% -19% -27				

PCP - pulmonary capillary pressure; MPAP - mean pulmonary artery pressure;

SVR - systemic vascular resistance; CO*- cardiac output; CI**- cardiax index;

DIG. - digitalis; DIUR. - diuretics; CHR. HF. - chronic heart failure;

CAD - coronary artery disease; PULM. HYPER. - pulmonary hypertension;

AMI - acute myocardial infarction; AC. HF. - acute heart failure; ° - dose titration;

c - control value; E - exercise test value; N - normal patients.

MPAP (mmHg)				SVR dynes s cm^{-5}		CO* / CI** L/min L/min/m^2	
1			24h	1	24h	1	24h
				^{c}1924/ -14%	NS	NS	, NS
						1,5	4h
						NS/NS*	
						NS/NS*	
						NS/NS*	
1-6			24h	1-6	24h	6	24h
^{c}35/ -23%			-13	NS	NS	5%**	NS
						90 min	
						NS	
						NS	
				0,5-6	24h	0.5-6	24h
				^{c}1860/ -18%	-15%	^{c}2.0**/ 30%	25%
				2	24h	2	24h
				NS	NS	NS	NS
2	4	12	24h	2	24h	2	24h
^{c}33%/NS	-27%	-18%	NS	NS	NS	NS	NS
				2 6 10 16	24h	2 6 10 16	24h
					NS		NS
2	4	6	24h				
^{c}38/-26% -29%	-29%	-19%					
-16% -16%	-13%						

that the arterial dilating effect was attenuated with the increased dose on day 2 of application.

99. In Lempereur et al. (69) (abstract), eight patients with chronic heart failure were assessed in an open trial with the nitroglycerin patch in the dose of 5–10 mg per 24 h. The pulmonary capillary pressure showed a decrease (51%), reaching maximal values between 2 and 10 h after application and lasting until 24 h after application; cardiac output and arterial blood pressure did not change significantly. Similar changes were observed during the administration of intravenous nitroglycerin in the dose of 30 µg/min.

100. In Bergbauer et al. (70, 71) (article), two groups of 10 patients with coronary artery disease and with slightly elevated pulmonary capillary pressure (12 and 13 mm Hg) were investigated at rest and during exercise with two doses of the nitroglycerin patch (5 and 10 mg per 24 h) in a placebo-controlled double-blind study. Both groups showed a decrease in pulmonary capillary pressure (5 mg, 30%; 10 mg, 39%) at rest and in mean pulmonary pressure both at rest and after exercise (50-watt work load) (5 mg, 22 and 13%; 10 mg, 30 and 25%) at 2 h after dosing. The cardiac index was also changed at rest (5 mg, not significant; 10 mg, 19% decrease) and at exercise (5 mg, 15% decrease; 10 mg, no significant increase–3%). There was no change in systemic arterial pressure and heart rate, except a significant drop induced by the 10-mg patch during 50-watt exercise. These results are supported by an echocardiographic study also carried out on 20 patients, using the same test design, on the 5 and 10 mg per 24 h nitroglycerin patch (71). The reduction in left ventricular diastolic and systolic diameter was shown at 2 h after acute dosing and partly attenuated after 4 weeks of continuous therapy (5 mg: LVDD by 5 and 5%; LVSD by 6 and 6%; 10 mg: LVDD by 8 and 4%; LVSD by 13 and 7%).

101. In Osterspey et al. (72) (article), three groups of 8 patients (24 patients) with coronary artery disease were investigated in an open study using the 5, 10, or 20 mg per 24 h nitroglycerin patch. They showed a decrease in mean pulmonary artery pressure 2 h after dosing at rest and during the exercise test (5 mg, 22 and 13%; 10 mg, 22 and 21%; 20 mg, 26 and 39%). These effects were dose dependent. The systemic arterial pressure and heart rate were not changed at any dosage. A comparison with a single dose of 20 mg 5-isosorbide mononitrate showed a decrease in mean pulmonary artery pressure at rest by 26% and during the exercise test by 30%, equivalent to the efficacy of the 20 mg per 24 h patch.

102. In Wiechmann et al. (73) (article), 30 patients with coronary artery disease were investigated in an open study with the nitroglycerin patch (10 mg per 24 h) at rest and with 3 min of 50-Watt exercise testing. No changes in systemic arterial pressure and heart rate were found. A decrease was observed in the pulmonary capillary

pressure from 16 mm Hg by 27 and 32% at rest and by 21 and 26% during exercise at 2 and 24 h after dosing without any change in systemic vascular resistance and cardiac output. The pulmonary artery pressure reverted to baseline values at rest and during exercise 2 h after removal of the patch.

When the patients were divided into two groups of 15 patients each according to the level of increase in mean pulmonary artery pressure during baseline exercise, the results showed two different hemodynamic responses concerning stroke volume. The group of patients with an increase in mean pulmonary artery pressure not above 35 mm Hg during exercise but before application of nitroglycerin patch showed no change in stroke volume induced by nitroglycerin patch. The other 15 patients, with baseline increase in pulmonary artery pressure above 35 mm Hg at exercise, achieved an increase in stroke volume, indicating that the nitroglycerin patch induced improvement of cardiac function.

103. In Vogt and Kreuzer (74) (article), 10 patients with acute heart failure due to coronary artery disease were assessed with the nitroglycerin patch (10 mg per 24 h) in an open protocol by hemodynamic monitoring 1, 2, 4, 6, 8, 10, 12, 16, 20, and 24 h after dosing. A decrease in elevated (24 mm Hg) pulmonary capillary pressure was shown, being maximum after 2 h (25%) and lasting for 16 h, as well as a reduction in the mean pulmonary artery pressure (21%) over 12 h. No changes were observed in the cardiac index, arterial blood pressure, and heart rate. A rebound hemodynamic deterioration appeared in 4 of the 10 patients after removal of the nitroglycerin patch 24 h after application.

104. In Yasky and Carosella (75) (abstract), 10 patients with chronic heart failure refractory to digitalis and diuretics were tested with the 10 mg per 24 h nitroglycerin patch in an open protocol and showed hemodynamic effects, which started 2 h after application and lasted for 24 h. A reduction in elevated (27 mm Hg) pulmonary capillary pressure (17 and 31%), in mean pulmonary artery pressure (19 and 27%), and in systemic vascular resistance (11 and 32%), with an increase in the cardiac index (15 and 30%), was observed. A marked rebound phenomenon occurred after removal of the patch.

105. In Daum and Heinl (76) (article), 10 patients with pulmonary hypertension due to chronic pulmonary disorders were investigated in an open acute and chronic trial with the 10 mg per 24 h nitroglycerin patch. Hemodynamic monitoring was carried out over 24 h before and after single patch application and after 4 weeks of continuous therapy at 2 and 6 h postdosing. A reduction was observed in the pulmonary capillary pressure (45, 67, 67, 56, and 33%) and in the elevated (30 mm Hg) mean pulmonary artery pressure (20, 30, 30, 27, and 13%) at 2, 6, 10, 14, and 24 h after dosing, and an increase was seen in the cardiac output (14, 22, and 10%) at 2, 6, and 10 h, but not at 14 and 24 h, after single patch application.

After 4 weeks of therapy, a sustained reduction in pulmonary capillary pressure (50 and 33%) and in mean pulmonary artery pressure (22 and 19%) was found at 2 and 6 h of monitoring, without further significant changes in the cardiac output.

106. In Reale and Motolese (77) (article), eight patients with coronary artery disease were assessed in a placebo-controlled, double-blind, randomized crossover study with the 10 and 20 mg per 24 h nitroglycerin patches and hemodynamic monitoring at rest, at 0, 2, 4, 6, 8, 12, and 24 h, and after the exercise test at 0, 4, and 24 h postdosing. A decrease in the systolic blood pressure and in the cardiac output was found with both patches over 24 h and a decrease in the pulmonary capillary pressure and in mean pulmonary artery pressure at 4 h postdosing in the rest, but these changes as well as those observed during exercise test, were not statistically significant.

107. In Packer et al. (78) (abstract), 11 patients with severe chronic heart failure were investigated in an open trial with 10–40 mg nitroglycerin patches with hemodynamic monitoring over 24 h postdosing, 2 h after patch removal and after oral isosorbide dinitrate (40 mg) given 2 h after patch removal. A decrease in mean arterial pressure (12%) and in systemic vascular resistance (14%) without change in the cardiac index was observed only at 1 h postdosing. A reduction in pulmonary capillary pressure was maintained, although attenuated, from 1 to 24 h (23 and 15%). Patch removal induced a slight increase in all parameters toward the baseline value. Isosorbide dinitrate administration induced an increase in the cardiac index (21%) and a decrease in pulmonary capillary pressure (35%) and in systemic vascular resistance (24%) at 2 h after dosing.

108. In Taylor et al. (79) (article), two groups of 24 patients with acute myocardial infarction (total, 48 patients) with and without acute heart failure were assessed in an open, randomized comparison trial between three doses of the nitroglycerin patch. The groups of eight patients were randomly allocated to receive a 10, 20, or 40 mg per 24 h nitroglycerin patch with hemodynamic monitoring at 15, 30, 60, 90, 120, 180, and 240 min postdosing. The patients with acute heart failure showed a dose-related reduction, systolic arterial pressure being greater than diastolic pressure in all three treatment groups. A dose-related reduction in pulmonary capillary pressure, with a maximum at 90 min and lasting over 240 min of monitoring (10 mg, 9%; 20 mg, 23%; 40 mg, 23%) was observed, but no changes in the cardiac output were found.

The patients without acute heart failure showed a reduction in mean arterial pressure, being maximal at 90 min and lasting over 240 min, without change in the cardiac output. A decrease in pulmonary capillary pressure sustained from 30 to 240 min after dosing was observed, being similar for all three nitroglycerin doses (27%).

Neither significant change in heart rate nor deleterious fall in blood pressure at the highest nitroglycerin patch dosage occurred in these two groups of patients with acute myocardial infarction.
109. In Olivari et al. (80) (article), the nitroglycerin patches were assessed in nine normal and in nine patients with chronic heart failure (four patients, NYHA class III; 5 patients, class IV) refractory to optimal therapy with digitalis, diuretics, and large doses of oral vasodilator drugs, in an open trial. Normal patients received the 5 or 10 mg per 24 h nitroglycerin patch and showed an increase in heart rate, in forearm blood flow, and in venous capacitance with a decrease in forearm vascular resistance between 2 and 4 h postdosing, but no change in systemic arterial pressure, cardiac index, or systemic vascular resistance during the 6 h of monitoring. Plasma norepinephrine levels increased at 2 h with no change in plasma renin activity.

The patients with heart failure showed no change in heart rate, systemic arterial pressure, or systemic vascular resistance, and stroke index was increased only at 6 h. The decrease in pulmonary capillary pressure (22%) and pulmonary vascular resistance (25%) persisted only for the first 6 h. The reduction in mean pulmonary artery pressure was maximal at 6 h (23%) and lasted with an attenuation by 24 h (13%). Removal of the nitroglycerin patch was followed by a significant rebound increase in pulmonary capillary pressure, mean pulmonary artery pressure, systemic and pulmonary vascular resistance, and mean arterial pressure and a decrease in stroke index. All variables returned to baseline values in the period of 2 h. Plasma norepinephrine and plasma renin activity did not change during 24 h of patch therapy or after its removal, meaning that this transient hemodynamic rebound was not related to stimulation of the sympathetic or renin-angiotensin systems.

110. In Verma et al. (81) (abstract), an open, randomized comparison study between the nitroglycerin patch (10 mg per 24 h) and intravenous isosorbide dinitrate (50–200 µg/kg per hr) was carried out in 16 patients with acute heart failure after acute myocardial infarction, with monitoring over 90 min of the therapy. Both nitrates elicited a similar decrease in pulmonary capillary pressure (20-mg patch and IV ISDN, 24%) and in mean arterial pressure (20-mg patch, 4%; IV ISDN, 8%) without change in the cardiac index at 90 min after dosing.

111. In Rajfer et al. (82) (article), nine patients with chronic heart failure (five patients, NYHA class III; four patients, class IV) were assessed in an open trial with the nitroglycerin patch (15–40 mg per 24 h) (three patients, 15–30 mg; six patients, 40 mg per 24 h) by hemodynamic monitoring at 0.5, 1, 1.5, 2, 4, 6, 8, 16, and 24 h after dosing. The nitroglycerin patch dosage was titrated to obtain the hemodynamic endpoint that had been previously achieved by

nitroglycerin infusion and averaged 2.6 µg/kg per minute. A nitroglycerin infusion was administered initially to establish a dose-response relationship for nitroglycerin and to estimate an equipotent dose of the nitroglycerin patch. The nitroglycerin patch showed a change in hemodynamic parameters with a peak at 6 h and sustained effects by 24 h after dosing and a decrease in pulmonary capillary pressure (25 and 17%) and in systemic vascular resistance (18 and 15%) with an increase in the cardiac index (30 and 25%).

After removal of the patch, heart rate and mean arterial pressure were unchanged. The hemodynamic variables returned to baseline values without rebound effect. There was a significantly greater decrease in pulmonary capillary pressure and mean arterial pressure with the nitroglycerin infusion compared with the nitroglycerin patch. There was no difference in the cardiac index or systemic vascular resistance, right atrial pressure, or heart rate between the two nitroglycerin formulations.

112. In Elkayam et al. (83) (abstract), 10 patients with chronic heart failure were tested in an open study with the 30–60 mg per 24 h nitroglycerin patch, with hemodynamic monitoring over 24 h.

The only hemodynamic variable showing a significant change was pulmonary capillary pressure, with a reduction in baseline value 30 mm Hg by 20% at 12 and 24 h after dosing. The authors explained that a 20% reduction in pulmonary capillary pressure was observed in 5 patients but did not last more than 10 h. The baseline values were again restored within 1 h after removal of the nitroglycerin patch.

113. In Jordan et al. (84) (article), 25 patients with chronic heart failure (NYHA class III and IV) were assessed with the nitroglycerin patch in two parts. In the first part, a hemodynamic effective dose, in the range of up to 60 mg per 24 h, was defined in eight patients. In the second part, a placebo-controlled, randomized double-blind trial was carried out in 15 patients (8 receiving the 60 mg per 24 h nitroglycerin patch and 7 with a placebo patch) with hemodynamic monitoring over 24 h. No significant effects on heart rate, mean arterial pressure, cardiac index, or systemic vascular resistance were established.

A major change was a reduction in pulmonary capillary pressure (36 and 28%) and a decrease in mean pulmonary artery pressure (27 and 18%), as well as in pulmonary vascular resistance (29 and 14%), being maximal at 4 h and lasting up to 12 h after dosing.

An additional investigation was carried out in this study. The plasma nitroglycerin levels were monitored during the trial, and high plasma concentrations were detected from 1 to 24 h (95). Despite persistently high plasma nitroglycerin concentrations, the pulmonary capillary pressure and other hemodynamic effects were not significantly changed by 18 h.

114. In Elkayam et al. (85) (article), 10 patients with chronic heart failure (NYHA class III and IV) were investigated in an open trial with the 90 mg per 24 h nitroglycerin patch by hemodynamic monitoring over 24 h. Plasma concentrations of catecholamines and renin were determined to be at baseline 2 and 24 h after patch dosing and 1 h after removal of the drug. No significant change was observed in heart rate, mean arterial pressure, cardiac index, or systemic and pulmonary vascular resistance. A significant decrease in elevated (27 mm Hg) pulmonary capillary pressure was found only at 2 h after dosing. Individual analysis of pulmonary capillary pressure revealed a 20% or greater reduction in the different time periods over 24 h in 8 of 10 patients. However, these effects were of short duration, being longer than 8 h in only 4 patients. There was no hemodynamic rebound during 2 h after removal of the nitroglycerin patch. No significant changes were found in serum catecholamine levels and renin concentration, indicating that hemodynamic attenuation is not a result of activation of a vasoconstrictive mechanism during continuous nitroglycerin patch therapy.

115. In Roth et al. (86) (abstract), an open study, the hemodynamic effect of the first and second doses of the 120 mg per 24 h nitroglycerin patch was compared in 11 patients with chronic heart failure who had demonstrated more than 20% reduction in pulmonary capillary pressure and were defined as responders to single patch administration. A significant reduction in right atrial pressure, pulmonary artery pressure (26, 29, 29, and 19%), and pulmonary capillary pressure (35, 39, 39, and 27%) lasting over 24 h (at 2, 4, 6, and 24 h) was found in these patients after the first patch application. A significant attenuation of these variables was demonstrated at 2, 4, and 6 h after the second patch application compared with the first day values (pulmonary artery pressure, 16, 16, and 13%; pulmonary capillary pressure, 16, 19, and 27%).

IV. MULTICENTFR STUDIES OF THE NITROGLYCERIN PATCH IN EUROPE

All multicenter studies conducted in Europe in patients with stable angina pectoris are presented in Table 5. The data are again described in a standardized way giving the name of the author, the nitroglycerin patch preparation, the dose per 24 h, the number of patients, and the duration of the trial. Therapeutic efficacy was estimated by the improvement in exercise capacity, by a decrease in angina attacks and sublingual nitroglycerin consumption, and by evaluation of treating physicians and the patients of overall subjective and objective evidence of antianginal improvement. All changes in the parameters are calculated as a percentage versus the values before therapy with the nitroglycerin patch.

Table 5 Multicenter Studies in Angina Pectoris in Europe

Author	Prepa-ration	Dose mg/24 hours	Other the-rapy	Pats. No.	Duration	Increase in exercise capacity
116. Garnier[87]	Trans-derm	5	BBL CAA	87	4 weeks	
117. Bridgman[88]	Trans-derm	5	BBL CAA NITRATE	2461	7-84 days 35 days 66% patients	°48% patients
118. Haehn[89]	Depo-nit	5	No	7880	4 weeks	
119. Letzel[90]	Trans-derm	5	BBL CAA	29457	3 weeks	
120. Garnier[91]	Trans-derm	5-10	BBL CAA	157	4 weeks	
121. Auer[92]	Trans-derm ISDN R	5 10 80 160	DIG	74 46 28 43 31	4 weeks 4 weeks	°45% ° 47%
122. Strano[93]	Depo-nit	5 10 5-10	BBL CAA	102 59 36 7	36 days	
123. Völker[94]	Depo-nit	10	DIG. DIUR.	409	2 weeks	°22% °°-38% 83% patients

SE - Side effects

Decrease in anginal attacks	Decrease in SL NTG comsumption	Positive efficacy estimated by physicians*/ patients**		Other results
-47%	-46% patients	°78%* °66%**		°Better than previous treatment
81% patients	-	73%* 83%**	SE 30%	°Decrease in anginal attacks and increase in exercise capacity
-69%	-69%	93%*	SE 20%	
° 3% °°21% ^{c} °52% °°30% ^{t} patients	-74%	93%* 88%**	SE 20%	c- control values t- values after 3 weeks of therapy °- no anginal attacks °°- attacks only at hard exercise
-61%	88% patients	°67%**		°Better than previous treatment
-65%	-66%	74%*/**		°Exercise test (working capacity Watt x min)
-52%	-51%	76%*/**		
-77% ° -76%	-80%	75%* 74%**	SE 26%	°Decrease in number of effort anginal attacks
-67%	-67%	88%* 92%**	SE 25%	°Working capacity (Watt x min) °°ST depression (exercise test)

116. In Garnier et al. (87) (article), a group of 29 specialists of internal medicine and general practitioners (Switzerland) investigated the antianginal efficacy of the 5 mg per 24 h nitroglycerin patch in an open trial in 87 patients with stable angina pectoris during 4 weeks of continuous therapy. The patients continued to receive previous therapy, except long-acting nitrates. A decrease in anginal attacks and in sublingual nitroglycerin consumption was significant after 2 weeks (30 and 38%) and even augmented after 4 weeks of therapy (47 and 46% of patients). Neither systolic nor diastolic blood pressure was changed, but a decrease in heart rate was significant after 4 weeks. The cutaneous tolerability was good. Cutaneous reddening or itching appeared at the end of 2 weeks in 7% and at 4 weeks only in 1% of patients. Other side effects (headache, nausea, and dizziness) occurred in 7% and in 1% of patients at the end of 2 and 4 weeks of therapy. After 4 weeks, the physicians evaluated the nitroglycerin patch as more effective than previous therapy in 78% of the patients, and 66% of patients had the same opinion. After 2 years, as shown by the answers returned to a written questionnaire, 60% of patients were still receiving the nitroglycerin patch with sustained antianginal efficacy.

117. In Bridgman et al. (88) (article), a group of 790 general practitioners (Great Britain) investigated in an open trial 2461 patients with stable angina pectoris on therapy with nitroglycerin patch (5 mg per 24 h). The duration of follow-up was from 7 to 84 days; 66% of patients were surveyed from 22 to 35 days. Concomitant therapy consisted of the β blockers, Ca antagonists, and long-acting nitrates. A decrease in anginal attacks was estimated in 81% of patients, and 48% of patients also achieved an increase in exercise capacity. A positive efficacy of the nitroglycerin patch was estimated by 73% of physicians and by 83% of patients. The majority of patients (70%) experienced no side effects; in 19% of patients occasional and transient side effects appeared, and 10% of patients felt them as persistent and troublesome. Headaches, dizziness, and faintness were the most important side effects, appearing in 24% of patients.

118. In Haehn (89) (article), a multicenter open study (1979 centers, Federal Republic of Germany) was carried out over 4 weeks of therapy with the nitroglycerin patch (5 mg per 24 h) in 7880 patients with stable angina pectoris. The patients did not receive any other concomitant therapy. A decrease in angina attacks per week (69%) and in sublingual nitroglycerin consumption (69%) was found. The number of patients without any anginal attacks per week increased by 16.5% and from one to two attacks per week in a further 43% of patients, while before therapy only 6.8% of patients had demonstrated from 0 to 2 anginal attacks per week. In 19.7% of patients, some side effects were observed: in 15.4% of cases,

headache; in 3.3% of cases, cutaneous reactions; and in 1.2%, dizziness. Nitroglycerin patch efficacy was evaluated by the physicians to be "very good" or "good" in 93% of patients, and they suggested continuing long-term therapy in 95% of patients. The patients estimated the nitroglycerin patch therapy as "very good" or "good" in 92% of cases.

119. In Letzel and Johnson (90) (article), a multicenter, open study (Federal Republic of Germany) was carried out in 29,457 patients with stable angina pectoris over 3 weeks of nitroglycerin patch (5 mg per 24 h) therapy; however, in 12.9% of patients the nitroglycerin dose was augmented to 10 mg per 24 h during the trial. All previous therapy (β blockers and Ca antagonists) was continued, except the long-acting nitrates. There was important improvement in the angina attacks per week: 52.3% of patients were without anginal attacks at the end of the third week compared with 3.1% at the beginning, 29.6% of patients had pains only with hard exercise compared with 21.4% before the trial, and 13.4% of patients had anginal attacks with daily activities compared with 40% of patients on previous therapy. Sublingual nitroglycerin consumption was decreased by 74%, with 52% of patients not consuming any short-acting nitrates in the third week of therapy compared with 13.5% before the trial. Side effects appeared in 20% of patients: in 13.7% as headache, in 2.6% as dizziness and nausea, and in 3.8% of patients as a cutaneous reaction. The nitroglycerin patch efficacy was estimated "very good" or "good" in 93% of patients by physicians and in 88% of causes by patients.

120. In Garnier and Kenzelman (91) (article), a multicenter, open study was conducted by 58 physicians (Switzerland) in 157 patients with stable angina pectoris with the nitroglycerin patch (5 mg, 79 patients; 10 mg per 24 h, 78 patients) during 4 weeks of therapy. The patients were on their previous therapy (β blockers and Ca antagonists), except that the long-acting nitrates were withdrawn. After 2 weeks of therapy, 43 patients were withdrawn from the study because of cutaneous intolerability (6.4%), headaches (5.7%), unsatisfactory efficacy (5.7%), general preferance for tablets (4.4%), difficulties in handling system (1.3%), and in 3.8% of cases, for reasons not related to patch therapy. After 4 weeks of therapy, 114 patients were still participating, with a decrease of 61% in anginal attacks per week and an 88% reduction in sublingual nitroglycerin consumption. Side effects were recorded in 36% of the total number of patients (157), with cutaneous reactions (erythema and itching) in 23% and headaches in 12% of cases. At the end of the study, 67% of patients expressed a preference for the nitroglycerin patch over oral long-acting nitrates.

121. In Auer (92) (article), a multicenter, open, randomized comparison study (Federal Republic of Germany) between the nitroglycerin patch (5 mg per 24 h) and two tablets of isosorbide dinitrate

(slow-release, 40 mg) was conducted in two periods of 4 weeks in 74 patients with stable angina pectoris. Therapeutic efficacy was estimated by exercise testing, number of angina episodes, and sublingual nitroglycerin consumption. The exercise capacity (watt × minute) was improved by both nitrates (patch, 45%; ISDN, 47%) at the end of 4 weeks. Anginal attacks (patch, 65%; ISDN, 52%) and sublingual nitroglycerin consumption (patch, 66%; ISDN, 52%) were · also reduced. The physicians and patients estimated therapy efficacy as "very good" or "good" for the nitroglycerin patch in 74% and for isosorbide dinitrate in 76% of cases. More patients expressed a preference for nitroglycerin patch therapy (68%) than for ISDN (32%). Overall evaluation did not show significant differences between the efficacy of the nitroglycerin patch and oral isosorbide dinitrate.

122. In Strano et al. (93) (article), a multicenter, open study was conducted in eight institutions (Italy) in 107 patients suffering from effort (51 patients) and/or rest stable angina pectoris (50 patients rest angina; 6 patients both angina). A total of 59 patients were treated with the 5 mg per 24 h nitroglycerin patch, 36 patients with the 10 mg per 24 h patch, and 7 reduced the dose from 10 to 5 mg per 24 h during the trial. The mean duration of treatment was 36.5 days, and 102 patients completed the study. Previous treatment (β blockers or Ca antagonists) was continued, except long-acting nitrates. The number of angina attacks during rest and with effort was reduced (78 and 76%), as well as sublingual nitroglycerin consumption, during rest by 77% and during exercise by 81%. Side effects appeared in 26% of patients: as headaches in 17% of cases, as tachycardia in 5% of cases, and as hypotension in 4% of patients. Cutaneous reactions occurred in 5% of patients without more serious problems with patch application. Physicians estimated the nitroglycerin efficacy as "very good" or "good" in 75% of patients, and the patients stated the same for effort angina in 76% and for rest angina in 71% of cases.

123. In Völker (94) (article), a multicenter, open trial was conducted in 216 centers (Federal Republic of Germany) in 409 patients with stable angina pectoris. The patients were investigated under therapy with the nitroglycerin patch (10 mg per 24 h) over 2 weeks, by exercise test, and by clinical follow-up. The patients continued to receive their previous therapy, except antianginal drugs. Exercise testing at the end of 2 weeks showed improvement in the working capacity (watt × minute) by 22%, a decrease in ST-segment depression in 76% of patients, by 38% with the comparable test and by 32% with the maximum exercise test. An improvement in ST-segment depression and/or work load (watt/minute) during the maximum exercise test was demonstrated in 83% of patients. The number of anginal attacks and sublingual nitroglycerin consumption per week decreased

the same, by 67%. The number of patients without pains (34%) or with one to two angina attacks per week (36%) was generally improved (70%) compared with the number (18%) before nitroglycerin patch treatment. Side effects appeared in 24.6% of patients, mainly as headaches (22%), and in 2.3% of cases as cutaneous reactions. The number and severity of headaches diminished over 2 weeks of therapy; at the end of second week it occurs only in 14% of the total number of patients at the beginning of patch application. At the end of the trial, 88% of physicians and 92% of patients judged the efficacy of nitroglycerin patch therapy as "very good" or "good."

V. OLD AND NEW DATA ABOUT NITROGLYCERIN PATCH EFFICACY

Several overviews have recently appeared discussing the problem of clinical efficacy of nitroglycerin patches in angina pectoris and congestive heart failure. Based on reviewed publications, the authors proposed the following conclusions (1,2,95–99):

1. The magnitude of nitroglycerin patch therapeutic effect in angina pectoris appears to be relatively modest and less than the maximum achievable with other nitrates, in "low" doses, that is, 5–10 mg per 24 h.
2. Antianginal efficacy does not provide continuous 24-h protection for the patient. It may be assumed that the nitroglycerin patch in an adequately high dose is likely to demonstrate antianginal and anti-ischemic benefit for 8–10 h after application.
3. Adequate dose requires the use of multiple patches, from 20 to 45 mg per 24 h, and should be documented by demonstrating a hemodynamic effect.
4. Acute antianginal efficacy completely disappears during continuous treatment, so intermittent therapy with nitrate-free intervals between two patch applications is recommended.
5. The nitroglycerin patch seems to be effective in congestive heart failure, but high doses of nitroglycerin patch are necessary. It is likely that the effects of the nitroglycerin patch persists in heart failure longer than in angina pectoris, but it seems clear the the desired nitrate effect does not last over 24 h.
6. The nitroglycerin patch therapy produces constant plasma levels over 24 h, which induces the rapid development of nitrate tolerance and during continuous patch administration.

These authors based their conclusions on a limited number of published clinical trials showing mostly modest efficacy and a short duration of action after nitroglycerin patch application.

Reichek (1) discussed 6 clinical studies, Abrams cited in his four reviews 11 (2), 10 (96), 9 (97), and 10 (98) trials, and Parker (99) reviewed 4 investigations. The major discussion concerned 11 clinical trials (3,12,21,22,40,46,57,62,68,80,82), and a total number of 18 publications were reviewed in these six overviews. Serious criticism about the clinical efficacy of nitroglycerin patch therapy was raised by these articles, but at the same time controversies appeared about the validity of these conclusions in explaining some beneficial findings. Scheidt (100) reviewed 13 acute and long-term clinical trials and tried to analyze the reasons for some obvious discrepancies among studies, in the different magnitude of efficacy and duration of action reported for nitroglycerin patch therapy.

Numerous new studies have appeared and give new possibilities for better understanding of nitroglycerin patch action. The aim of this chapter is to present all published clinical trials in angina pectoris and congestive heart failure, as well as multicenter studies in Europe, available up to spring 1986, and to analyze the variability of nitroglycerin patch responses regarding efficacy and duration of action.

A total number of 94 publications with 123 trials are presented. All acute and long-term (semichronic and chronic) studies in angina pectoris accounted for 96 studies. There were 47 acute studies with 674 patients and 49 chronic trial with 895 patients. The total number of patients studied was smaller, since 17 acute studies with 321 patients were also investigated during chronic follow-up. Altogether, there were only 30 acute studies with 353 patients, only 32 chronic studies with 574 patients, and 17 combined acute and chronic studies with 321 patients, a total of 1248 patients with angina pectoris (Tables 1, 2, and 3).

A. Summary of Acute Nitroglycerin Patch Trials in Angina Pectoris

All 47 acute studies could be divided into 43 positive and 4 negative studies. The positive studies were those demonstrating a positive efficacy early (1–12 h) and/or late (12–24 h) after dosing and negative studies those without proven efficacy in either period (Table 1).

Acute positive studies demonstrated different durations of nitroglycerin patch action. In 8 studies with 125 patients, positive early efficacy was shown, constituting 17% of all acute studies, but nothing could be said about the action in later periods since it was not tested (Table 1.1). In 15 studies with 140 patients (32% of all acute studies) an early efficacy was found with attenuation of the effects 8–14 h after dosing (Table 1.2). In 20 studies with 353 patients (42.5% of all acute studies), a 24-h duration of nitroglycerin patch action was proven (Table 1.3). Four studies with 56 patients (8.5% of all acute studies) showed a complete absence of efficacy: 2 studies over 24 h, 1 study from 1–8 h, and 1 study at 22 h, which were the periods of testing (Table 1.4). All together, 38 acute studies were made over 24 h. In 20 studies (53% of all tested studies), a sustained 24-h duration of action was maintained; in 15 studies (39%) action was limited to the first 8–14 h, and in 3 studies (8%) there was no significant effect at all. ·

B. Summary of Semichronic and Chronic Nitroglycerin Patch Trials in Angina Pectoris

There were a total of 49 semichronic or chronic clinical trials in angina pectoris found; 33 studies, or 67% of the total number, demonstrated a positive efficacy in 669 patients and 16 negative studies, or 33%, with 226 patients showed no significant action at any part of the day (Tables 2 and 3).

Semichronic and chronic positive studies covered a period of follow-up from 2 days to 12 months, with 15 studies from 14 to 28 days and 10 studies from 2 to 12 months. The 16 chronic positive studies (33% of all chronic studies) with 276 patients demonstrated a 24-h duration of action during 2 days to 12 months of continuous nitroglycerin patch therapy. Thirteen of the 16 studies were conducted from 2 to 12 days; 3 studies were followed for 3–12 months. These studies showed a sustained efficacy at 1, 2, 3, 5, 8, and 24 h after dosing during long-term treatment.

In 10 studies with 263 patients (20% of all chronic studies), an early efficacy (2, 3, 4, 5, and 7 h after dosing) was observed, without any data about the action 12 h after patch application. These studies were conducted in 7 cases from 14 to 28 days and in 2 cases from 2 to 6 months.

In 7 studies with 130 patients (14% of all studies), positive efficacy was shown but the time of testing was not indicated. However, these are studies with the greatest number of long-term follow-ups: in 3 studies, 1–2 months and in 2 studies, 5 months.

In 16 studies, a negative efficacy was demonstrated. In 8 studies testing was carried out over 24 h; in the remaining 8 studies testing was from 2.5 to 8 h or the time after dosing was not indicated. Most of these studies (14) were conducted from 2–14 days, and only 2 investigations were followed up from 1–2 months of continuous patch therapy.

Of the total 24 chronic studies, 24 h testing was carried out, demonstrating in 16 studies (67%) sustained efficacy over 24 h and in 8 trials (33%) complete absence of significant effect.

In 17 studies with 321 patients, acute investigation was continued by semichronic and chronic patch therapy, with 15 studies positive and 2 studies negative in acute testing.

In 12 of 17 studies (70.5%) with 274 patients, positive acute patch efficacy was sustained and confirmed in 4 cases from 7 to 21 days, in 4 cases from 1 to 2 months and in 4 trials from 3 to 12 months of long-term follow-up. In 9 of these studies, a positive 24 h duration of patch action was found in acute studies, maintained over 24 h in 6 long-term studies (67%) with 134 patients, and in 3 chronic studies only early (2 h after dosing), not 24 h efficacy, was tested, so nothing could be said about the later period.

In 5 studies with 47 patients, a negative chronic efficacy was found. In 3 trials, a positive acute efficacy was established 2.5, 4, 8, and 14 h after dosing without positive effects during 2–14 days of patch administration, but 2 trials showed negative efficacy in acute investigation as well as in chronic long-term follow-up from 14 days to 2 months.

Of interest is that 12 trials (80%) of 15 with positive acute efficacy and long-term follow-up maintained significant benefit during continuous nitroglycerin patch therapy, even in 67% of cases with 24 h duration of action. However, in 3 (20%) of 15 trials a positive acute efficacy could not be demonstrated after repeated patch application.

C. Summary of Hemodynamic Studies with the Nitroglycerin Patch

A total of 19 hemodynamic studies and 277 patients with coronary artery disease, acute or chronic heart failure, and pulmonary hypertension are reviewed.

In 18 studies (95% of all studies) with 269 patients, some positive efficacy was observed, but only 1 trial did not demonstrate significant hemodynamic effect.

In most studies (14 or 74% of the total), hemodynamic monitoring was performed over 24 h, with 9 trials (64% of tested studies) demonstrating sustained efficacy over 24 h, and 4 trials (29%) showing at 2, 12, or 16 h after dosing a significant loss of action. In 1 study (7%) no significant change was seen over 24 h after patch application.

In 3 studies with 24 h positive efficacy, acute investigation was continued by continuous patch therapy. In 1 study, a day 2 patch application showed an attenuated but significant effect at 2, 4, and 6 h of testing, and 2 studies demonstrated maintained efficacy at 4–6 h of testing at the end of 4 weeks and 3 months of therapy. The testing was not performed in the later period in either study.

In the remaining 5 of 19 studies, a significant hemodynamic effect was established 1.5, 2, 4, and 8 h after dosing without data for the later period since no further testing was planned.

D. Summary of Multicenter Studies in Europe

A total number of eight multicenter studies with 40,627 patients with angina pectoris were performed with nitroglycerin patch therapy of from 2 to 4 weeks of duration. Significant improvement was detected: a decrease of 47-77% of anginal attacks and a reduction of 51-80% of sublingual nitroglycerin consumption. Positive efficacy was estimated by 73-93% of treating physicians and by 66-92% of patients. Side effects were detected in 20-30% of patients, but they were mostly transient and mild.

It is of interest to emphasize the similarity of findings in different studies, which proves the good and reliable antianginal efficacy of nitroglycerin patch therapy.

E. Analysis of Differences Between Positive
   and Negative Trials

Since a significant beneficial antianginal and anti-ischemic efficacy of the nitroglycerin patch is proved by many trials, as well as the absence or very rapid attenuation of efficacy in the others, a major question is the reason for these differences. The possible reasons included trial design, experimental testing endpoints, the kind of nitroglycerin patch preparation, and the dose of nitroglycerin patch. Since all these variables can influence a final research result independently of differences in pathophysiological mechanisms of the illness itself, they will be analyzed using the data of the trials presented previously.

1. Trial Design

Analysis of the trial designs revealed in most studies great effort by investigators to conduct the research according to meticulously controlled protocols, so only 23 of 96 clinical trials (24%) with angina pectoris patients were performed in an open protocol (21% of all acute and 27% of all chronic trials).

In 16 of 20 acute 24-h positive studies (80%), a placebo-controlled and/or double-blind design was performed (12 studies were placebo controlled, double-blind, randomized crossover; 2 trials were placebo controlled and double-blind).

In 14 of 15 (93%) acute studies with early positive but late negative efficacy, a placebo-controlled and/or double-blind protocol was planned (12 studies, placebo controlled, double-blind, randomized crossover; 2 cases, placebo controlled double-blind).

Of 4 acute negative studies, 2 (50%) were performed in a placebo-controlled, double-blind, randomized crossover manner.

In 23 of 33 (70%) chronic positive studies, a placebo-controlled and/or double-blind protocol was designed (11 studies, placebo controlled, double-blind, randomized crossover; 1 trial, placebo controlled double-blind).

In 13 of 16 (81%) chronic negative studies, a placebo-controlled and/or double-blind design was performed (12 studies, placebo controlled, double-blind, randomized crossover).

Slight differences are seen in the percentage of controlled studies between acute 24-h positive studies and acute studies with early positive/late negative efficacy, 80 versus 93% of trials, as well as between chronic positive and chronic negative studies, 70 versus 81% of trials. However, these differences cannot influence significantly the acute 24-h positive findings and chronic positive results, since they were conducted with much larger patient samples than trials showing acute early positive/late negative efficacy or chronic negative effects (353 versus 140 patients; 669 versus 226 patients).

There was no information about a nitrate-free interval in any of the chronic positive or negative studies of angina pectoris.

The influence of trial design on differences in hemodynamic studies is not possible to analyze since an open protocol was planned in 15 of 19 trials, but only in 4 cases were investigations carried out in a placebo-controlled and double- or single-blind manner.

2. Experimental Testing Endpoints

The antianginal and antiischemic efficacy of nitroglycerin patches was estimated by multistage treadmill, bicycle, and climbing step exercise tests in acute and chronic trials with angina pectoris patients. Antianginal efficacy and cardiovascular functional capacity were estimated by maximum exercise time and/or maximum work load (watt/minute) and/or working capacity (watt × minute) and/or time to onset of angina pectoris, as well as in chronic trials by the number of angina episodes and the amount of sublingual nitroglycerin consumption. Anti-ischemic efficacy was measured by a decrease in the maximum ST-segment depression, by a reduction in the sum of ST-segment depressions, and by the time to the onset of ST-segment depression of 1.0 mm.

In 11 of 20 acute 24-h positive trials (55%) and in 7 of 15 acute studies with early positive/late negative efficacy (47%), the data are assessed for both exercise parameters. It seems that acute 24-h positive trials are more rigorously tested, accounting for a much larger number of patients, compared with acute early positive/late negative studies (353 versus 140 patients), which supports the accuracy of the 24-h efficacy results.

In 18 of 33 chronic positive studies (54%) and in 9 of 16 chronic negative studies (56%), both exercise parameters were detected; angina episodes and nitroglycerin consumption were followed in 22 of

33 chronic positive studies (67%) and in only 5 of 16 chronic negative trials (31%). Although the number of anginal episodes and the amount of sublingual nitroglycerin consumption are discounted by some authors, which is perhaps reflected in chronic negative studies, these parameters are additional proof of antianginal improvement in patients investigated during long-term treatment. They also attest to the importance of more precise exercise test findings, since they are demonstrated on a large number of patients (514) in clinically controlled trials.

Hemodynamic efficacy is best measured with several variables that give information about preload and afterload changes. It is of interest to note that 12 of 19 studies with hemodynamic monitoring over 24 h had data for at least three of the following variables: pulmonary capillary pressure, mean pulmonary artery pressure, systemic vascular resistance, and cardiac output, which supports the accuracy of measurements. The remaining 7 of a total of 19 studies, except 1, were described by two or by one hemodynamic parameter.

3. Dose of Nitroglycerin Patch

In 38 of a total number of 47 acute studies (81%) of angina pectoris patients, the 5 and 10 mg per 24 h nitroglycerin patch was administered: in 22 studies (47%), the 5-mg patch and in 16 trials (34%), the 10-mg patch.

The 5 or 10 mg per 24 h nitroglycerin patch was applied in 10 and 9 of 20 acute 24-h positive studies (50 and 45%) and in 6 and 3 of 15 acute early positive/late negative studies (40 and 20%). In a further 6 acute early positive/late negative trial (40%), higher doses (15-30 mg per 24 h) of nitroglycerin patch were administered.

It is worthwhile to mention that a patch of 5 and 10 mg per 24 h did not elicit a significant fall in arterial blood pressure in many acute studies; nevertheless, they demonstrated important positive efficacy. This means that antianginal and anti-ischemic nitroglycerin performance should not be documented by hemodynamic changes since these parameters are not obligatorily correlated.

In 41 of a total of 49 chronic studies (84%), the 5 and 10 mg per 24 h nitroglycerin patches were used: in 25 studies (51%) the 5-mg patch and in 16 trials (33%) the 10-mg patch.

The 5 or 10 mg per 24 h nitroglycerin patch was administered in 19 and 12 of 33 chronic positive studies (58 and 36%) and in 6 and 3 of 16 chronic negative studies (37 and 19%). Higher doses, from 10 to 22.5 mg per 24 h, were applied only in 2 chronic positive trials (6%), but in chronic negative trials, higher doses were administered, in 4 studies (25%) from 15 to 20 mg and in 1 trial (6%) 30 mg per 24 h. A 2.5 mg per 24 h nitroglycerin patch was applied in another 2 chronic negative studies (13%).

These data show that 5 and 10 mg per 24 h nitroglycerin patches were administered in 95% of acute studies with 24 h duration of action and in 94% of chronic studies with positive efficacy for angina pectoris. In contrast, these doses were applied in only 60% of acute studies with early positive/late negative efficacy and in 56% of chronic negative studies. However, higher doses were applied in 40% and in 31% of these studies, suggesting that nitroglycerin patch of 15 mg or more per 24 h could induce complete attenuation of positive acute efficacy and complete absence of the effects in long-term treatment of patients with angina pectoris.

The eight multicenter studies were performed in four trials with 5 mg, in three studies with a dose from 5 to 10 mg, and one study with a 10 mg per 24 h nitroglycerin patch. The positive findings of antianginal efficacy in these trials support the beneficial actions of the 5 and 10 mg patch in chronic clinical studies.

The 5 or 10 mg per 24 h nitroglycerin patch was administered in 11 of 19 hemodynamic studies (58%); in another 8 studies (42%), higher doses, from 15 to 120 mg per 24 h, were applied.

In the hemodynamic trials with efficacy over 24 h in five of nine cases (56%) a dose from 5 to 10 mg was administered, and in another four studies (44%) a higher dose was needed: in three cases 15–40 mg and in one case a 120 mg per 24 h nitroglycerin patch. One study was negative over 24 h with the 10 mg per 24-h patch.

The four hemodynamic studies with early positive/late negative efficacy were performed in one case with the 10-mg patch (2–16 h duration of action) and in three cases with 30–90 mg per 24 h of nitroglycerin (2 and 12 h duration of action).

Of the five hemodynamic studies positive from 1 to 8 h after dosing, without data in later period, in four cases (80%) a dose from 5 to 10 mg per 24 h of nitroglycerin was also administered.

These data indicate that 24 h hemodynamic efficacy was effected in 80% of cases with a dose from 5 to 40 mg; however, in 50% of cases these effects were induced by the 5–10 mg per 24 h nitroglycerin patch. Attenuation of early positive efficacy was related in 75% of cases after higher administered doses, with nitroglycerin patch in the range from 30 to 90 mg per 24 h.

4. Nitroglycerin Patch Preparations

The four preparations of nitroglycerin patch used in the studies reviewed were Transderm,* Deponit, Nitro-Dur, and Nitrodisc.

---

*All CIBA patch preparations are arbitrarily named Transderm for easier comparison.

In 47 acute studies, the different patch preparations were administered as follows: Transderm in 16 studies, 34%; Deponit in 19 trials, 40%; Nitro-Dur in 8 studies, 17%; and Nitrodisc in 4 investigations, 9%.

Transderm, given in 16 acute studies, induced in 5 studies (31%) 24 h positive efficacy, in 4 studies (25%) early positive/late negative efficacy, in 5 studies (31%) early positive/late not studied efficacy, and in 2 studies (13%) negative efficacy.

Deponit, given in 19 acute studies, effected in 10 studies (53%) 24 h positive efficacy, in 6 studies (32%) early positive/late negative efficacy, in 2 studies (10%) early positive/late not studied efficacy, and in 1 study (5%) negative efficacy.

Nitro-Dur, administered in eight acute studies, induced in four studies (50%) 24 h positive efficacy, in three studies (38%) early positive/late negative efficacy, and in one study (12%) early positive/late not studied efficacy.

Nitrodisc, applied in four acute studies, effected in one study 24 h positive efficacy, in one study early positive/late negative efficacy, and in two studies early positive/late not studied efficacy.

In 48 chronic studies,* the patch preparations were applied as follows: Transderm in 25 studies, 52%; Deponit in 17 studies, 35%; Nitro-Dur in 5 studies, 10%; and Nitrodisc in 1 study, 2%.

Transderm, given in 25 studies, induced in 13 studies (52%) positive efficacy and in 12 cases (48%) negative efficacy.

Deponit, applied in 17 studies, effected in 15 studies (88%) positive efficacy and in 2 trials (12%) negative efficacy.

Nitro-Dur, administered in five studies, induced in three studies (60%) positive efficacy and in two studies (40%) negative efficacy.

Nitrodisc was applied in one study and induced positive efficacy.

These data show that Transderm therapy induced in 31% of studies acute 24 h positive efficacy and in 52% of trials chronic positive effects, but Deponit administration effected in 52% of trials acute 24 h positive action and in 88% of cases chronic positive effects. These findings suggest that the formulation of nitroglycerin patch preparation (see Chapter 2) may influence their performance in acute and chronic administration.

VI. CONCLUSIONS

In this review, a total of 94 publications with 124 trials are presented. The 115 clinical trials of angina pectoris and congestive heart failure with 1525 patients and eight multicenter studies in

---

*The name of the patch preparation was not noted in one study.

Europe with 40,627 patients are reviewed. The following conclusions could be defined based upon the data from this documentation.

A significant antianginal and anti-ischemic efficacy of nitroglycerin patch therapy in angina pectoris was demonstrated in 43 acute studies with 618 patients and in 33 chronic trials with 669 patients. However, no significant effects were observed in 4 acute studies with 56 patients and in 16 chronic trials with 226 patients.

The 24 h duration of nitroglycerin patch action was shown in 20 acute trials with 353 patients and in 16 chronic studies with 276 patients. This beneficial efficacy was sustained from several days to 12 months of continuous nitroglycerin patch administration. These data show that acute nitroglycerin patch application induced in 67% of patients a significant sustained action over 24 h and in 26% of patients an efficacy significantly attenuated after the first 12 h. In 7% of patients, a complete absence of any effect was observed.

Chronic nitroglycerin patch application induced in 70% of patients a significant efficacy maintained over 24 h. In 30% of patients, no beneficial effects could be detected over 24 h during long-term therapy.

It is concluded that the nitroglycerin patch induces a significant antianginal and anti-ischemic efficacy after single and repeated administration in angina pectoris. There are obviously subsets of patients with efficacy sustained over 24 h and during long-term therapy, those with rapid attenuation of positive acute efficacy over 24 h and during repeated administration, and finally others with no significant beneficial response, in either single or repeated administration.

The beneficial efficacy of single and long-term patch administration is achieved in the greatest number of patients with angina pectoris with a dose of 5 and 10 mg per 24 h of nitroglycerin. However, the data suggest that doses higher than 15 mg per 24 h of nitroglycerin patch may induce a complete attenuation of positive acute efficacy or complete absence of action in long-term treatment.

The nitroglycerin patch demonstrated significant hemodynamic improvement, mainly of preload parameters, in coronary artery disease and in acute or chronic heart failure. This improvement was maintained in 67% of patients over 24 h after a single application, but in 28% of patients these effects were attenuated 10–12 h after dosing. No efficacy could be observed in 5% of patients. The data for long-term therapy are too few to allow any conclusion.

A positive hemodynamic efficacy maintained over 24 h could be achieved in most patients with a dose in the range 5–40 mg per 24 h, and in about half of patients, it could be induced with a nitroglycerin patch dose from 5 to 10 mg per 24 h. It seems that doses higher than 40 mg per 24 h may induce rapid attenuation of early positive efficacy; however, this assumption needs more data to be proved.

This overview of complete documentation of clinical nitroglycerin patch performance gives essentially different conclusions than most earlier reviews of this topic. It may be concluded that nitroglycerin patch therapy in angina pectoris has important antianginal and anti-ischemic efficacy sustained over 24 h and during long-term therapy. This efficacy may be achieved with a nitroglycerin patch of 5 and 10 mg per 24 h as the optimal dose in most patients.

The nitroglycerin patch influences important hemodynamic improvement sustained over 24 h in coronary artery disease and in acute or chronic heart failure after a single nitroglycerin patch application at a dose of 5–40 mg per 24 h; however, in about half the patients a dose of 5–10 mg per 24 h may induce a beneficial effect.

The contributions of this review to the problem of nitroglycerin therapy are the evidence of many clinical trials that the nitroglycerin patch is effective in angina pectoris and in congestive heart failure in the greatest part of the patient population and that relatively low doses are necessary. However, a controversy remains as long as the reasons for the absence of an effect and the cause of a rapid attenuation of primarily beneficial nitroglycerin patch response in some patients are unexplained. This phenomenon is observed in investigations with similar trial protocols, with the same testing methodology, the same dosage, and the same patch preparation, so these variables have a secondary influence. The problems are related to different patients' nitroglycerin sensitivity, to nitroglycerin resistance, and to the development of nitrate tolerance.

However, the most important problem is a definition of patient subsets founded on the pathophysiological mechanisms that play a major role in the etiology of objective and subjective symptoms of the illness that is called stable angina pectoris. This approach could help us to define the indications for nitroglycerin administration based on functioning pathophysiological mechanisms and nitroglycerin's ability to affect it.

The transdermal delivery of nitroglycerin is an interesting concept, and it seems to be beneficial in a great many patients with coronary artery disease. Further investigations should develop this nitrate delivery system to its full and defined clinical application.

REFERENCES

1. N. Reichek, Long-acting nitrates: Relative utility of nitroglycerin patches, *Am. J. Med.*, 76(6A): 63 (1984).
2. J. Abrams, The brief saga of transdermal nitroglycerin discs: Paradise lost? *Am. J. Cardiol.*, 54: 220 (1984).
3. M. Hollenberg and M. Go, Clinical studies with transdermal nitroglycerin, *Am. Heart J.*, 108: 223 (1984).
4. P. Kenedy, Langzeitanwendung eines transdermalen Nitroglycerin bei stabiler Angina pectoris in Klinik und Praxis, *Herzmedizin*, 9: 71 (1986).

5. G. Reiniger, F. Kraus, J. Dirschinger, R. Blasini, and
    W. Rudolph, Hochdosierte transdermale Nitroglycerintherapie:
    Wirkungsverlust innerhalb von 25 Stunden, *Herz*, *10*: 157
    (1985).

6. A. Zeiher, H. Drexler, T. Bonzel, H. Wollschläger, M. H.
    Hust, H. Löllgen, and H. Just, Wirksamkeit verschiedener
    kutan applizierbäre Nitroglycerin-Präparationen bei koronarer
    Herzkrankheit, *Schweiz. Med. Wochenschr.*, *114*(Suppl. 16):
    70 (1984).

7. M. Bassan, The wide variability of the effective dose of Nitro-
    derm patches (abstract), *Israel J. Med. Sci.*, *20*: 742 (1984).

8. G. Nyberg, Antianginal and anti-ischemic effects (immediate and
    1 and 3 h post-dose) of sublingual, buccal and transdermal
    nitroglycerin (abstract), *Br. J. Clin. Pharmacol.*, *19*: 559P
    (1985).

9. G. Colombo, G. Favini, S. Aglieri, G. Pollavini, and C. de Vita,
    Nitroderm TTS in exercise-induced angina pectoris—a random-
    ized double-blind study, *Int. J. Clin. Pharmacol. Ther.*, *23*:
    211 (1985).

10. M. Goldstein, P. Vandermoten, G. Berkenboom, E. Stoupel,
    J. Sobolski, and S. Degre, Evaluation of the efficacy of Nitro-
    derm TTS 10, once a day, and isosorbide dinitrate SR 20 mg
    b.i.d. in patients with stable angina pectoris (abstract), *Eur.
    Heart J.*, *8*(Suppl. 1): 103 (1985).

11. G. Müller, Unterschiedliche Dosierungen von transdermalen
    Nitroglycerin in Abhängigkeit vom Schweregrad der koronaren
    Herzkrankheit, *Münch. Med. Wochenschr.*, *129*: (1986)
    (in press).

12. J. O. Parker and H. L. Fung, Transdermal nitroglycerin in
    angina pectoris, *Am. J. Cardiol.*, *54*: 471 (1984).

13. M. A. James, P. R. Walker, M. Papouchado, and P. R. Wilkin-
    son, Efficacy of transdermal glyceryl nitrate in the treatment
    of chronic stable angina pectoris, *Br. Heart J.*, *53*: 631 (1985).

14. P. Sellier, J. P. Demarez, P. Audouin, B. Payen, P. Corona,
    and P. Ourbak, Nitroglycerin patches (5 and 10 mg) in angina
    pectoris: Dose—effect relationship (abstract), *Eur. Heart J.*,
    6(Suppl. I): 113 (1985).

15. U. Thadani, D. C. Brady, S. J. Klutts, D. R. Goins, J. L.
    Anderson, E. G. Olson, S. F. Hamilton, and S. M. Teague,
    Dose titration and duration of effects of transdermal nitroglyc-
    erin patches in angina pectoris (abstract), *Circulation*, *72*(Suppl.
    III): III–431 (1985).

16. N. Reifart and W. D. Bussmann, Placebo kontrollierte doppel-
    blind Studie zur antiischämischen Wirksamkeit und Wirkdauer
    von transdermalen Depot nitraten, *Z. Kardiol.*, *75*(Suppl. 3):
    83 (1986).

17. C. Gohlke-Bärwolf, P. Betz, and H. Roskam, Wirkung und Wirkdauer eines transdermalen Nitrates Deponit 10 auf die Belastungsischämie: Eine Computer - Belastungs - EKG - Analyse, in *Depot Nitrat* (T. Meinertz, E. Jänchen, A. Schrey, et.), Vaw, München, p. 66 (1985).

18. M. H. Mertens, H. Ohlmeir, M. Möller, and S. Engelbart, Vergleichende Untersuchung dreier verschiedener Nitroglycerinpflaster zur Ermittlung der antiischämischen Wirkung und Wirkdauer im Akutversuch, *Herz Kreislauf*, 19(Suppl. 1): 18 (1986).

19. E. Lönne and J. Chvatik, Nachweis der Wirkung und Wirkdauer von Deponit 10 in einem Doppelblindversuch, in *Depot-Nitrat* (T. Meinertz, E. Jänchen, A. Schrey, ed.), Vaw, München, p. 57 (1985).

20. G. Reiniger, R. Blasini, U. Brügmann, and W. Rudolph, Nitroglycerin patches in coronary artery disease: Can tolerance development be avoided through an interval therapy? (abstract), *Circulation*, 72(Suppl. III): III-431 (1985).

21. N. Reichek, C. Priest, D. Zimrin, T. Chandler, and M. St. John Sutton, Antianginal effects of nitroglycerin patches, *Am. J. Cardiol.*, 54: 1 (1984).

22. N. Reichek, C. Priest, D. Zimrin, T. Chandler, N. Berger, P. Douglas, and M. St. John Sutton, Anginal effects of nitroglycerin over 24 hours: Role of the method of administration (abstract), *Circulation*, 70(Suppl. I): II-90 (1984).

23. M. A. B. Naafs, A. C. De Boer, R. W. Koster, C. W. Klasen, and A. J. Dunning, Exercise capacity with transdermal nitroglycerin in patients with stable angina pectoris, *Eur. Heart J.*, 5: 705 (1984).

24. G. Müller, Antianginöse Wirksamkeit und Wirkdauer von akut und chronisch verabreichtem Depot-Nitrat bei Patienten mit koronarer Herzkrankheit im Doppelblindvergleich mit Placebo, *Herz Kreislauf*, Sonderheft "Stellenwert des transdermalen Depotnitrates in der Therapie der koronaren Herzkrankheit," 12 (1985).

25. J. Weisbort, N. Meshulam, M. Benjamini, F. Zerikier, and D. Brunner, Effects of short- and long-term treatment with transdermally and orally administered nitroglycerin (a double-blind crossover study), *Z. Kardiol.*, 75(Suppl. 3): 96 (1986).

26. D. Hey, Antianginöse und antiischämische Wirkung von Deponit 5 im Vergleich mit einem anderen transdermalen therapeutischen System, *Z. Allg. Med.*, 62: 364 (1986).

27. H. P. Krepp, Wirksamkeit eines neuen Depot-Nitrates: Eine Doppelblindstudie mit Nitroglyzerin-Pflaster bei Koronarkranken, Wissenschaftliche Dokumentation Deponit, 1986.

28. Dž. E. Rezaković, Jr., S. Lakatoš, J. Štalec, and L. Pavičić, Acute and chronic efficacy of low-dose nitroglycerin patches in stable angina pectoris, Z. Kardiol, 75(Suppl. III): 90 (1986).

29. A. J. Georgopoulos, A. Markis, and H. Georgiadis, Therapeutic studies with Nitroderm TTS, in New Horizons in Nitrate Therapy (W. D. Bussmann and S. H. Taylor, eds.), Medizin Verlag, Munich, 1984, p. 7.

30. R. H. Thompson, Clinical use of transdermal delivery devices with nitroglycerin (abstract), Circulation, 68(4, II): III-407 (1983).

31. G. Sabin and S. Görlitz, Interindividueller Vergleich der Wirkung von 1 Deponit 5 bzw. 2 Deponit 5. Belastungs-EKG, Echokardiographie, Rechtsherzkatheter, (abstract 7), 3-Forum Depot Nitrat, Feb. 21-22, 1986, Flims, Switzerland.

32. B. Cerri, F. Grasso, M. Cefis, and G. Pollavini, Comparative evaluation of the effect of two doses of Nitroderm TTS on exercise-related parameters in patients with angina pectoris, Eur. Heart J., 5: 710 (1984).

33. M. Fazio, S. Novo, A. Giannola, L. Adamo, G. Allaimo, and A. Strano, Effects of transdermal application of trinitroglycerin on exercise performance and thallium stress scintigraphy in patients with effort angina pectoris (abstract), Eur. Heart J., 5(Suppl.): 1368 (1984).

34. P. Pucci, G. Zambaldi, G. Cerisano, and P. Roccanti, Valutazione di un nuovo preparato di nitroglicerina percutanea nell angina da sforzo, G. Ital. Cardiol., 13: 167 (1983).

35. P. H. Krepp, Wirkdauer über 24 Stunden von Deponit 10 akut und nach 7 Tagen im Vergleich zu Placebo in der Auswaschund Auslassphase, Herz Kreislauf, 19(Suppl. 1): 3 (1986).

36. P. Wagner, Die antianginöse Wirkung von Deponit 10 bei Patienten mit Koronarer Herzerkrankung und stabiler Angina pectoris, Herz Kreislauf, Sonderheft "Stellenwert des transdermalen Depot-Nitrats in der Therapie der Koronaren Herzkrankheit," 16 (1985).

37. S. Scardi, F. Pivotti, F. Fonda, C. Pandullo, M. Castelli, and G. Pollavini, Effect of a new transdermal therapeutic system containing nitroglycerin on exercise capacity in patients with angina pectoris, Am. Heart J., 110: 546 (1985).

38. W. Heepe, Transdermales Nitroglycerin (10 mg/24 Std) im placebokontrollierten Akutversuch und während einer offenen Therapie über 12 Monate bei stabiler Angina pectoris, Herz Kreislauf, 19(Suppl. 1): 30 (1986).

39. G. Schiavoni, M. Mazzari, G. Lanza, A. Frustaci, R. Mongiardo, and F. Pennestri, Evaluation of the efficacy and the length of action of a new preparation of slow release nitroglycerin for

percutaneous absorption (Nitro-dur, Sigma-Tau) in angina pectoris caused by exercise, *Int. J. Clin. Pharmacol. Res.*, *2*(Suppl. 1): 15 (1982).

40. M. J. O'Hara, N. S. Khurmi, M. J. Bowles, S. W. Duffy, C. W. Robinson, and E. B. Raftery, Is transdermal nitroglycerin effective for the treatment of stable angina pectoris? (abstract), *JACC*, *5*: 506 (1985).

41. R. S. Kohli, M. J. O'Hara, N. S. Khurmi, C. W. Robinson, A. Lahiri, and E. B. Raftery, Transdermal dose titration with glyceryl trinitrate patches—an objective study with angina pectoris (abstract 550). Cardiovascular Pharmacotherapy International Symposium, April 22-25, 1984, Geneva.

42. W. Schneider, O. Michel, M. Kaltenbach, and W.-D. Bussmann, Antianginöse Wirkung von transdermal appliziertem Nitroglycerin in Abhängigkeit von der Pflastergrösse, *Dtsch. Med. Wochenschr.*, *110*: 87 (1985).

43. Dž. E. Rezaković, Wirksamkeit von Nitroglycerin-Pflaster bei stabiler Angina pectoris in einer doppelblinden placebokontrolierten klinischen Studie über 2 Wochen, *Herz Kreislauf*, Sonderheft "Stellenwert des transdermalen Depotnitrats in der Therapie der koronaren Herzkrankheit," 7 (1985).

44. A. S. Kapor, N. S. Dang, and R. D. Reynolds, Sustained effects of transdermal nitroglycerin in patients with angina pectoris, *Clin. Ther.*, *7*: 674 (1985).

45. H. Löllgen, H. Wollschläger, E. Lindel, A. Zeiher, and G. Dietlein, Orale oder transdermale Nitrattherapie bei koronarer Herzerkrankung, *Med. Prax.*, *79*: 48 (1984).

46. A. Georgopoulos, A. Markis, and H. Georgiadis, Therapeutic efficacy of a new transdermal system containing nitroglycerin in patients with angina pectoris, *Eur. J. Clin. Pharmacol.*, *22*: 481 (1982).

47. H. A. Wester and N. Mouselimis, Zur therapeutischen Wirksamkeit des transdermalen Systems mit Nitroglycerin im Vergleich zu Nifedipin, *Z. Kardiol.*, *73*: 510 (1984).

48. P. R. Imhof, P. Müller, A. J. Georgopoulos, and B. Garnier, Nitroderm TTS versus oral isosorbide dinitrate: A double-blind trial in patients with angina pectoris, *Acta Ther.*, *11*: 155 (1985).

49. C. Martines, Comparison of the prophylactic anti-anginal effect of two doses of Nitroderm TTS in out-patients with stable angina pectoris, *Curr. Ther. Res.*, *36*: 483 (1984).

50. H. Höhfeld, Langzeittherapie mit Deponit 5 mit stabiler Angina pectoris über 6 Monate mit Placebo-Auslassversuch, *Herz Kreislauf*, *19*(Suppl. 1): 26 (1986).

51. Dž. E. Rezaković, Langzeittherapie über 6 Monate mit Nitroglycerin Pflaster bei stabiler Angina pectoris, *Herz Kreislauf*,

Sonderheft "Stellenwert des transdermalen Deponitrats in der Therapie der koronaren Herzkrankheit," 20 (1985).

52. W. E. Shell, Mechanism and therapy of silent myocardial ischemia and the effect of transdermal nitroglycerin, *Am. J. Cardiol.*, 56: 231 (1985).

53. R. Greco, Efficacy of new transdermal nitroglycerin patch in patients with stable angina pectoris (abstract 03140), Tenth World Congress of Cardiology, Washington, D.C., 1986.

54. E. Agabiti-Rosei, M. L. Muiesan, G. Romanelli, C. Pastori, G. Fiori, L. Muratori, A. M. Zuarini, C. Postorini, S. Borziani, L. B. Bozzi, S. Marchetti, and G. Pollavini, Nitroderm TTS in exercise-induced angina pectoris: A multicenter study (abstract 369), Cardiovascular Pharmacotherapy, International Symposium, April 22–25, 1984, Geneva.

55. K. Midtbó, A comparative study of transdermal nitroglycerin versus placebo in the treatment of stable angina pectoris, in *Transdermal Nitroglycerin Therapy* (W. D. Bussmann and A. Zanchetti, eds.), Hans Huber, Bern, 1985, p. 35.

56. P. Giani, D. Alberti, M. R. Castelli, G. Ferrario, V. Giudici, M. Landolina, R. Roccaforte, and M. Radice, Efficacy and tolerability of Nitroderm TTS and metoprolol slow release in patients with stable exercise-induced angina pectoris (abstract 538), Cardiovascular Pharmacotherapy International Symposium, April 22–25, 1984, Geneva.

57. R. H. Thompson, The clinical use of transdermal delivery devices with nitroglycerin, *Angiology*, 34: 23 (1983).

58. J. A. Salerno, M. Previtali, M. Chimienti, P. Verdecchia, C. Panciroli, E. Marangoni, C. Kleray, S. de Servi, and P. Bobba, Nitroglycerin-transdermal therapeutic system in vasospastic angina at rest. A preliminary report (abstract 1320), Ninth World Congress of Cardiology, June 20–26, 1982, Moscow.

59. S. Lin and J. T. Flaherty, Crossover from intravenous to transdermal nitroglycerin therapy in unstable angina pectoris, *Am. J. Cardiol.*, 56: 742 (1985).

60. K. Dickstein and H. Knutsen, A double-blind multiple crossover trial evaluating a transdermal nitroglycerin system vs. placebo, *Eur. Heart J.*, 6: 50 (1985).

61. R. K. Mahapatra, B. Hunter, J. E. Barnhill, K. D. Stottlemyer, and D. E. Cloyd, Acute titration with Transderm-Nitro in angina pectoris. Nitroglycerin treatment revisited (abstract), *Clin. Res.*, 32: 187A (1984).

62. P. A. Crean, P. Ribeiro, F. Crea, G. J. Davies, D. Ratcliffe, and A. Maseri, Failure of transdermal nitroglycerin to improve chronic stable angina: A randomized, placebo-controlled, double-blind, double crossover trial, *Am. Heart J.*, 108: 1494 (1984).

63. B. Subramanian, N. S. Khurmi, M. J. O'Hara, M. J. Bowles, and E. B. Raftery, Anti-anginal efficacy of transdermal nitroglycerin: Assessment by a double-blind, randomized, crossover trial, in Transdermal Nitroglycerin Therapy (W. D. Bussmann and A. Zanchetti, eds.), Hans Huber, Bern, 1985, p. 42.

64. A. Petersen, E. H. Frandsen, and J. Videbaek, Prophylactic treatment with transdermal nitroglycerin in severe angina pectoris (abstract 1366), Ninth European Congress of Cardiology, Düsseldorf, 1984.

65. M. Sullivan, M. Savvides, N. Abouantoun, E. B. Madsen, and V. Froelicher, Failure of transdermal nitroglycerin to improve exercise capacity in patients with angina pectoris, JACC, 5: 1220 (1985).

66. N. C. Jackson, B. Silke, P. Lee, M. Hafizullah, S. P. Verma, G. Reynolds, and S. H. Taylor, Dose-response studies with a transdermal formulation of nitroglycerin in angina pectoris (abstract), Br. J. Clin. Pharmacol., 19: 561P (1985).

67. G. Noseda and B. Pfister, Haemodynamic investigations with Nitroderm TTS in chronic heart failure, in New Horizons in Nitrate Therapy (W. D. Bussmann and S. H. Taylor, eds.), Medizin Verlag, Munich, (1984), p. 120.

68. D. N. Sharpe and R. Coxon, Nitroglycerin in a transdermal therapeutic system in chronic heart failure, J. Cardiovasc. Pharmacol., 6: 76–82 (1984).

69. P. Lempereur, D. El Allaf, and J. Carlier, Haemodynamic effects of transdermal nitroglycerin (Nitroderm TTS) in patients with severe congestive heart failure (abstract 4), Cardiovascular Pharmacotherapy, International Symposium, April 22, 1984, Geneva.

70. M. Bergbauer, G. Sabin, and G. Börsch, Wirkung von transdermalem Depot-Nitroglyzerin bei Patienten mit hämodynamisch wirksamer koronarer Herzkrankheit unter Berücksichtingung der Dosis, Herzmedizin, 7: 106 (1984).

71. M. Bergbauer, G. Sabin, and P. Plassmann, Langzeiteffekte transdermal applizierten Nitroglyzerins bei koronarer Herzkrankheit: Echokardiographische Messungen, Herzkreislauf, 7: 347 (1984).

72. A. Osterspey, W. Jansen, T. Ulbrich, P. Simon, M. Tauchert, and H. H. Hilger, Wirkung von Nitroglycerinpflastern auf Hämodynamik und Belastbarkeit von Patienten mit koronarer Herzkrankheit, Dtsch. Med. Wochenschr., 109: 714 (1984).

73. H. W. Wiechmann, P. Schuster, and G. Trieb, Transdermale Nitroglycerin-applikation mittels eines neuen therapeutischen Systems: Häemodynamische Effekte bei Patienten mit koronarer Herzkrankheit, Herzmedizin, 7: 189 (1984).

74. A. Vogt and H. Kreuzer, Hämodynamische Wirkungen und Wirkdauer von Deponit 10 bei Patienten mit kongestiver Herzinsuffizienz, Z. Kardiol., 75(Suppl. 3): 86 (1986).

75. Y. Yasky and C. Carosella, Haemodynamic response to nitroglycerin (NG) (Nitroderm TTS 10 or 20 cm2) in patients with congestive heart failure (C. HF) (abstract 42), Cardiovascular Pharmacotherapy, International Symposium, April 22–25, 1984, Geneva.

76. S. Daum and K. W. Heinl, Transdermales Nitroglycerin in der Behandlung der pulmonalen Hypertonie, Z. Kardiol., 75(Suppl. III): 115 (1986).

77. A. Reale and M. Motolese, Haemodynamic changes induced over 24 hours by two different doses of transdermal nitroglycerin: A double-blind, placebo-controlled study in coronary patients, in Transdermal Nitroglycerin Therapy (W. D. Bussmann and A. Zanchetti, eds.), Hans Huber, Bern, (1985), p. 24.

78. M. Packer, N. Medina, and M. Yushak, Rapid attenuation of haemodynamic efficacy of continuous transcutaneous nitroglycerin in severe heart failure: Lack of cross-tolerance to isosorbide dinitrate (abstract), Circulation, 70: II–113 (1984).

79. S. H. Taylor, S. P. Verma, B. Silke, G. Reynolds, and N. C. Jackson, Haemodynamic effects of transdermal nitroglycerin in acute myocardial infarction, in Transdermal Nitroglycerin Therapy (W. D. Bussmann and A. Zanchetti, eds.), Hans Huber, Bern, (1985), p. 56.

80. M. T. Olivari, P. F. Carlyle, T. B. Levine, and J. N. Cohn, Haemodynamic and hormonal response to transdermal nitroglycerin in normal subjects and in patients with congestive heart failure, JACC, 2: 872 (1983).

81. S. P. Verma, B. Silke, G. Reynolds, N. C. Jackson, A. Richmond, and S. H. Taylor, A randomized haemodynamic comparison of isosorbide dinitrate (ISDN) infusion and transdermal nitroglycerin (NTG-TTS) in left ventricular failure following acute myocardial infarction (abstract 325), Cardiovascular Pharmacotherapy International Symposium, April 22–25, 1985, Geneva.

82. S. I. Rajfer, F. J. Demma, and L. I. Goldberg, Sustained beneficial haemodynamic responses to large doses of transdermal nitroglycerin in congestive heart failure and comparison with intravenous nitroglycerin, Am. J. Cardiol., 54: 120 (1984).

83. U. Elkayam, B. Henriquez, L. Weber, D. Tonnemacher, and S. H. Rahimtoola, Lack of haemodynamic effect of high-dose transdermal nitroglycerin in severe heart failure (abstract), Circulation, 70(Suppl. II): 455 (1984).

84. R. A. Jordan, A. Henry, M. A. Wilen, and J. A. Franciosa, Transdermal nitroglycerin in heart failure (abstract), Circulation, 70: II–114 (1984).

85. U. Elkayam, A. Roth, B. Henriquez, L. Weber, D. Tonnemacher, and S. H. Rahimtoola, Haemodynamic and hormonal effects of high-dose transdermal nitroglycerin in patients with chronic congestive heart failure, Am. J. Cardiol., 56: 555 (1985).

86. A. Roth, D. Kulick, L. Freidenberger, and U. Elkayam, Early tolerance to haemodynamic effects of sustained nitrate therapy with high-dose transdermal nitroglycerin in patients with severe chronic heart failure (abstract), JACC, 7: 27A (1986).

87. B. Garnier, P. Imhof, F. Spinelli, and H. Jost, Feldstudie: Die Behandlung der Angina pectoris mit einem neuen transdermalen therapeutischen System von Nitroglycerin (Nitroderm TTS) unter Praxisbedingungen, Schweiz. Rundsch. Med. (Prax.) 71: 511 (1982).

88. K. M. Bridgman, M. Carr, and A. B. Tattersall, Post-marketing surveillance of the Transderm-Nitro patch in general practice, J. Int. Med. Res., 12: 40 (1984).

89. K. D. Haehn, Ergebnisse einer multizentrischen offenen Studie mit Deponit 5 zur symptomatischen Behandlung der Angina pectoris, in Depot-Nitrat (T. Meinertz, E. Jänchen, and A. Schrey, eds.), VaW, Munich, 1985, p. 130.

90. H. Letzel and L. C. Johnson, Therapie der Angina pectoris mit Nitroderm TTS, Med. Welt, 35: 326 (1984).

91. B. Garnier and R. Kenzelman, Utility of Nitroderm TTS in general practice, in New Horizons in Nitrate Therapy (W. D. Bussmann and S. H. Taylor, eds.), Medizin Verlag, Munich, 1985, p. 131.

92. B. Auer, Angina pectoris, Nitratpflaster oder orales Isosorbiddnitrat—Ein Vergleich, Münch. Med. Wochenschr., 128: S. 27 (1986).

93. A. Strano, S. Novo, C. Minneci, and R. Immordino, Multicenter-Studie zur Ermittlung der für eine ausreichende Angina pectoris—Reduzierung efordlichen transdermalen Nytroglycerin-Dosen, Herz Kreislauf, 19(Suppl. 1): 8 (1986).

94. K. Völker, Belastbarkeit, Verträglickeit und Akzeptanz während einer zwei-wochigen Untersuchung mit Deponit 10 an 878 Patienten mit Angina pectoris, Herz Kreislauf, 19(Suppl. 1): 38 (1986).

95. R. J. Jordan, L. Seth, P. Cassebolt, M. Hayes, M. M. Wilen, and J. Franciosa, Rapidly developing tolerance to transdermal nitroglycerin in congestive heart failure, Ann. Intern. Med., 104: 295 (1986).

96. J. Abrams, Nitrate delivery system in perspective, Am. J. Med., 76(6A): 38 (1984).

97. J. Abrams, Transcutaneous nitroglycerin—ointment or disc? Am. Heart J., 108: 1597 (1984).

98. J. Abrams, Transdermal nitroglycerin and nitrate tolerance, *Ann. Intern. Med.*, *104*: 424 (1986).
99. J. O. Parker, Efficacy of nitroglycerin patches: Fact or fancy? *Ann. Intern. Med.*, *102*: 548 (1985).
100. S. Scheidt, Update on transdermal nitroglycerin: An overview, *Am. J. Cardiol.*, *56*: 3I (1985).

11

Transdermal Delivery of Clonidine

G. S. PERLMUTTER, ESTER PARAN,* BONITA FALKNER,
CAROL M. BIES,† T. FAGAN, ROBERT R. CHASE, and
DAVID T. LOWENTHAL‡ / Hahnemann University Hospital
and Hahnemann University School of Medicine, Philadelphia,
Pennsylvania

I. INTRODUCTION

The relationship between prolonged hypertension and major cardio-vascular disease has been well established over the years, and thus new approaches in regard to prevention and treatment of hypertension have emerged.

Clonidine, a central α-receptor agonist, has gained popularity in . the treatment of all grades of essential hypertension. Clonidine, historically, has been administered in the oral form, but recently a new system has been developed to administer this antihypertensive medication transdermally. The clonidine transdermal therapeutic system (TTS) is advantageous as compared to oral therapy in that a steady-state plasma concentration of clonidine can be maintained. This enables therapeutic dosage to be reduced to weekly intervals.

*Present affiliation: Soroka Medical Center, Ben Gurion University of the Negev, Beersheba, Israel.
†Present affiliation: Lock Haven Hospital, Lock Haven, Pennsylvania.
‡Present affiliation: The Mount Sinai Medical Center, New York, New York.

Moreover, a reduction of both frequency and intensity of side effects as well as an improvement in patient compliance has been associated with the transdermal administration of clonidine. Therefore, clonidine TTS may prove to be a viable alternative to oral therapy for the treatment of hypertension.

II. MECHANISM OF ACTION

It has been well established that central catecholaminergic neurons play an important role in the regulation of systemic arterial blood pressure. Stimulation of specific α-adrenergic receptors in the brain leads to a reduction of blood pressure as well as heart rate. Clonidine reduces blood pressure via this central mechanism of action; it inhibits sympathetic outflow from the central nervous system by stimulating α-adrenergic receptors in the vasomotor center of the medulla as well as the nucleus tractus solitarius. Stimulation and activation of peripheral α-adrenergic receptors is not clinically significant. The hypotensive effect of clonidine is associated with a decline in peripheral vascular resistance and a minimal fall in heart rate. Initially, cardiac output is reduced; however, during prolonged therapy it tends to return to baseline levels. In addition, the reduction in sympathetic outflow from the central nervous system results in a decrease in the input to the juxtaglomerular cells of the kidney, leading to a fall in plasma renin concentration. This reduction in plasma renin concentration also plays an important role in the antihypertensive effects of this drug because the generation of angiotensin II, a powerful endogenous vasoconstrictor, is suppressed.

III. PHARMACOKINETICS

Clonidine is readily absorbed following oral administration, and blood pressure reduction is evident within 30–60 min. Peak plasma levels, as well as maximum effect, are attained within 2–3 hr (1). The antihypertensive effect of clonidine is present for at least 6–8 hr subsequent to oral ingestion. The mean biological half-life is estimated to range between 8 and 13 hr (1–4).

Clonidine is suitable for transdermal administration because of its inherent physical properties, which include its low molecular weight, high lipid solubility, and effectiveness at very low plasma concentrations (1,5,6). Major advantages of this transdermal route include the ability to deliver the drug directly into the general circulation and thus, unlike orally ingested drugs, bypass the portal system and the liver. Therefore, any "first-pass" effect may be avoided (7). In addition, this route of administration enables continuous "infusion" of drug during a predetermined period of time. The drug delivered by the device diffuses through the skin, is transported away by underlying capillaries, and is carried into the systemic circulation. The rate of drug released from such a transdermal system is usually a small fraction of the amount that the skin can absorb (4). Hence, the rate of drug transported into the general circulation is fairly constant even when variations in skin permeability are encountered (4). Thus, continuous and constant plasma drug concentrations can be achieved transdermally.

In contrast, conventional dosage forms, such as tablets and capsules, inevitably provide a peak in the plasma drug concentration after each dose and a trough prior to the following dose (7). This results in wide fluctuations in plasma drug concentrations.

Finally, the transdermal delivery system avoids the unreliability of gastrointestinal drug absorption due to variable acidity, motility, and food content in the gastrointestinal tract, which may cause further variations in plasma drug concentrations.

Clonidine TTS provides rate-controlled, continuous administration of the drug for a full 7 days. Although initially the release of clonidine from the transdermal system is rapid (the first 24 hr), the drug release rate remains constant thereafter (4). Increasing rates of drug input can be accomplished by increasing the area of the system applied to the skin. After application, plasma levels of clonidine slowly increase and a steady state is achieved in approximately 3 days. The maximum antihypertensive effect is also achieved at this time. This steady state remains constant throughout the remainder of time during which the transdermal therapeutic system is worn. Again, a proportionate increase in steady-state plasma concentration of clonidine may be achieved by increasing the surface area of the clonidine TTS delivery system (4, 8–10). After removal of the patch, the plasma drug level can be expected to remain constant for approximately 8 hr and then decline with an elimination half-life reported to be about 21 hr (4).

An estimated 70% of clonidine is excreted unchanged in the urine, while the remaining 30% is believed to be metabolized by the liver. These metabolites have no significant pharmacological activity (2, 3, 11). Accumulation of clonidine does not occur with chronic administration in normal patients. However, in renal-insufficient patients, the elimination half-life is prolonged, and no replacement of clonidine is necessary after dialysis (3). When patients with renal insufficiency are treated with oral clonidine and are then transferred to TTS, there is no loss of blood pressure control or of plasma clonidine concentration.

IV. PHARMACOLOGICAL EFFECTS

Oral clonidine therapy has been shown to be extremely effective for the treatment of hypertension due to its ability to cause a substantial reduction in blood pressure. Studies in man have demonstrated that this reduction in blood pressure is similar in supine, sitting, and standing positions (Figs. 1–3) and may also be associated with a mild fall in heart rate (1). However, it is important to note that clonidine does not inhibit sympathetic reflexes that are initiated by standing, and thus orthostatic hypotension does not pose a significant problem with this medication (2,8,11). Recently, numerous studies have shown that transdermally administered clonidine produces the same hemodynamic effects, although the onset of action as well as the peak plasma drug concentration differ between these two routes of administration.

The cardiovascular effects of clonidine include decreases in arterial pressure, heart rate, and peripheral vascular resistance. Clonidine reduces renovascular resistance without changing renal blood flow or glomerular filtration rate (11). Renin production is suppressed (2,12). As mentioned earlier, the cardiovascular effects of clonidine are due to its ability to decrease sympathetic outflow from the central nervous system. Many studies have demonstrated that the hypotensive effects of both oral and transdermal clonidine parallel reductions in the concentration of circulating norepinephrine (9,11,15). In addition, patients with the greatest elevation of plasma norepinephrine levels seem to exhibit the greatest reduction

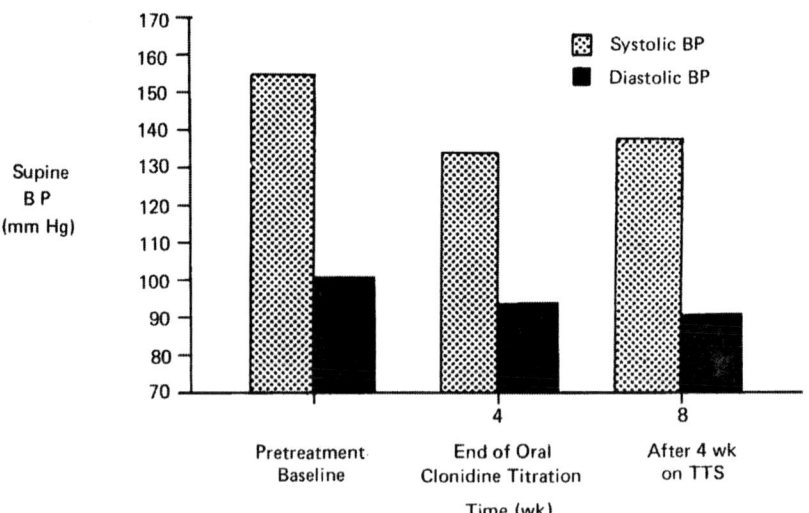

Figure 1 Blood pressure response in the supine position at baseline, after oral clonidine and during transdermal clonidine.

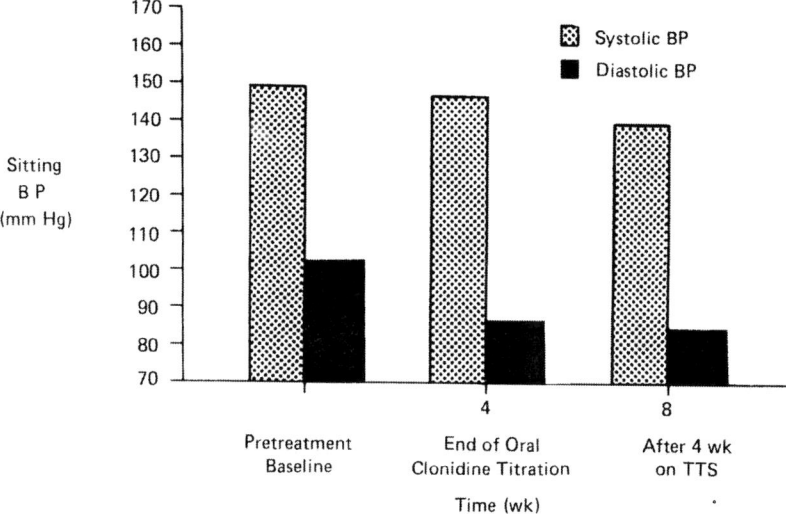

Figure 2   Blood pressure response in the sitting position at baseline, after oral clonidine and during transdermal clonidine.

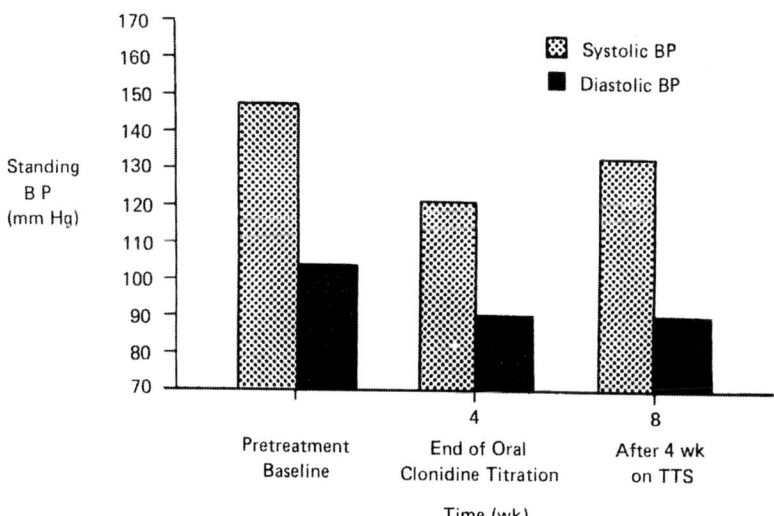

Figure 3   Blood pressure response in the standing position at baseline, after oral clonidine and during transdermal clonidine.

of blood pressure during long-term sympathetic inhibition with clonidine (9,14). Clonidine appears to have no effect on circulating
epinephrine (8).

When administered transdermally, smaller doses of clonidine are
needed to produce the same reduction in blood pressure as that
necessary with oral therapy (4,12,16,17). This is due to an achievement of a steady-state plasma drug concentration, which remains
constant throughout the transdermal application of this medication.
In contrast, the "peak-and-trough" profile associated with oral therapy provides daily variations of plasma drug concentrations. Therapeutic plasma levels of clonidine TTS approximate trough values
achieved during oral administration (4,12,17). Therefore, plasma
drug concentrations needed during transdermal clonidine therapy
are significantly less than those necessary during oral administration
of this antihypertensive medication, and this remains a major benefit
of clonidine TTS. It is important to note that the reduction in blood
pressure achieved via oral therapy is fully maintained when changing
to the clonidine transdermal delivery system (12,17,18).

Studies in adolescent hypertensives receiving clonidine TTS show
adequate control and normalization of blood pressure comparable to
the stabilization of blood pressure noted during oral clonidine treatment.

The effect of antihypertensive treatment on blood pressure during physical exercise is an important factor to be considered when
choosing an appropriate medication. While clonidine decreases sympathetic tone and blood pressure during resting conditions, the normal
response to both dynamic (aerobic) and static (isometric) exercise
remains intact (9,13,14).

Finally, certain antihypertensive medications are known to alter
lipid profiles that tend to enhance the risk of cardiovascular disease.
However, recent studies have reported either no significant changes
in lipid profiles (9) or changes in these profiles that would be considered favorable (increase in high-density-lipid/cholesterol level
and decrease in low-density lipid/cholesterol level (19).

V. ADVERSE EFFECTS

The most common adverse reactions associated with oral clonidine
therapy include dry mouth (xerostomia), drowsiness, sedation, and
constipation. Clonidine reduces salivary flow, and this appears to
be due to the central effect of the drug. The xerostomia is often
accompanied by dry eyes, dry nasal mucosa, and parotid gland swelling. Although the incidence of these side effects may approach 50%,
they usually diminish as therapy is continued. Rarely, clonidine
may cause central nervous system side effects, which include vivid
dreams, nightmares, insomnia, anxiety, and depression. Raynaud's

phenomenon as well as sexual disturbances have been reported to occur subsequent to clonidine administration (5).

Clonidine TTS therapy is also associated with the adverse effects above; however, the frequency as well as the severity of these side effects seem to be reduced (4,12,17,20). As stated previously, clonidine transdermal patches maintain constant plasma drug concentrations well below the peak levels seen during oral administration. This, theoretically, would be expected to reduce the adverse reactions experienced by patients using this form of therapy. Clinical studies support this theory (8,15,20). Moreover, systemic side effects, such as dry mouth and drowsiness, appear to be less pronounced when patients change from oral to transdermal therapy (8).

One of the most common adverse effects associated with transdermally administered clonidine is the development of local skin reactions to the clonidine preparation. Reports of such dermatological reactions range in incidence between 5 and 42% (6,12,17,21,23).

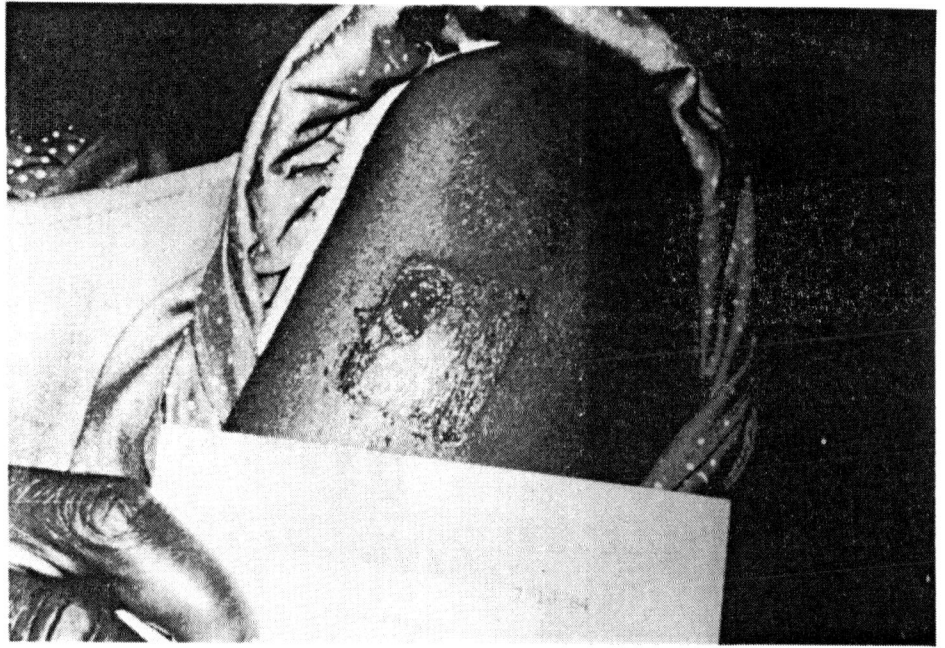

Figure 4   Excoriating ulcer in reaction to transdermal clonidine in a patient with chronic renal insufficiency who previously tolerated oral clonidine well.

These reactions vary in severity from mild erythema and pruritus to vesiculation and inflammatory infiltration of the skin beneath the transdermal patch. Rarely, development of a generalized maculopapular rash has been reported to occur following transdermal clonidine therapy. The vast majority of these skin reactions are mediated via a delayed type IV hypersensitivity reaction (allergic contact dermatitis), which may be confirmed with patch testing utilizing components of the clonidine transdermal device. In some of these patients the allergic reaction is due to clonidine specifically, while in other patients a specific component of the transdermal system (polyisobutylene) functions as the allergen (22,24).

Several patients with proven sensitization to the clonidine device have been challenged and treated with oral clonidine for periods of up to one year. Of these, only one patient developed a reaction which was characterized by a maculopapular rash (Figs. 4 and 5). However, this patient had severe renal impairment with clonidine levels significantly above the normal therapeutic range (25). No adverse skin reactions were seen in the adolescent hypertensive

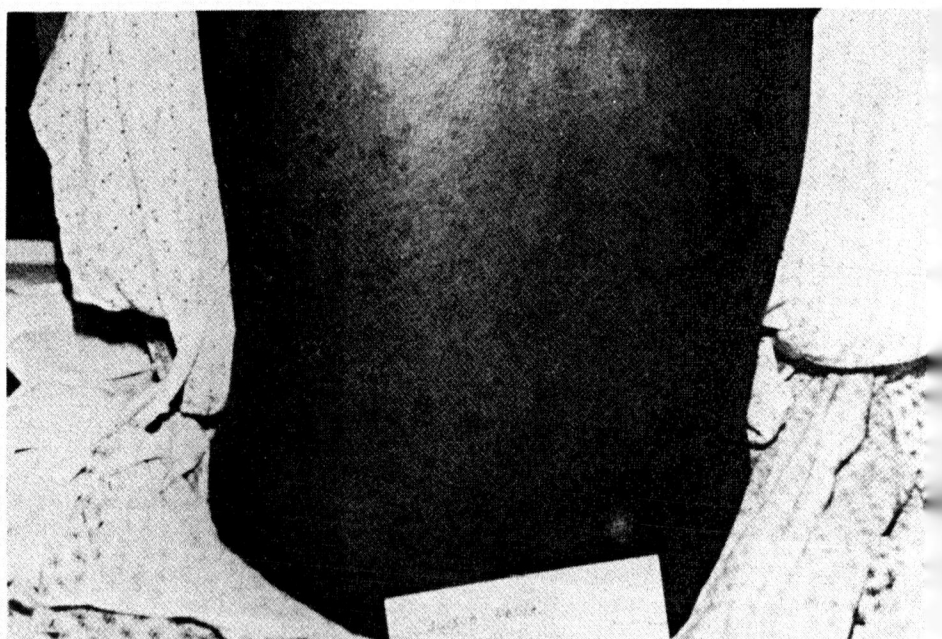

Figure 5   Erythema multiforme reaction to oral clonidine, 0.1 mg twice daily, begun 3 days following removal of transdermal clonidine. Plasma clonidine concentration at time of diagnosis was 11 ng/ml. Reaction cleared with diphenhydramine, 50 mg every 12 hr.

patients. Furthermore, there have not been any reported incidences of clonidine-induced anaphylaxis in 10 years of clinical studies involving oral clonidine or in recent studies involving clonidine TTS (21,24). Ninety percent of the dermatological reactions reported to be associated with clonidine TTS materialize within the initial 20 weeks of treatment. Even though the reactions, in general, have not been severe and have usually disappeared after cessation of therapy, the full significance of these effects has not yet been determined.

Abrupt withdrawal of oral clonidine is associated with a rapid return of blood pressure to the pretreatment baseline. A catecholamine-like withdrawal reaction is likely to occur in patients who have been receiving large doses of clonidine. Withdrawal from clonidine TTS seems to result in a much less dramatic reaction or no reaction at all (18). Symptoms of this syndrome include headache, nervousness, abdominal pain, diaphoresis, tachycardia, and a rapid rise in blood pressure. This reaction is believed to be the result of sympathetic overactivity and can be reversed by resuming clonidine therapy, or by administering an α-adrenergic antagonist or a combination of an α- and β-adrenergic antagonists (labetalol). The exact incidence of this syndrome is uncertain and can be avoided by discontinuing the drug gradually over 2-4 days.

VI. CONCLUSIONS

Research over the past few years has led to the development of a revolutionary transdermal drug delivery system that can steadily deliver a drug to the surface of skin for periods of up to 7 days following a single application. Recently, clonidine, a centrally acting antihypertensive, has been utilized in such a system. Clonidine TTS is available as small, flexible, self-adhesive skin patches from which clonidine may exert its pharmacological effects.

The efficacy of both oral and transdermal clonidine therapy for the treatment of essential hypertension has been well established in numerous clinical studies. The therapeutic effects achieved with clonidine TTS can be expected to be comparable to those seen during oral therapy. However, both dosage and plasma drug concentration associated with transdermal clonidine application are well below those seen with therapeutic oral therapy. This would explain the reduction of systemic side effects experienced by patients being treated with clonidine TTS. Local skin reactions reported during transdermal clonidine therapy are primarily mild and are characterized by erythema and pruritus at the transdermal therapeutic system site. However, more severe reactions consisting of vesiculation and inflammatory infiltration have been known to occur with varying frequency. More data from larger groups of patients are necessary to assess the long-term dermatological effects of clonidine TTS and the clinical relevance of such allergic reactions. In summary, the convenience of once-a-week medication for the treatment of hypertension can be expected to significantly enhance patient compliance. The steady-state plasma concentrations of clonidine produced by the rate-controlled transdermal delivery system, along with good control of blood pressure at relatively low plasma drug concentrations, make clonidine TTS an effective and well-tolerated alternative to conventional oral clonidine therapy.

REFERENCES

1. C. T. Dollery, D. S. Davies, G. H. Draffean, et al., Clinical pharmacology and pharmacokinetics of clonidine, *Clin. Pharmacol. Ther.*, *19*: 11–17 (1976).
2. J. R. DiPalma, *Basic Pharmacology in Medicine*, 2nd ed., McGraw-Hill, New York, 1982.
3. D. T. Lowenthal, S. D. Saris, B. Falkner, et al., Pharmacodynamics and pharmacokinetics of oral and transdermal clonidine in chronic renal insufficiency, in *Low Dose Oral and Transdermal Therapy of Hypertension* (M. A. Weber, J. I. M. Drayer, and R. Kolloch, eds.), Steinkopff, Darmstadt, Germany, 1985.
4. J. E. Shaw, Pharmacokinetics of nitroglycerin and clonidine delivered by the transdermal route, *Am. Heart J.*, *108*: 217–222 (1984).
5. H. Groth, H. Vetter, J. Knusel, et al., Clonidine through the skin in the treatment of essential hypertension: Is it practical? *J. Hypertension*, *1*(Suppl. 2): 120–122 (1983).
6. H. Groth, H. Vetter, J. Knusel, et al., Transdermal clonidine in essential hypertension: Problems during long-term treatment, in *Low Dose Oral and Transdermal Therapy of Hypertension* (M. A. Weber, J. I. M. Drayer, and R. Kolloch, eds.), Steinkopff, Darmstadt, Germany, 1985.
7. D. D. Breimer, Rationale for rate-controlled drug dleivery of cardiovascular drugs by the transdermal route, *Am. Heart J.*, *108*: 196–199 (1984).
8. M. D. Schaller, J. Nussberger, B. Waeber, et al., Transdermal clonidine therapy in hypertensive patients, *JAMA*, *253*: 233–235 (1985).
9. R. Kolloch, H. Finster, A. Overlack, et al., Low dose oral and transdermal application of clonidine in mild hypertension: Hemodynamic and biochemical correlates, in *Low Dose Oral and Transdermal Therapy of Hypertension* (M. A. Weber, J. I. M. Drayer, and R. Kolloch, eds.), Steinkopff, Darmstadt, Germany, 1985.

10. R. G. A. van Wayjen, A. van den Ende, R. G. L. van Ol, et al., Pharmacokinetics of transdermally delivered clonidine, in *Low Dose Oral and Transdermal Therapy of Hypertension* (M. A. Weber, J. I. M. Drayer, and R. Kolloch, eds.), Steinkopff, Darmstadt, Germany, 1985.

11. *Boodman and Gilman's The Pharmacological Basis of Therapeutics*, 7th ed. (A. G. Gilman, L. S. Goodman, T. W. Rall, and F. Murad, eds.), Macmillan, New York, 1985.

12. M. A. Weber and J. I. M. Drayer, Clinical experience with rate-controlled delivery of antihypertensive therapy by a transdermal system, *Am. Heart J.*, 108: 231–235 (1984).

13. D. T. Lowenthal, M. B. Affrime, B. Falkner, et al., Potassium disposition and neuroendocrine effects of propranolol, methyldopa and clonidine during dynamic exercise, *Clin. Exp. Hypertension Theory Pract.*, A4: 1895–1911 (1985).

14. D. T. Lowenthal, D. Dickerman, S. D. Saris, et al., The effect of pharmacologic interaction on central and peripheral alpha-receptors and pressor response to static exercise, *Ann. Sports Med.*, 1: 100–104 (1983).

15. E. L. Bravo, M. D. Cressman, and M. A. Pohl, Cardiovascular and neurohumoral effects of long-term clonidine monotherapy in essential hypertensive patients, in *Low Dose Oral and Transdermal Therapy of Hypertension* (M. A. Weber, J. I. M. Drayer, and R. Kolloch, eds.), Steinkopff, Darmstadt, Germany, 1985.

16. J. I. M. Drayer, M. A. Weber, and D. D. Brewer, A multicenter study on the use of transdermal clonidine in patients with essential hypertension, in *Low Dose Oral and Transdermal Therapy of Hypertension* (M. A. Weber, J. I. M. Drayer, and R. Kolloch, eds.), Steinkopff, Darmstadt, Germany, 1985.

17. S. Popli, G. Strok, T. S. Ing, et al., Transdermal clonidine for hypertensive patients, *Clin. Ther.*, 5: 624–626 (1983).

18. P. Balansard, T. Danays, A. Baralla, et al., Antihypertensive action of Catapres-TTS, in *Low Dose Oral and Transdermal Therapy of Hypertension* (M. A. Weber, J. I. M. Drayer, and R. Kolloch, eds.), Steinkopff, Darmstadt, Germany, 1985.

19. C. Diehm and H. Morl, Lipid metabolism and antihypertensive treatment, in *Low Dose Oral and Transdermal Therapy of Hypertension* (M. A. Weber, J. I. M. Drayer, and R. Kolloch, eds.), Steinkopff, Darmstadt, Germany, 1985.

20. M. A. Weber, J. I. M. Drayer, D. D. Brewer, et al., Transdermal continuous antihypertensive therapy, *Lancet*, 2: 9–11 (1984).

21. H. Maibach, Clonidine-irritant and allergic contact dermatitis assays, *Contact Dermatitis*, 10: 211–214 (1983).

22. H. Groth, H. Vetter, J. Knuesel, et al., Allergic skin reactions to transdermal clonidine, Lancet, 2: 850–851 (1983).

23. J. C. Boekhorst, Allergic contact dermatitis with transdermal clonidine, Lancet, 2: 1031–1032 (1983).

24. H. Maibach, Clonidine transdermal delivery system: Cutaneous toxicity studies, in Low Dose Oral and Transdermal Therapy of Hypertension (M. A. Weber, J. I. M. Drayer, and R. Kolloch, eds.), Steinkopff, Darmstadt, Germany, 1985.

25. D. T. Lowenthal, internal communication, Boehringer-Ingelheim, 1984.

12

Transdermal Delivery of Bupranolol

INGE WEISS, HANS-MICHAEL WOLFF, GÜNTER CORDES, and
WILLI CAWELLO / Schwarz GmbH, Monheim, West Germany

I. INTRODUCTION

The transdermal route of application offers considerable advantages
especially for treatment of chronic diseases: whereas multidose oral
application often leads to unwanted fluctuations of plasma levels,
transdermal application allows plasma levels to be kept constant over
the application period. For drugs undergoing extensive first-pass
metabolism after oral administration, dosage may be reduced considerably under transdermal treatment. For example, the transdermal
application route is of special interest for potent β-adrenoceptor
blocking agents such as bupranolol, a drug that has been reported
to be subject to an extensive first-pass metabolism (>90% in humans)
(1).

This chapter describes results from three in vivo absorption
studies with bupranolol: one experiment conducted in rabbits to
gain baseline information about the effects of the transdermally administered β-adrenergic blocking agent and two studies in human
volunteers, where pharmacokinetic and pharmacodynamic effects were
investigated.

II. TRANSDERMAL ABSORPTION OF BUPRANOLOL IN RABBITS

The objective of the study in rabbits was to obtain information about the onset of action, the intensity and duration of action, and the bioavailability of transdermally absorbed bupranolol. The design of the study included transdermal application via an adhesive-type transdermal therapeutic system (TTS) containing 2.5 and 5.0 mg of bupranolol in comparison to intravenous application of 2.5 and 5.0 mg of bupranolol·HCl. The parameter measured was the increase in heart rate after intravenous application of isoprenaline (0.25 µg/kg) compared to heart rate at rest.

A. Test Material

Included in this study were three male rabbits (chinchilla bastards CHB) with an average weight of 2.2 kg. The animals were obtained from Ivanovas, in West Germany.

Each test patch contained 0.64 mg of bupranolol per square centimeter, and the patch sizes were 4.1 and 8.2 cm^2, corresponding to drug contents of 2.5 and 5.0 mg, respectively. The adhesive base was the same for both the test and placebo TTS.

B. Methods

Test patches were applied to a skin area of the lumbar region; the skin had been shaved and depilated 24 hr before application. The patches were left in place for 24 hr. After removal of the patches, the absorbed dose of bupranolol was estimated by the "difference method," that is, determination by high-performance liquid chromatography (HPLC) of the total drug content in the patches before and after application (samples from the same batch).

Effects were compared to the intravenous infusion of 2.5 and 5.0 mg of bupranolol·HCl per 24 hr. Infusion was performed at a constant rate over 24 hr through an indwelling catheter into the ear vein of the animal. The isoprenaline challenge to test the degree of β-adrenergic blockade was done by intravenous injection of 0.25 µg/ kg body weight. The injection was given via the ear vein catheter. Heart rate at rest was monitored via electrocardiogram during a nonapplication period of about 1 hr, a 24-hr application period, and a 4-hr postapplication period. Between 5 and 20 hr after application, no data were recorded. Heart rate at rest was measured at intervals of 30 min over a period of 30 sec; isoprenaline was injected immediately afterward and the resulting tachycardia was monitored. The difference between heart rate at rest and the maximum after isoprenaline-induced tachycardia was compared to the respective difference before bupranolol application, calculated in percent inhibition, and served as a quantitative parameter for evaluating the effect of β-adrenergic blockade. Total effect was determined by comparing the area under the inhibition curves with 5 mg of intravenous bupranolol·HCl serving as a 100% standard. The area between 5 and 20 hr postapplication was interpolated.

C. Results

Effect profiles are depicted in Figures 1, 2, and 3, with the time profile for inhibition in percent given in the upper part of the graphs and the time profile of heart rate (HR) before and after isoprenaline challenge outlined below.

Figure 1 demonstrates the dramatic decrease in isoprenaline response under infusion of bupranolol·HCl. In the untreated animals, injection of 0.25 μg of isoprenaline per kilogram of body weight caused an increase in heart rate of about 90 beats/min above heart rate at rest. After 1 hr of treatment, 25% inhibition was found. Steady state was reached after about 3 hr, the inhibitory effect being 80-86%. This effect was kept up until infusion was stopped, and it decreased to 20% within 4 hr after termination of the infusion.

As can be seen from Figure 2, application of one test patch containing 5.0 mg of bupranolol led to comparable effects. The inhibitory effect started, with a somewhat less rapid increase, reaching steady state between 3 and 5 hr after application. The maximal effect of 80% inhibition was kept up until the patches were removed after 24 hr. The decrease after removal of the patches was similar to the decrease after termination of infusion.

Both graphs (Figs 1 and 2) show essentially the same behavior of the two curves: upon onset of β-adrenergic blockade, the response curve to the isoprenaline challenge rapidly declines from a starting level of approximately 100 beats/min above the rest rate to about 20 beats/min above the rest level, with both curves then running parallel as long as treatment is continued. Termination of treatment results in an almost immediate rise of the response curve.

Figure 3 illustrates the results under placebo treatment: both curves remained unchanged over the test period; no inhibitory effect could be observed. A slight increase in percentage action of isoprenaline, which is expressed in the upper part of the graphic by the inhibition going down to about 20%, must be ascribed to the nervous regulation of the animal.

Upon application of a 2.5-mg patch and infusion of 2.5 mg, the same effect profiles were found, although, in accordance with the smaller dose applied, less pronounced effects were observed.

Since the drug content of a transdermal system is not necessarily identical with the dose applied, results can be evaluated only after dose correction. For this purpose the areas under the inhibition

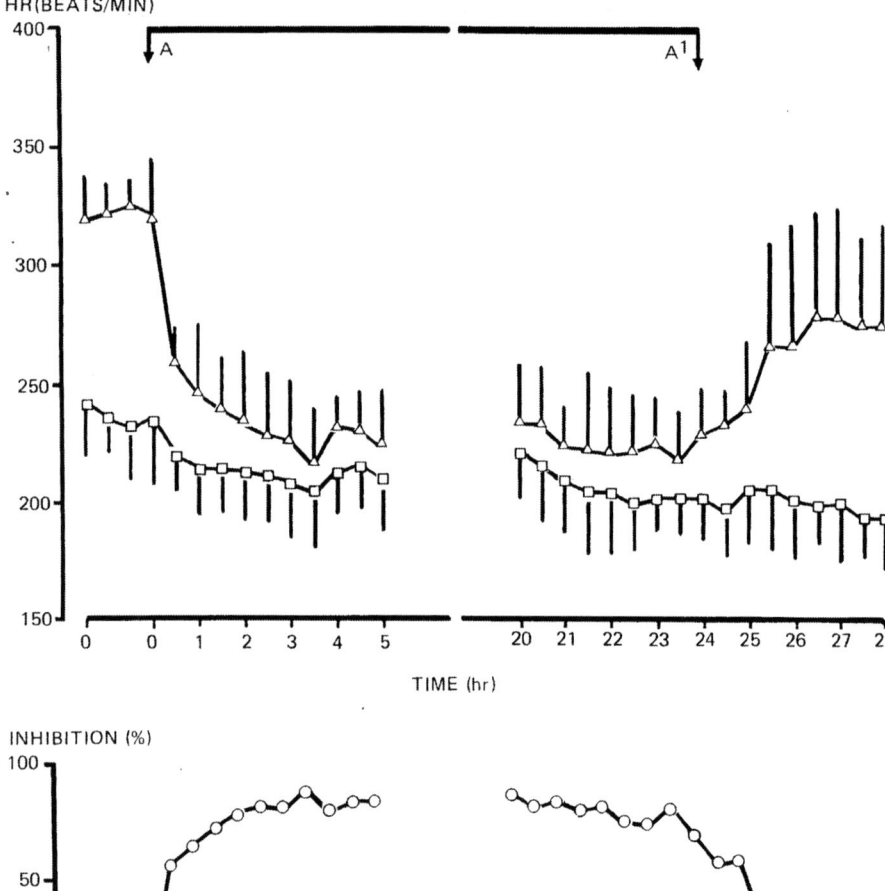

Figure 1   Pharmacodynamic effect of bupranolol·HCl in the rabbit, administered at an infusion rate of 5 mg/24 hr. Top: heart rate (HR) profile before (□) and after (△) isoprenaline challenge; A–A[1], 24-hr administration of the infusion data represent mean ±SEM; n = 3. Bottom: inhibition profile.

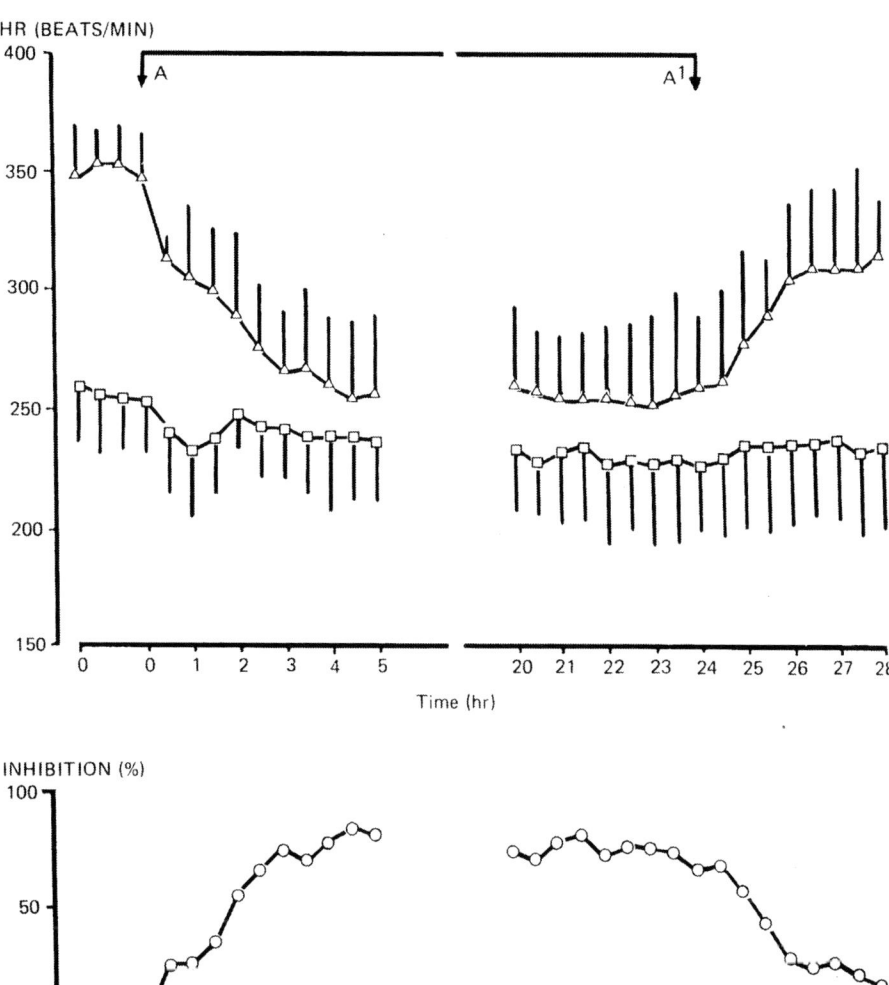

Figure 2 Pharmacodynamic effect of transdermally applied bupranolol in the rabbit; bupranolol content of the 8.2-cm^2 transdermal system was 5 mg. Symbols and conditions as in Figure 1.

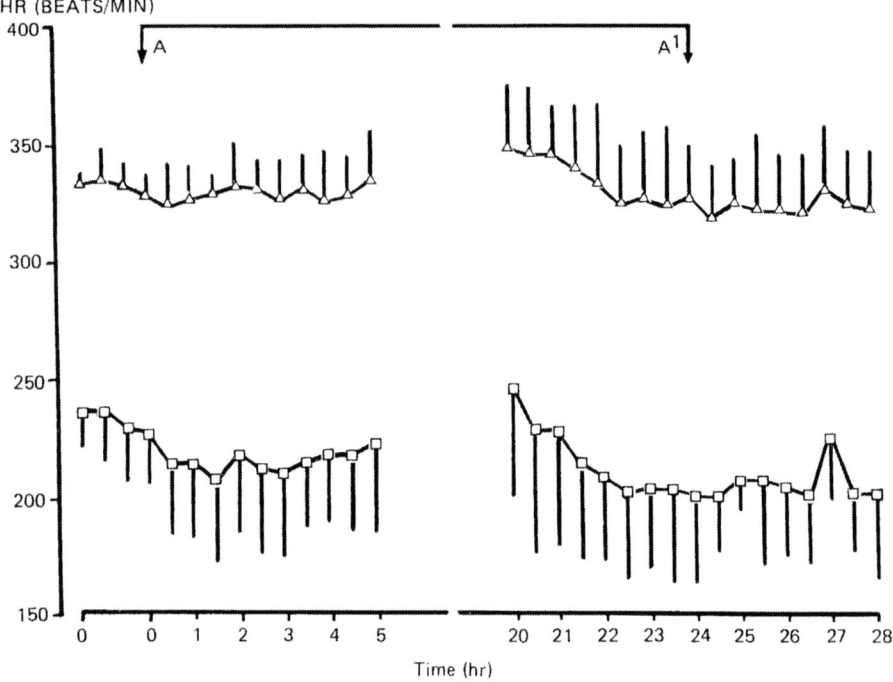

Time (hr)

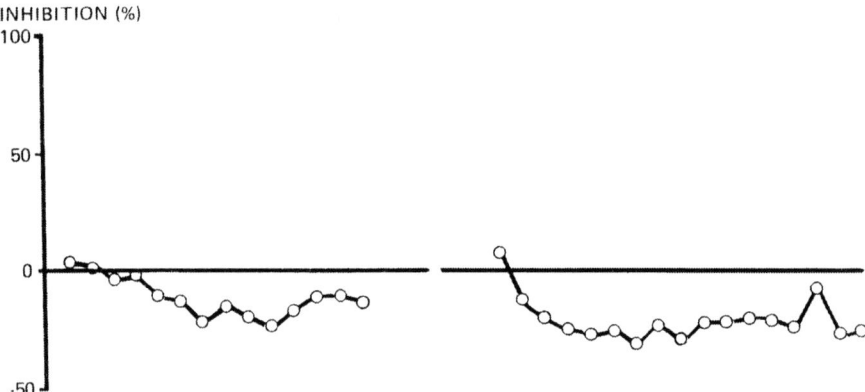

Figure 3 Heart rate during placebo application in the rabbit. Symbols and conditions as in Figure 1.

curves (AUC) were calculated, with the area under the 5-mg infusion curve set as a standard of 100%. The following relations between applied dose and AUC values were obtained:

	AUC (%)
Infusion of 5.0 mg bupranolol·HCl/24 hr:	100
Patch containing 5.0 mg bupranolol/8.2 cm^2:	86
Infusion of 2.5 mg bupranolol·HCl/24 hr:	85
Patch containing 2.5 mg bupranolol/4.1 cm^2:	53

The estimated uptake from the patches was 1.5 mg for the 2.5-mg patch and 2.8 mg for the 5.0-mg patch. After dosage correction, the bioavailability was 97% for the 2.5-mg patch and 88% for the 5.0-mg patch, indicating that practically the entire amount of drug released from the patch was systemically available.

III. PHARMACOKINETIC AND PHARMACODYNAMIC STUDIES IN HUMAN VOLUNTEERS

The study was conducted with the aim of getting information about the plasma levels that can be reached in humans and the characteristics of the plasma level curve on repeated application of a bupranolol-TTS. At the same time, the effect was measured by isoprenaline challenge and by bicycle ergometry. To get an idea about the degree of β-receptor blockade a radioreceptor assay was performed. Six healthy volunteers participated in the study.

A. Material and Methods

Each volunteer received one bupranolol TTS (25 cm^2; drug content 30 mg), which was fixed at the frontal chest wall. After 24 hr and 48 hr the TTS was removed and a fresh patch was applied.

Test patches were of essentially the same composition as those applied in the rabbit study; that is, the drug was incorporated in a self-adhesive matrix consisting of a mixture of polyisobutylene and resin. The drug content was 1.2 mg/cm^2.

The in vitro release from the test patches was determined at 16.1 mg/24 hr/25 cm^2. Release had been determined using the rotating-bottle apparatus described in NF XIII (receptor medium: 80 ml of phosphate buffer pH 5.5, 34°C). Determination of the amount of drug released had been performed by HPLC. The in vitro release profile is shown in Figure 4.

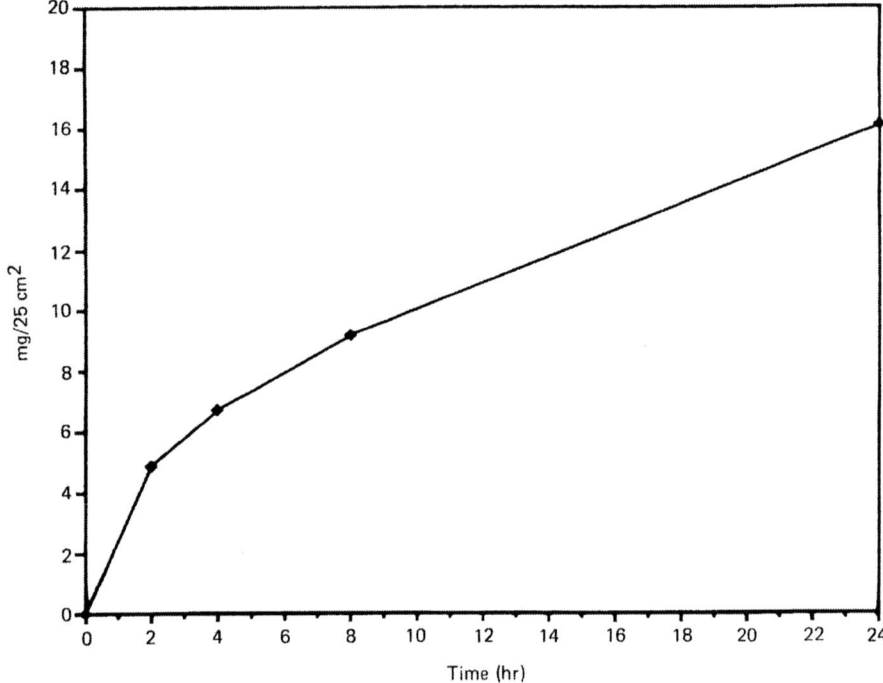

Figure 4 In vitro release profile of bupranolol from patches containing 30 mg/25 cm^2 (rotating-bottle apparatus).

The estimated mean ($\pm$ SD) in vivo drug release from the patches applied was 12.74 $\pm$ 1.84 mg/24 hr. Determination of the in vivo release was performed by the "difference method" as explained above. Blood was sampled at 6, 12, 24, 36, 48, 60, and 72 hr. Samples were divided in two portions; one was used for determination of plasma levels by radioimmunoassay (RIA), and the other portion was used for receptor binding studies. Receptor binding studies were performed by Dr. A. Wellstein, and a detailed report of the complete work has been submitted for publication (2). For details of the radioreceptor assay, see Wellstein et al. (3).

Response to isoprenaline challenge was determined by injecting 0.0025–0.3 μg of isoprenaline per kilogram of body weight at intervals of 5 min. Heart rate should have returned to rest level between injections. Exercise-induced tachycardia was measured after 5 min of bicycle ergometry (75% maximum workload).

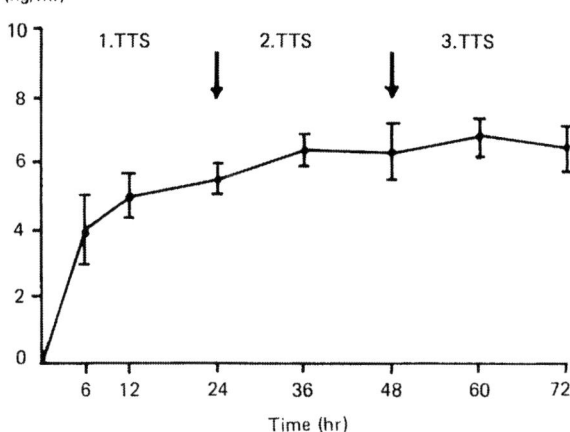

Figure 5 Plasma levels in human volunteers during transdermal application of bupranolol from patches containing 30 mg/25 cm^2 (patches were changed at points indicated by arrows).

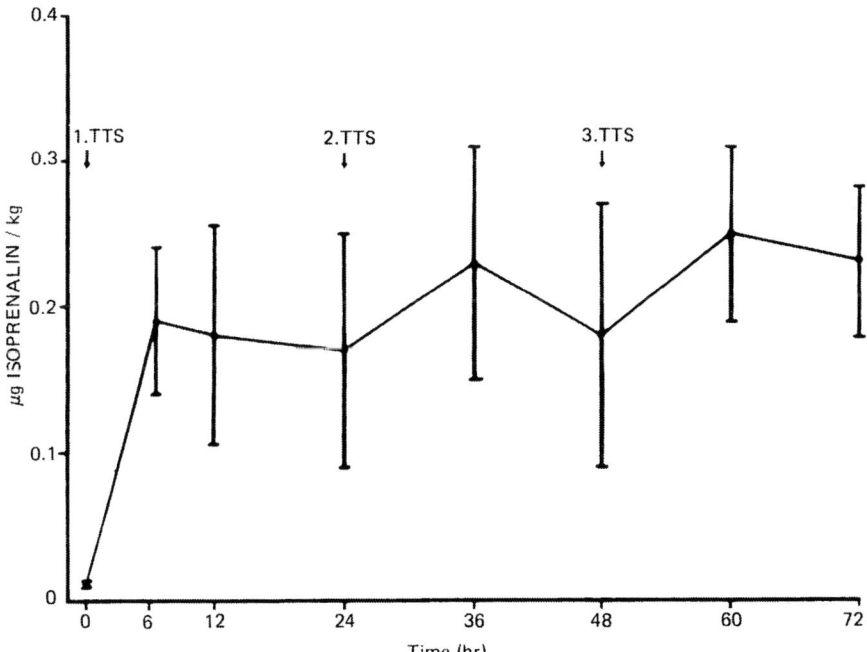

Figure 6 Mean dose of isoprenaline (μg/kg) necessary to induce an increase in heart rate by 20 beats/min during application of bupranolol patches in human volunteers: patch size, 25 cm^2; bupranolol content 30 mg.

B. Results

Figure 5 shows the time profile of bupranolol plasma concentrations as determined by RIA. Steady state was reached between 6 and 12 hr postapplication and kept up until the end of the test period.

As summarized in Figures 6 and 7, the plasma levels observed were sufficient to induce in the pharmacodynamic parameters significant changes that were sustained over the test period.

Figure 6 illustrates the effect profile in isoprenaline-induced tachycardia. The dose of isoprenaline that caused a rise in heart rate by 20 beats/min increased from 0.01 μg/kg before application to 0.19 μg/kg at 6 hr after application, remaining constant until the end of the test, thus indicating a constant degree of β-adrenergic blockade. This was confirmed by considerable reduction of tachycardia after bicycle ergometry: as demonstrated in Figure 7, exercise-induced tachycardia was inhibited by about 20 beats/min once steady state had been reached between 6 and 12 hr after application.

To get an idea about the degree of receptor blockade, a radioreceptor assay was performed. Bupranolol is a nonselective β-adrenoceptor antagonist, with K_i values of 6–15 nmol/L in the presence of human plasma (2).

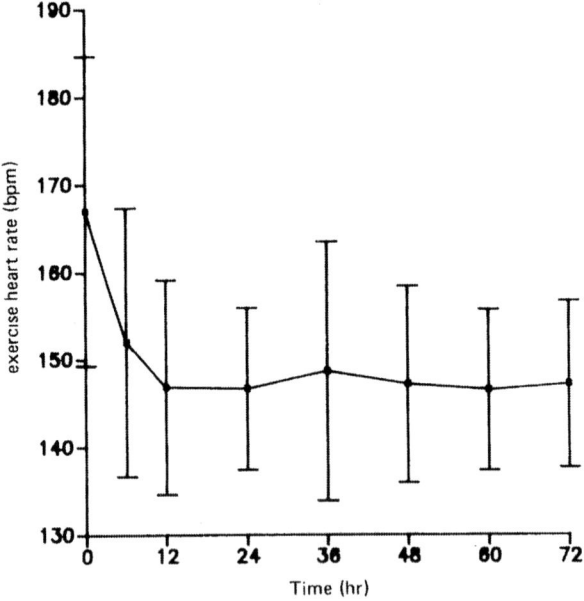

Figure 7   Postexercise heart rate in the persons tested during application of TTS containing 30 mg/25 cm^2.

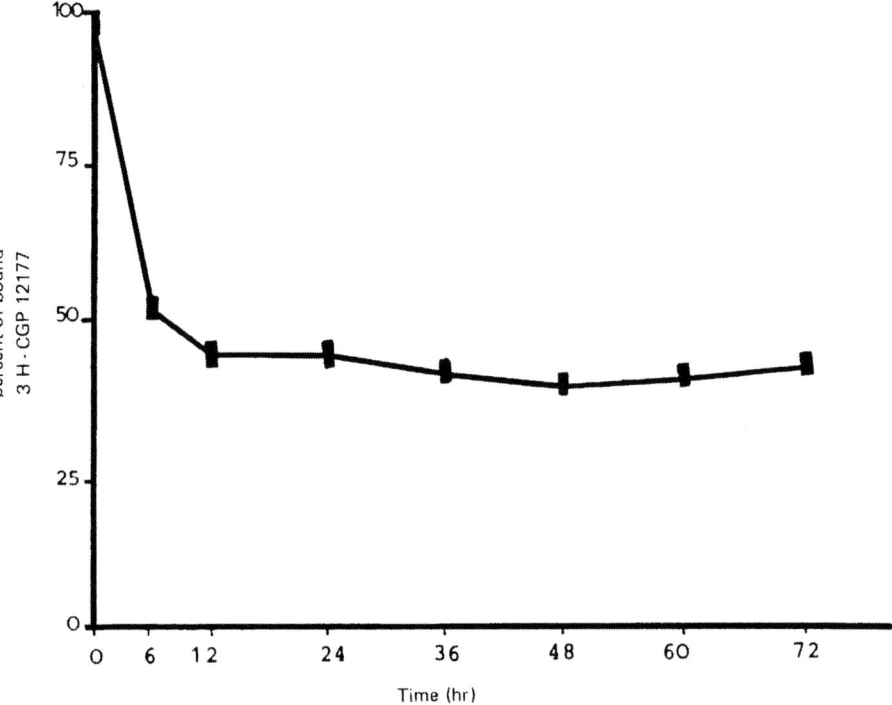

Figure 8   Effects of plasma samples from the persons tested on in vitro β-adrenoceptor binding of the radioligand ³H-CGP 12177 at rat reticulocyte membranes.

Figure 8 summarizes the effect of plasma samples on the in vitro β-adrenoceptor binding of the radioligand ³H-CGP 12177 at rat reticulocyte membranes (β₂-adrenoceptors). From these data a receptor occupancy of about two-thirds of the β-adrenergic receptors can be calculated, which remained fairly unchanged over the test period (2).

IV. EVALUATION OF PHARMACODYNAMIC EFFECTS COMPARED TO PERORAL PROPRANOLOL

To be able to evaluate the effects described above, we compared the effects of one 25-cm² bupranolol test patch to those of two 80-mg doses of orally administered propranolol. Four volunteers participated in the study; the application period was 24 hr. The mean in vivo release (±SD) from the patches was found to be 11 mg/24 hr.

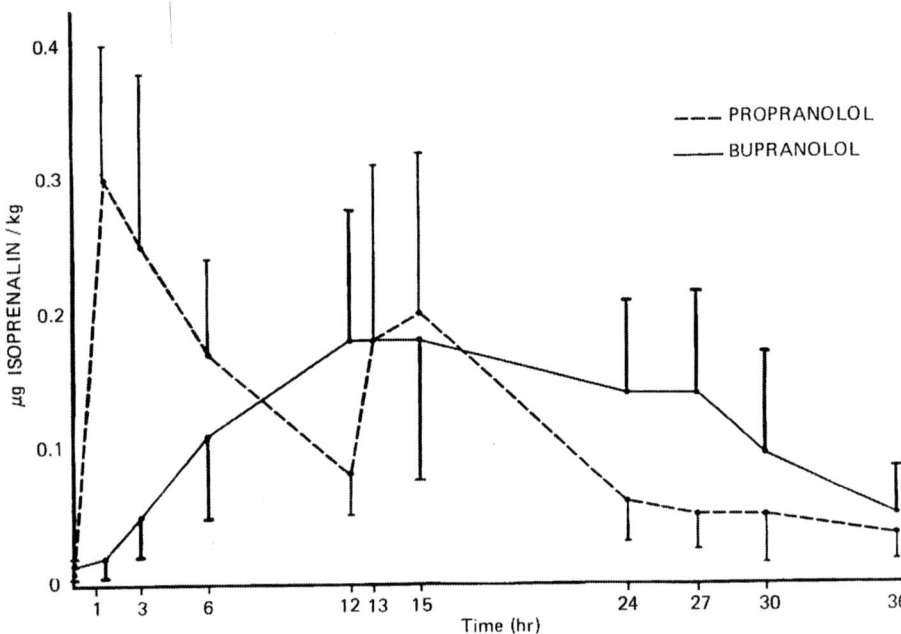

Figure 9   Mean dose of isoprenaline (µg/kg) necessary to induce ΔHR ≈ 20 under treatment with one test patch containing 30 mg/ 25 cm² bupranolol compared to 2 × 80 mg of oral propranolol·HCl.

Propranolol tablets were administered at intervals of 12 hr, each tablet containing 80 mg of propranolol·HCl.

The effects of the treatments were evaluated from the inhibition of isoprenaline-induced tachycardia as summarized in Figure 9. The graph gives a more detailed picture of the effect profile of transdermally delivered bupranolol in man, confirming the data gained from the 3-day study reported above. Compared to the bupranolol patches, the effects observed under treatment with oral propranolol· HCl varied considerably during the test period, with maxima found between 1 and 3 hr postapplication and minima observed at 12 hr postapplication. Figure 9 illustrates that the effect of 11 mg of transdermally absorbed bupranolol is almost in the range of effect of two 80 mg doses of oral propranolol·HCl. Comparing the areas under the curves from 0 to 24 hr, the effect may be considered to be roughly comparable to 80% of propranolol action. These data will have to be further investigated in long-term studies.

V. SUMMARY

The results from our pilot studies indicate bupranolol to be a promising candidate for transdermal delivery. Upon application on a relatively small area (25 cm^2 in human volunteers), bupranolol penetrated in sufficient amounts to produce pronounced pharmacological effects. By comparison to the therapeutically effective dose of 2 × 80 mg of oral propranolol, the effect of the transdermally absorbed amount of bupranolol could be shown to be in the therapeutic range. Plotting of effects versus time yielded remarkably steady effect profiles, very similar to those observed during intravenous administration. The main difference was a considerable lag time (about 3–5 hr in rabbits, around 6 hr in humans), probably due to the process of penetration through the skin. Once steady state had been reached, effects could be kept at steady-state level for as long as 3 days by changing the test patches every 24 hr.

The results obtained from the rabbit study showed bioavailability to be about 90%. Thus, transdermal delivery might turn out to be the way to overcome the severest problem in oral bupranolol administration: the poor bioavailability of the drug due to extraordinarily high first-pass metabolism.

We feel the results obtained from these initial studies must be considered very encouraging with respect to the feasibility of transdermal administration of bupranolol. Further investigations will give more detailed informations about the various aspects of transdermal β-adrenoceptor blocking therapy with bupranolol, including the determination of skin irritation in relation to drug release rate and vehicle effects.

ACKNOWLEDGMENTS

The authors wish to thank Dr. H. Küppers, Department of Medical Research, and Dr. K. Müller, Department of Pharmacokinetics, Schwarz GmbH, Monheim, for their scientific and technical assistance, and Dr. A. Wellstein, Pharmacology Center, Goethe University Clinic, Frankfurt, for permission to present part of the results of his receptor binding studies.

REFERENCES

1. A. R. Waller, L. F. Chasseaud, R. Bonn, T. Taylor, A. Darragh, R. Girkin, W. H. Down, and E. Doyle, *Drug Metab. Disposition, 10:* 51 (1982).
2. A. Wellstein et al., *Eur. J. Clin. Pharmacol., 31:* 419 (1986).
3. A. Wellstein, D. Palm, G. Wiemer, M. Schäfer-Korting, and E. Mutschler, *Eur. J. Clin. Pharmacol., 27:* 545 (1984).

ENGINEERING AND MANUFACTURING OF TRANSDERMAL THERAPEUTIC SYSTEMS

13

Development of Processes and Equipment for Rate-Controlled Transdermal Therapeutic Systems

JOHN W. DOHNER / *Alza Corporation, Palo Alto, California*

I. INTRODUCTION

Recent years have witnessed the introduction of a new dosage form to the pharmaceutical industry—the controlled-release transdermal drug delivery system. Such transdermal systems are now commercially available to treat angina, hypertension, and motion sickness. The rationale for, and advantages of, transdermal delivery of drugs have been the subject of numerous papers. Less has been published on engineering, development, and production of these dosage forms (1). This chapter defines critical engineering activities relating to the scaleup and commercial production of controlled-release transdermal products, referencing products Alza Corporation has developed and commercialized for major pharmaceutical firms.

II. TRANSDERMAL PRODUCTS DEVELOPED AT ALZA

Four transdermal products developed at Alza are currently commercially available: Catapres-TTS®, Transderm®-Nitro, Transderm®-Scop, and Estraderm®.

Catapres-TTS will be marketed by Boehringer Ingelheim for the treatment of mild to moderate hypertension. The dosage form contains the drug clonidine, which it delivers into the bloodstream at a controlled, predetermined rate for 7 days. The product (Fig. 1) consists of five layers:

1. *Backing substrate*, an impermeable substrate that protects the product during use on the skin.
2. *Drug reservoir*, an adhesive layer containing most of the system's drug.
3. *Control membrane*, a polymeric film that controls the rate at which drug leaves the system and enters the body.
4. *Contact adhesive*, a hypoallergenic adhesive designed to hold the product next to the skin for 7 days.
5. *Release liner*, a plastic substrate that protects the product in the package. The user discards the liner when applying the system.

Catapres-TTS is fabricated using technologies adopted from the adhesives and coatings industry. It is currently manufactured at Alza for Boehringer.

Transderm-Nitro (Fig. 2) is marketed by Ciba-Geigy for the prevention and treatment of angina. The patch is worn on the chest and delivers nitroglycerin for 24 hr. The drug reservoir of Transderm-Nitro consists of a gel or ointment sealed into the product using liquid filling and sealing technology.

Transderm-Scop delivers scopolamine for 3 days to prevent motion sickness. This system is manufactured by Alza and marketed by Ciba-Geigy. Transderm-Scop and Catapres-TTS share similar manufacturing technologies.

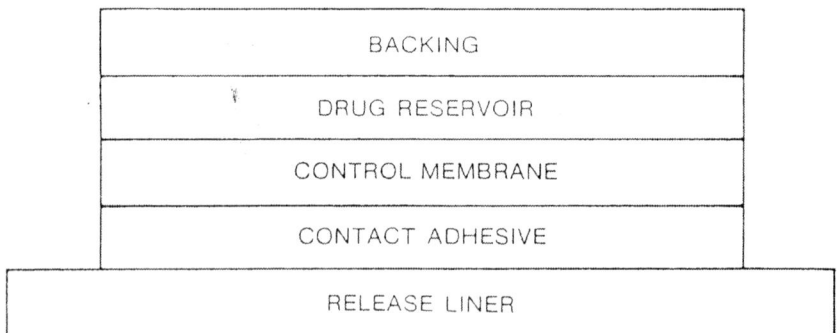

Figure 1   A transdermal therapeutic system multilaminate: Catapres-TTS.

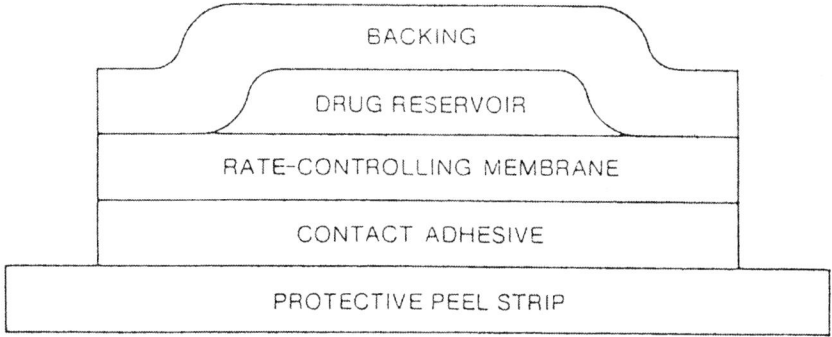

Figure 2 A transdermal therapeutic system illustrating the form-fill-seal approach: Transderm-Nitro.

Estraderm delivers estradiol for the treatment of peri- and post-menopausal disorders. The product uses manufacturing technology similar to that of Transderm-Nitro.

Each of these transdermal products contains a control membrane. As resistance from the membrane increases, the percentage of control offered by the system increases, thereby minimizing intra- and inter-person variability. Thus, drug is administered at a more predictable, precise rate. Physical and chemical properties of the membrane can be designed to achieve particular levels of system control.

III. MANUFACTURING PROCESSES AND EQUIPMENT

Large-scale production of new pharmaceutical dosage forms, such as transdermal products, requires manufacturing technologies that are new to, or modified from, the traditional pharmaceutical industry. Large-scale production processes and equipment have been developed to make each of the transdermal products described above. A qualitative description of those processes is presented here.

Alza has designated Catapres-TTS and Transderm-Scop as "multilaminate" products, referring to the layers that are coated and laminated together. Figure 3 shows the manufacturing process flowchart for multilaminate products. Multilaminate products comprise three substrates, held together by two layers of drug-containing adhesives that are prepared and coated at Alza. The first manufacturing step involves processing the drug into the physical/chemical form required for incorporation into the transdermal product. Next, the adhesive coating solutions are prepared. Adhesive components,

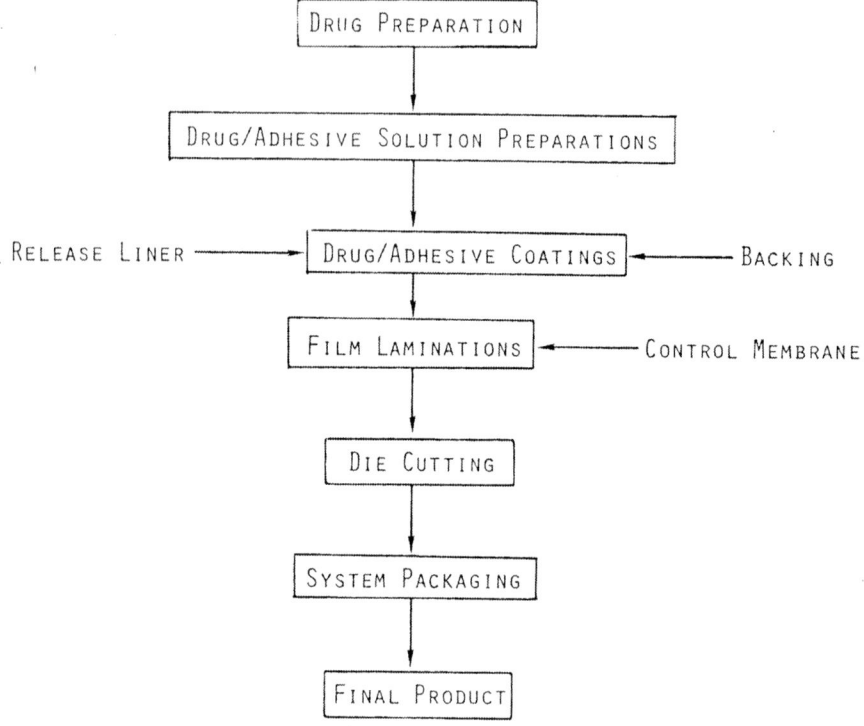

Figure 3   Multilaminate transdermal dosage form manufacturing process flow diagram.

excipients, and drug are mixed with a solvent until a uniform solution or dispersion is achieved. The mixing step is carefully controlled because the product composition is determined here. The adhesive compositions are deposited as thin films onto moving substrates, which then pass through a series of drying ovens to remove solvent. After drying, the adhesive films and other layers are laminated together to form the five-layer product consisting of release liner + contact adhesive + control membrane + drug reservoir + backing substrate. The laminate is then printed and die-cut into the final dosage form. The film coating and laminating steps are probably the most critical to final dosage form performance. Precise coating thicknesses and a wrinkle-free laminate require accurate control of process variables.

Transderm-Scop and Catapres-TTS are packaged in individual foil pouches. Dosage forms pass over an inspection table and are automatically inserted into a continuously moving web of pouch stock.

The pouch stock is then sealed around the dosage form. Individual pouches are cut from the web and shingled on a conveyor. Pouches are loaded, with patient and physician inserts, into cartons or blisters, which are sorted into units for shipment.

Alza designates Transderm-Nitro and Estraderm as "Form-Fill-Seal" products, based on the manufacturing process and equipment used to fill and seal the drug ointment into the product. Figure 4 illustrates the process employed to manufacture this type of dosage form design. A laminate of release liner + contact adhesive + control membrane is prepared and fed into packaging-type equipment, where discrete portions of drug gel are deposited onto the web, covered with the backing, and sealed using heat and pressure. Individual systems are die-punched from the web and collected for packaging, where they are loaded into foil pouches and subsequently into cartons for shipment.

The multilaminate and form-fill-seal processes are highly automated and run with a minimum of direct labor. The processes are continuous, and batch sizes on the order of a million units are typical.

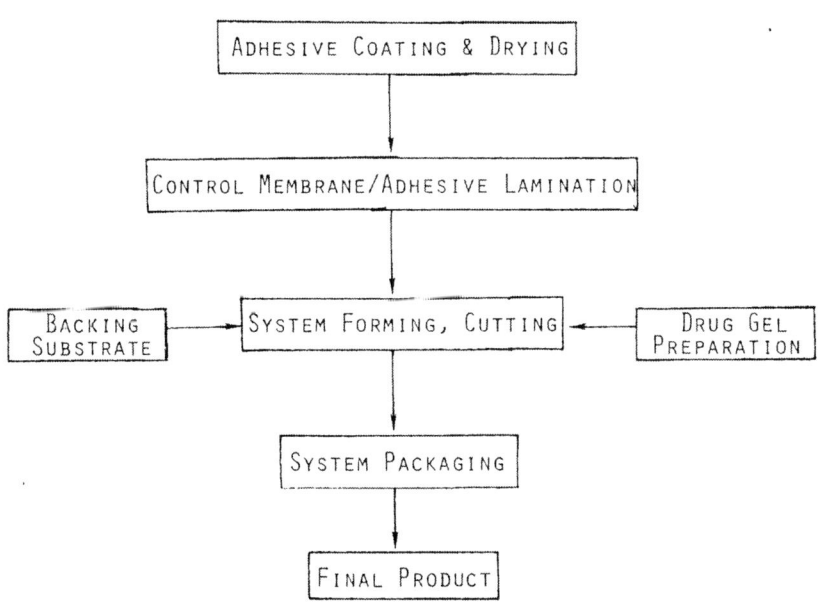

Figure 4   Form-fill-seal process flow diagram.

IV. ENGINEERING DEVELOPMENT OF TRANSDERMAL SYSTEMS

After a transdermal product's technical and functional feasibility have been established, an engineering development phase can be initiated. This phase requires a significant commitment of time and money to achieve commercial production of a marketable product. The primary goal of this effort is to develop economical manufacturing processes, equipment, and facilities that will consistently produce transdermal products with desired performance attributes. The time and cost of such a development program depends on many facturs: product complexity, desired performance attributes, novelty of the processes and equipment required, experience of the engineering development group, targeted sales prices and volumes, and the thoroughness that goes into defining the product as it comes from research. Whether the development effort is straightforward or complex, the activities required are similar. These activities are typical in the engineering development and scaleup of any pharmaceutical product, although certain tasks relate specifically to transdermal products. Subsequent sections summarize critical activities.

A. Development of Product Circumscription

The engineering development effort should start by documenting everything that is known about, and desired of, the product. Alza calls this listing a "product circumscription." The better defined and complete a circumscription is, the more accurately engineering costs can be projected, and hence the more smoothly activities will progress. Elements of a product circumscription should include the following.

1. *Desired attributes and specifications.* What physical, chemical, and pharmaceutical properties should the product have, and over what ranges can these properties vary? What tests are used to quantify these properties?
2. *Formulation and components.* What is the system composition as it comes from research? What special materials are involved?
3. *Manufacturing directions.* How is the product made? What in-process checks and controls are used? What are the recommended settings for critical process variables?
4. *Packaging configuration.* How should the proposed product be packaged? What alternates are desired?
5. *Marketing information.* What are the anticipated production volumes? What manufacturing cost is acceptable?

The product circumscription is an evolutionary document. Initially it may comprise a few pages. As development continues, it will grow and eventually provide the backbone for an NDA filing (if the drug is an ethical product) and a technology transfer document, to be passed on as responsibility for the product moves from engineering to production.

B. Process Design

Design of a commercial manufacturing process can proceed once the product has been initially defined with regard to its purpose and market. The process scale should be sized consistently with projected sales volumes: an economical process designed to produce 20 million transdermal products yearly may not be economical at 2 million units per year, and may not be feasible at 200 million units per year.

The principal unit operations required can be listed in a flow diagram (see Figs. 3 and 4). Each unit operation should show materials added and removed, projected batch sizes, and anticipated processing rates and yields. After the flow diagram has been tentatively defined, its technical feasibility should be established. Although answering all questions of large-scale feasibility is impractical, critical process steps should be modeled or tested on a small scale to ensure their applicability to the product.

Procurement of equipment can proceed once a reasonably accurate process flow diagram has been defined. As with process design, depending on the equipment complexity, it may be preferable to develop the equipment in stages—from feasibility demonstration, to pilot-scale unit, to commercial unit. This is especially true for transdermal manufacturing equipment, much of which is new to, or significantly modified from, the pharmaceutical industry. At this time alternate plans must also be developed to locate the commercial production site. Should production be done "in-house," or should all or part of it be contracted to manufacturing firms with experience in, and equipment for, carrying out the desired operations?

In-process tests and testing locations should be specified. Alza has found that extensive in-process testing, early in the development phase, can provide a valuable understanding of critical processes and variables. When the processes are well defined and have been shown to be reliable and reproducible, certain in-process tests may become unnecessary. Generally, though, in-process testing costs less than finished-product testing, and it occurs at a time when corrective measures can be taken to change a process.

C. Materials Selection

Transdermal dosage forms require specialized materials that are generally new to the pharmaceutical industry—substrates, membranes, and adhesives. Vendors must be selected for these materials, specifications agreed on, and raw material testing procedures developed. Desired attributes of critical materials used for transdermal products developed by Alza are discussed next.

1. Rate-Controlling Membranes

Rate-controlling membranes are films that control the rate of drug flux from the dosage form. Tight physical and chemical specifications will ensure reproducible drug release rates between lots. Transdermal products have been made with microporous membranes and with dense polymeric membranes.

2. Backing Substrates

Backing films must be flexible, and they must provide a good bond to the drug reservoir, prevent drug from leaving the dosage form through the top, and accept printing.

3. Release Liners

The release liner should permit easy peel by the user and yet should not interfere with the functionality of the product. Cost must be compatible with a "disposable" concept because the liner is thrown away.

4. Drug Reservoir Components

Components of the drug reservoir must be compatible with the drug and must allow for drug transport at the desired rate. If an ointment, the drug reservoir must possess desired viscosity attributes to ensure a reliable manufacturing process. If an adhesive, the drug reservoir must possess the desired adhesive and cohesive properties to hold the system together.

5. Contact Adhesive Components

The contact adhesive materials must provide desired adhesive and cohesive properties, possess the desired drug solubility and permeability characteristics, and be skin compatible.

6. Packaging Substrates

Transdermal systems may require special packaging materials. Those used on transdermal products developed by Alza include a moisture barrier and an easily printable exterior surface. Product stability in the packages should be tested.

D. Development of Quality Control Procedures

All new technologies require new tests and test procedures to confirm that the product performs as specified. Typical tests for transdermal products measure drug release rate, drug content, and adhesive properties.

1. Drug Release Rate

The in vitro drug release test is the most important performance test for a transdermal dosage form. The data can be expressed either as the cumulative amount of drug released over time or as the release rate of drug during specified time intervals. Testing intervals provide information on the initial release of drug from the contact adhesive, and the constant release of drug from the reservoir through the control membrane and adhesive. In vivo, the initial release of drug from the system saturates the skin beneath the dosage form and quickly brings plasma levels of drug up to a therapeutically effective concentration. After the initial release of drug, the control membrane offers the primary resistance to drug flow from the reservoir. This steady rate of drug release maintains plasma drug concentrations within the therapeutic window throughout the specified lifetime of the system.

Alza has developed specialized automated testing equipment to measure the in vitro rate of drug release over time. Systems are placed on holders and agitated in test tubes filled with appropriate test media for predetermined time intervals. At the end of each interval, the holders automatically advance to the next set of tubes.

The average in vitro drug release rate for 11 production lots of a typical multilaminate transdermal dosage form (Table 1) indicates high reproducibility of system performance.

Table 1   In Vitro Drug Release from 11 Consecutive Production Lots of a Typical Transdermal Product

Time interval	In vitro drug release rate (μg/hr $\pm$ SD)	Coefficient of variation
1st	51.2 $\pm$ 1.8	3.5
2nd	11.9 $\pm$ 1.1	9.2
3rd	9.2 $\pm$ 0.8	8.9
4th	8.3 $\pm$ 0.6	7.6

The release rate test has proved to be reliable for demonstrating the performance of dosage forms in a controlled environment. In vitro testing and in vivo performance have shown good correlation.

2. Drug Content

The test for drug assay of a dosage form is standard to the pharmaceutical industry. The difference between transdermal and conventional oral dosage forms, however, is that drug content per se does not greatly affect the performance of this dosage form. The total amount of drug in the reservoir of a transdermal dosage form does not dramatically affect the magnitude of the drug release rate; rather, it determines the duration of drug delivery. Both Transderm Scop and Catapres-TTS contain excess drug; that is, after in vivo wearing of the product for the specified lifetime, a certain amount of drug remains and is discarded with the dosage form. Thus, drug assay is not as critical a parameter of dosage form functionality as it is for other pharmaceutical products. It is, however, important that the actual drug content be within specified limits of the value shown on the product label. With a target content of 1.5 mg, an average drug content of 1.56 ± 0.05 mg and a coefficient of variation of 3% was found for 11 production lots of a transdermal dosage form. These data indicate the reproducibility of the manufacturing process.

3. Adhesive Properties

Effective, continuous transdermal drug delivery requires that the dosage form maintain intimate contact with the skin. Products developed by Alza maintain contact with an adhesive. In addition, the other layers of the product are bonded together by adhesives. Thus, a measurement of adhesive forces demonstrates that the dosage form possesses the proper characteristics to maintain an integral structure and to adhere to the user on wearing. For example, the force required to peel the release liner from a typical system is 5 g/cm, which indicates the ease with which the user will be able to remove the liner and use the product. For reference, using the same test, the force required to peel the liner from a Band-Aid adhesive bandage is approximately 200 g/cm. The adhesive quality of the contact adhesive can be measured by placing the system against a reference surface and measuring the force required to peel it away. Adhesion tests are not as quantitative as other tests performed on transdermal dosage forms, but they do indicate the qualitative behavior of systems during use.

E. Characterization Experiments

Characterization experiments are the core of the engineering development activities. These studies, which elucidate the relationship between process variables and product attributes, are performed most economically at a relatively small scale and involve statistical design to maximize the quality and quantity of data obtained. For each process step, controlled or independent variables are defined. Desired attributes or responses that can be measured (dependent variables) are listed. The relationship between process variables and measured responses can be tabulated (2) in an "influence matrix," shown, typically, in Table 2. Using background knowledge, theoretical analyses, or designed experiments, each blank is filled in with "strong," "medium," "weak," or "none" to indicate the expected influence of a particular variable on the response. To quantify the effects, squares showing greater degrees of influence are studied in detail with statistically designed experiments.

Because designed experiments typically require repetitive studies, small-scale characterization studies should be done to use less material and time. If the small-scale or pilot-scale experiment is reasonably similar in concept to the commercial-scale process, the relative degree of influence will hold, although some of the exact quantification may need repeating. Once the small-scale experiments have been done, the engineer can more effectively plan the few large-scale experiments required.

The data obtained can optimize the process (i.e., maximize the production rate of product meeting desired quality attributes), set realistic specifications for product attributes, and set allowable ranges for process variables. Well-planned, documented experiments can contribute heavily to a formal process validation program.

Table 2 Influence Matrix for Film Coating Process

Process variables	Measured responses				
	Drug content	Release rate	Residual solvent	Adhesive properties	Etc.
Variable 1					
Variable 2					
Variable 3					
Variable 4					
Variable 5					
Etc.					

A final note on characterization experiments is that the engineer should ensure a good supply of high-quality analytical testing support. Accurate, reproducible analytical results are crucial to successful interpretation of the data.

F. Process and Equipment Scaleup

The timing for scaleup should be carefully integrated into an overall program, or master schedule, which involves other critical items such as the regulatory process and the market introduction dates. Alza generally scales up in stages. The first stage reaches a level where the NDA can be filed. The process at the NDA stage represents the commercial process at the pilot-plant level. Significant process changes should not occur during the subsequent final scaleup to commercial production. The final scaleup can take place while the NDA approval proceeds; in this way a full-scale manufacturing process will be available coincident with the NDA approval.

Scaleup activities involve processes, equipment, and facilities. Influences of certain critical process variables on product attributes must be confirmed and quantified and optimum throughput rates established. Equipment is either purchased or fabricated in-house. Since transdermal dosage forms are new, the larger scale equipment generally differs from that available at most pharmaceutical facilities. Each transdermal product currently on the market has required a significant equipment development effort to achieve commercial-scale production. As more products are developed, equipment developed for one product probably will be useful for other products, thereby reducing the per-product capital expenditure.

The commercial-scale process and equipment, when available, are established in a facility adequately designed to support the required level of commercial production. Because the products are new, production space generally must be created. If outside converters are used, special efforts may be necessary to ensure compliance with the FDA's Good Manufacturing Practice (GMP) guidelines. Adhesive converting houses often do not have facilities and procedures adequate for pharmaceutical processing.

The final step of scaleup requires revision of the manufacturing documents to make them compatible with the large-scale process, equipment, facility, and production personnel.

G. Validation and Technology Transfer

Although some validation activities are ongoing throughout the engineering development phase, the large-scale process validation phase starts when the commercial-scale process, equipment, and facility are in place. While the work can go on simultaneously with a technology transfer from engineering to production, the validation program should be an engineering responsibility. The validation program should aim to prove that the manufacturing process is controlled, and that when the written procedures are followed, product meeting desired quality specifications can be reproducibly produced.

One approach to validation involves the manufacture of a series of product batches at target process settings. The process is frequently sampled and tested at the intermediate and finished-product stages. Control charts are created showing the measured values for each attribute tested. If the observed results show reproducible product performance, the process is considered to be validated. This type of validation program is not costly because control charts are a normal part of current quality control programs, and the validation efforts only involve extra testing and analysis.

A more rigorous approach to validation involves challenging the process and proving that acceptable product can be made, as long as process settings remain within the specified ranges. For specific experiments, products can be made using the extremes of stated process variable ranges to provide "worst-case" performance. If the product thus produced has acceptable quality attributes, the process, including specified ranges for variables, is validated. This type of validation experiment is more rigorous and useful, but it also is more expensive because it involves a number of large-scale experiments: for example, if product fabrication requires three processes, if two variables are important for each process, and if a high and a low limit for each variable must be validated, validation would require 12 experiments. Judicious selection of variables can reduce this number somewhat, but validation still represents a commitment of engineering and analytical testing personnel.

Prior to steady-state commercial production, responsibility for the product moves from engineering to production or operations. This move requires a carefully planned training program. Personnel with a background in adhesives, coating, printing, and other film-converting operations offer skills required for transdermal dosage form production. Alza utilizes a series of production demonstration runs (PDRs) to effect technology transfer and personnel training. Engineering personnel perform the first PDR or set of PDRs, supervised by engineering personnel and observed by production personnel. Production personnel perform the second PDR or set of PDRs, supervised by engineering personnel. Production personnel perform and supervise the third PDR or set of PDRs, with engineers observing. The engineering responsibility is thus phased out as production personnel become trained. The number of PDRs required is a function of the process complexity and the degree of training required.

V. COMMERCIAL PRODUCTION OF TRANSDERMAL SYSTEMS

Market introduction of a transdermal product requires a coordinated effort between technical, regulatory, and marketing functions. Probably the single most critical responsibility falls to the group charged with producing commercial product to supply market demand. Commercial production can take place in-house, or it can be contracted, at least initially, to a manufacturer experienced in transdermal production. Ideally, the initial commercial manufacturing site should be determined early in the engineering development phase. In this manner, production technology can be smoothly transferred from engineering to commercial production at a timely point.

Regardless of where commercial manufacturing is done, certain prerequisites should be met by the production group to ensure a reliable supply of product. Most importantly, the manufacturing group should have a proven record of pharmaceutical production, preferably with transdermal systems. Such experience does exist in the industry. Alza, for example, has produced more than 100 commercial lots of Transderm Scop for Ciba-Geigy and more than 20 lots of Catapres-TTS for Boehringer Ingelheim. Knowledge gained from this extensive experience is invaluable in assuring a smooth startup and steady production.

Engineering abilities should be evaluated. Process engineering, equipment engineering, and industrial engineering expertises all contribute significantly to efficient production startup and are important to the successful resolution of production problems that may arise once production is under way. The production engineering staff should be evaluated for its experience in developing specialized manufacturing processes and equipment and for its ability to design cost-efficient material handling and production operations.

A strong quality control group is essential. Such a group should be capable of ensuring GMP compliance and should also anticipate problems related to transdermal system production. They should actively participate in the specification setting process, with a knowledge of what attributes are important and how tightly they can be controlled. Alza's quality control group is responsible for GMP compliance, intermediate and finished-product testing, production documentation, and records storage, as well as maintenance and evaluation of control charts to monitor routine production.

The largest contributor to the manufacturing cost of a transdermal product is the package. Therefore, efficient packaging design, equipment, and experience are important. If significant production is anticipated, packaging operations should be highly automated and streamlined. Packaging personnel should be familiar with pouching and cartoning equipment and should have the capabilities to provide special controls and automated inspection equipment. Although aseptic packaging is not required for current transdermal products, the packaging facility should clearly meet GMP requirements typical for tablet packaging operations.

Extensive analytical testing capabilities are very useful, both to develop test methods for measuring system performance and for troubleshooting unanticipated production problems that invariably arise, especially during the initial phases of production. Sophisticated, modern analytical equipment should be available on site, not only to routinely quantify system attributes, but also to quantitatively analyze the chemical and physical composition of each layer in a transdermal system.

Production personnel should have experience with, and an understanding of, adhesives and web handling, two major components of current transdermal systems. A knowledge of adhesive and substrate suppliers, meaningful raw material testing to ensure incoming material quality, and the ability to resolve production problems common to the film-converting industry are essential. Production personnel with film-converting (lamination, extrusion, coating, printing, etc.) backgrounds are a major asset to the successful production of transdermal products.

Validation experience with both processes and equipment should be examined. Regardless of what was done during engineering scaleup, a significant validation effort at the commercial production level will be required. It is important to know which processes the validation effort should concentrate on, and how the validation can most efficiently proceed.

If production is contracted, the manufacturing firm should provide effective technology transfer of both processes and equipment to the pharmaceutical company owning the product, if production is brought in-house. Technology transfer would include personnel training and production startup assistance.

VI. SUMMARY

Transdermal products already on the market have proved the technical and economical success of this pharmaceutical dosage form. Four products developed by Alza Corporation for Ciba-Geigy and Boehringer Ingelheim utilize polymeric membranes to control the flux of drug leaving the system. Manufacturing processes and equipment have been developed to produce these systems economically and in large volume.

The engineering development phase is important in the product development cycle for transdermal products. At this phase, the production process is scaled up from laboratory level to commercial production. Components of the engineering development phase have been described. When engineering development is complete, technology transfer to commercial production occurs. Whether production is done in-house or contracted to a manufacturer experienced in transdermal production, those responsible for the commercial production should secure the presence of a number of functional support groups. Proper support by these groups will ensure a high probability of successful, large-volume transdermal system manufacture.

REFERENCES

1. J. E. Shaw and J. W. Dohner, Transdermal dosage forms, *Proceedings of Interphex, 1984*, Brighton, UK, 1984.
2. P. J. Von Doehren, F. St. John Forbes, and C. D. Shively, An approach to the characterization and technology transfer of solid dosage form processes, *Pharm. Technol.*, *6*(9): 139 (1982).

14

Development of Processes and Technology for Adhesive-Type Transdermal Therapeutic Systems

HANS-MICHAEL WOLFF / Schwarz GmbH, Monheim, West Germany
HANS RAINER HOFFMANN / LTS Lohman Therapie-Systeme
GmbH & Co. KG, Neuwied, West Germany
GÜNTER CORDES / Schwarz GmbH, Monheim, West Germany

I. INTRODUCTION

Pressure-sensitive adhesives are important components of transdermal therapeutic systems (TTS): by guaranteeing sufficient contact between the drug release area and the skin, they fulfill a crucial precondition for drug delivery. Additionally, in preparations in which the adhesive layers cover the whole application area, the drug must pass through such layers, and this event may become a rate-determining step.

Depending on its capacity to absorb drug molecules, the adhesive may act as a drug reservoir, too, and may store a loading dose (1). These possible functions are combined in a galenical* concept that is characterized by incorporation of the total amount of drug into self-adhesive films having one or more layers. This represents the basic idea of adhesive-type transdermal systems offering some important practical advantages related to the manufacture of such systems.

---

*Galenical = technological.

A. Manufacturing Method

Since known coating technologies can be employed during all stages of development, a considerable portion of know-how and equipment already available for the production of medical adhesive tapes can be transferred to the manufacture of transdermal systems.

B. Feasibility of Adjusting Dosage Strengths

Flexible dosing, which may be necessary for individual requirements, is achievable by punching or cutting systems of the desired size out of the original tapelike laminate on the basis of a linear relation between the size of the transdermal system and the bioavailable dose of drug.

One typical example of the adhesive-type transdermal therapeutic systems is marketed under the tradename Deponit®. This multilayered patch was developed by Schwarz/Lohmann for the controlled transdermal delivery of nitroglycerin. Published results of in vitro and in vivo release studies concerning this system (2) have shown good agreement with the original concept of TTS, which demands an effective control mechanism for drug delivery during the whole application period.

In the following, some features of the galenical design and manufacturing process of the Schwarz/Lohmann system are described, illustrated by the structure and concept of the Deponit system. Determinations of in vitro and in vivo drug release were performed as described in Ref. 2.

II. GALENICAL STRUCTURE OF THE DEPONIT SYSTEM

The cross section of a Deponit system can be divided into three main components (Fig. 1):

1. A flexible polyester foil about 20 μm thick, representing the carrier foil for the drug-loaded film
2. A multilayered adhesive film loaded with nitroglycerin, approximately 350 μm thick, simultaneously representing the drug reservoir and the release control system
3. An aluminized and siliconized polyester foil about 100 μm thick, representing a protective foil that can be peeled off before application.

Component 2 is characterized by:

1. Its content of lactose as a hydrophilic ingredient in a skin-compatible, water-insoluble, adhesive mass of a base consisting

THICKNESS COMPONENT

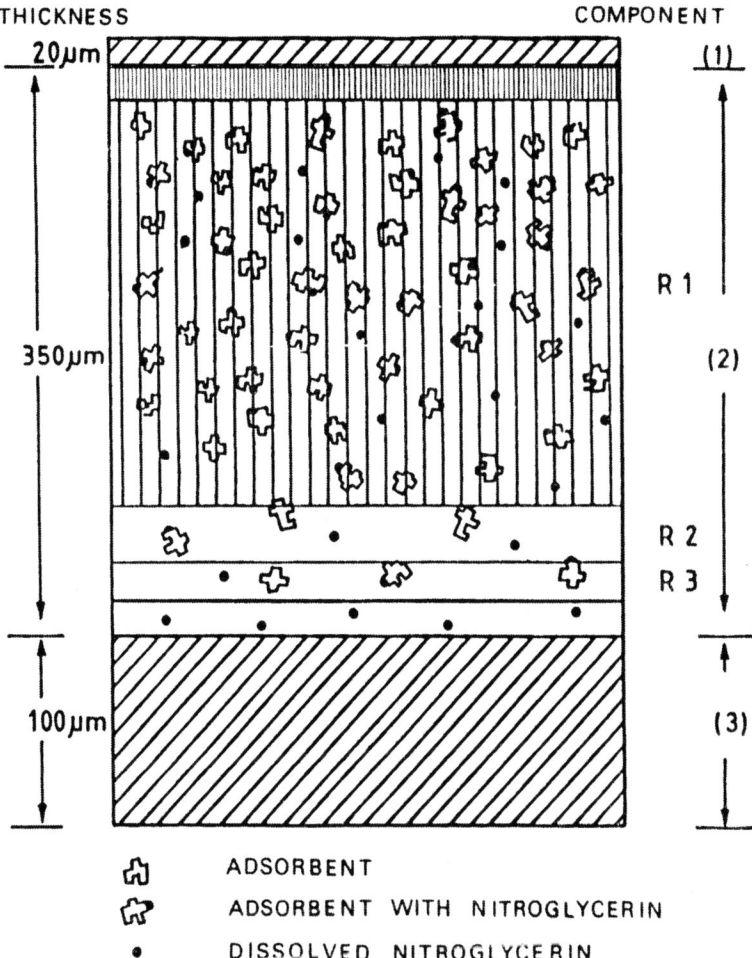

ADSORBENT

ADSORBENT WITH NITROGLYCERIN

• DISSOLVED NITROGLYCERIN

Figure 1   Cross-sectional view of Deponit, an adhesive-type multi-layered transdermal therapeutic system (Schwarz/Lohmann); R1–R3 represent the drug reservoir layers containing different amounts of nitroglycerin and lactose.

of polyisobutylene (PIB) and resin with absorbed and dissolved nitroglycerin

2. A nitroglycerin-lactose concentration gradient that rises step-wise toward the carrier foil (1), built up by distinct drug dispersion or reservoir zones (R1-R3, Fig. 1)

As described in Ref. 2, the scanning electron microscope image of the TTS cross section revealed no particular structural elements such as cavities or micropores besides the suspended lactose crystals.

III. MANUFACTURING PROCESS

The production of a TTS according to the Lohmann/Schwarz system is subdivided into five steps:

1. Preparing the individual matrix solutions
2. Coating the individual matrix layers
3. Building the multilayer laminate
4. Separating units of the multilayer laminate
5. Packaging

A. Preparing the Individual Matrix Solutions

To begin, each matrix raw material is dissolved in an organic solvent. In this way one obtains a so-called standard or stock solution for each raw material. Hence, primarily the following raw materials are possible: base polymers, softening agents, tackifiers, and resorption agents. After determination of solid content and other decisive quality parameters, the matrix solution is prepared from the stock solution by mixing it with ingredients specified by the formulation. In the last step the calculated amount of active agent and eventually other nonsoluble additives (e.g., inert fillers) are added.

The quality-determining parameters of a matrix solution or suspension thus obtained are checked once again. The number of matrix solutions or suspensions to be manufactured determines the building of the TTS. In the system described here at least three matrix solutions of different compositions are necessary. In the case of Deponit, five different solutions/suspensions are used.

B. Coating the Individual Matrix Layers

The individual layers are made by coating the solutions/suspensions described above on a smooth web and removing the solvent by drying. Preferably this process is done on a coating machine, which consists of two main units: the coating head and the dryer section. Generally the substratum to be coated is a paper or film web.

Figure 2 schematically shows the coating machine. Depending on the viscosity, the solid content, the flowability, and the surface tension of the matrix solution or suspension and the solvent, different coating units are used. Commonly used are roll coaters, coating heads, and knife systems.

In the coating unit the solvent-based formulations are coated onto the appropriate web. To guarantee a uniform and reproducible ' coating, the unit must work very precisely. For example, the nip in the roll coater must be exactly adjustable within 0.001 mm to achieve the required cross-direction (CD) and machine direction (MD) coating exactness of ±1 g/m^2. Such an accuracy is absolutely necessary to obtain the desired release profile of each matrix layer.

Because solvents and eventually active agents evaporate to some extent in the coating unit, this unit must be totally encased and hermetically closed to the surrounding environment. For this reason, the casing of the coating unit is directly connected to the drying system.

The solvent is evaporated from the adhesive mass by running the coated web through a drying channel. A modern unit of this kind consists of several sections and works according to the following principle. Highly cleaned, hot fresh air or inert gas is blown onto the adhesive mass, still containing considerable amounts of solvent, through nozzles that can be adjusted to control outlet speed. The drying medium (air or inert gas), loaded with solvent and eventually with active agents, is exhausted. A combustion unit may be

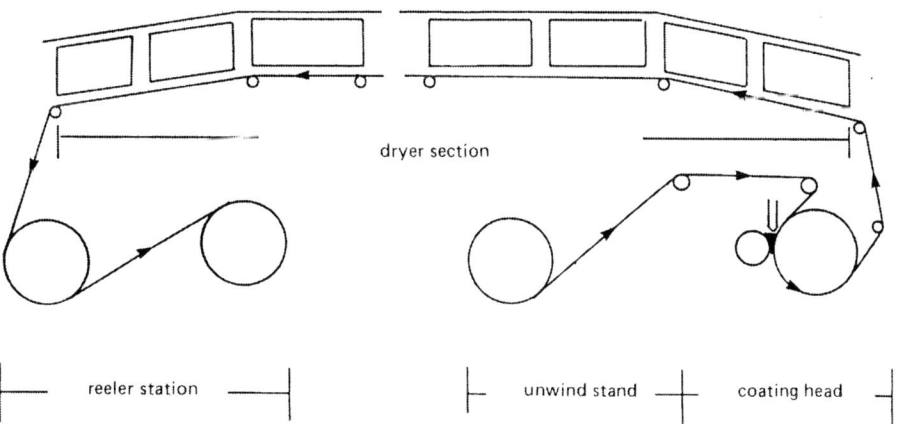

Figure 2 Schematic representation of a coating machine illustrating the main components.

considered as an emission control. In the case of inert gas, only a solvent recovery system can be used.

Each section of the drying unit is adjustable as far as temperature and air guiding is concerned, to control the retention of solvent and the eventual loss of active agent in the matrix during its run through the unit. The parameters under which the drying process must be conducted are to be experimentally determined for each matrix solution and/or suspension, depending on composition.

The weblike substratum is moved through the drying channel with aid of a transport system. Mechanical systems based on cranked shafts or conveyor belts are most commonly used as well as air-pillow systems mounted in the so-called floating-type drying channel.

The coating and drying processes influence quality. They must be extensively monitored by using various controlling devices. For example, continual monitoring of the coating weight, drying temperature, web speed, and air circulation is a must. Any deviation from the standard values must cause corresponding corrections. Cosmetic defects like pin-holes, creases, bubbles, and entrapped dirt must be identified and marked as to their effects on the following manufacturing steps.

To allow the production process to run uninterrupted, the web materials are used in form of jumbo rolls. The web is removed from these rolls in the unwind stand and is led through the coating and drying system to a reeler station mounted at the outlet of the drying channel.

Further requirements are necessary to wind the coated web itself. Simply, for this purpose, a differential release paper or film web is used. The ratio of the release levels is decisive for avoiding the unwanted transfer of the adhesive layer to the reverse side of the web.

Another possibility is to use an intermediate sheet, which protects the surface of the manufactured matrix layer. Depending on the peel characteristics of both materials one can, analogous to the example above, remove the original web (transfer of the matrix layer) or the additional intermediate sheet if necessary.

The speed of the unroll station, the coating unit, the transport system in the drying unit, and the winder must exactly by synchronized. Only in this way can it be guaranteed that the quality of the individual layers is not negatively influenced by varying web tensions. State of the art requires an edge-control system, since "misrun" of the web can result in incalculable quality risks and production problems.

C. Building the Multilayer Laminate

The building of a multilayer matrix system ensues from pressing the separately manufactured individual layers together, a process called lamination. Here two matrix layers, each adhering to one side of the web, are laminated together, coated side up. After the removal of a carrier material from the two-layer laminate thus obtained, a third layer, with the laminated side to the laminated side of the two-layer laminate, is pressed. This procedure is repeated until the final laminate is complete. It is most logical to begin the entire laminating process with one of the two outer layers. This procedure is carried out mechanically through use of a laminating unit. Here the manufacturer may use a counterrotating roll system, wherein the line pressure between the rolls can be exactly and reproducibly adjusted.

The adjustment of the laminating pressure is especially important because it must, on the one hand, assure sufficient adhesion of the two sides to be laminated, and, on the other hand, not be too high, since excessive pressure could destroy the extremely sensitive matrix layers, which are only a few micrometers thick.

The rolls can be cooled or heated. The laminating unit itself can be integrated into the overall coating process between the drying unit outlet and the winding station, or it can be operated as a separate aggregate. In the latter case, winding and unwinding systems are needed before and after the laminating station. At the conclusion of the laminating procedure, the finished system exists as a bulk product in the form of wide rolls.

Figure 3 schematically shows the building of the multilayer Deponit matrix.

D. Separating Units of the Multilayer Laminate

The bulk product, in jumbo rolls, is first subjected to longitudinal slitting if this is necessary. The cutting equipment is constructed so that one cutting unit is located between a winding unit and an unwinding unit.

The slitting itself occurs automatically upon unwinding the bulk product. The width of the roll is product-specified.

In a subsequent procedure the individual TTS units are punched or cut from the narrow rolls. Of decisive importance here is surface precision of the finished system, since this is in direct proportion to the release rate (ratio) of the active agents.

Modern machines for separating adhesive systems offer—in addition to the actual punching procedure—a number of further technical possibilities. For example, when the final carrier film and/or the final liner (masking film) has not been introduced during the coating process, the necessary material can be applied shortly before or shortly after the actual punching procedure. Furthermore, there exists the possibility of imprinting both materials. In addition, it is possible to apply the liner (masking film) with necessary release aids.

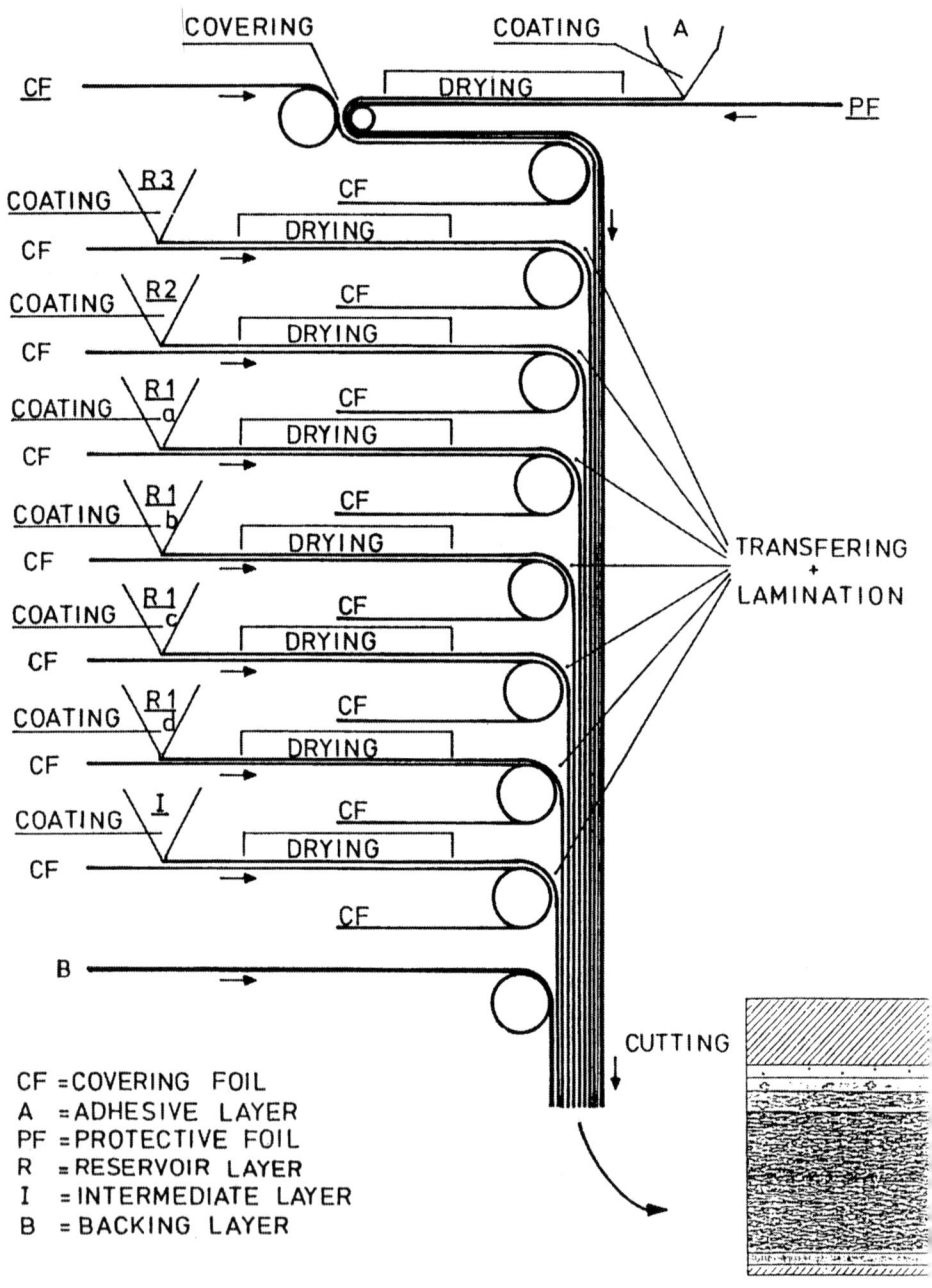

Figure 3   Schematic illustration of the Deponit manufacturing process.

E. Packaging

Packaging follows the separation of the adhesive TTS units. The
primary packaging—in most cases sealed, four-cornered pouches—
as well as the packaging in the cardboard boxes, is done with
machines that are usual in the industry.

IV. COMMENTS ON GALENICAL DESIGN

The galenical possibilities for the development of an adhesive-type
TTS with the desired adhesion, cohesion, stability, and drug release profile can be described by the modification of the physicochemical properties of all three main components (i.e., the carrier
foil, the drug-loaded adhesive film, and the protective foil). Naturally the drug-containing adhesive is the most important component,
bearing crucial variables that must be optimized as described in the
sections that follow.

A. Chemical Nature of the Self-Adhesive
   Polymer Film

Polymers used customarily in patch technology, such as polyacrylates,
rubber, and silicone elastomers, can be principally used in a transdermal system, too, if sufficient chemical compatibility of the polymer—drug mixture can be established. In the case of nitroglycerin,
a lipophilic, reactive, volatile substance, the polymers of choice
must be chemically inert as far as possible, and especially stable
against oxidation and (cyclo)-addition reactions. In the case of
Deponit, a low water absorption capacity and permeability of the
adhesive film have proved to be of advantage with respect to the
relevance of in vitro release studies.

The reactivity of nitroglycerin can be demonstrated when this
substance is incorporated in adhesives prepared on the basis of
natural rubber: intensive changes of color from yellow to black may
be visible within a few days.

Sufficient chemical inertness and an extremely high resistance to
the uptake of water are guaranteed by chemical pure, high-molecular-
weight polyisobutylene, the favored base for the Deponit system.
The capacity of the adhesive to absorb humidity may be advantageous
with respect to skin nonirritation and adhesion/cohesion properties,
and diffusity of the polymer matrix, but greater amounts of incorporated water unavoidably lead to a decrease of drug volume concentration, possibly resulting in decreased thermodynamic activity
of the drug. In cases of substances with poor water solubility, it
can be assumed that this negative effect is further reinforced by an
additional decrease of the drug solubility in the constituents of the
polymer film.

B. Chemical Nature and Content of Plasticizers

Figure 4 illustrates the in vitro nitroglycerin release from PIB-based adhesive films with identical galenical structure and drug concentration, but different tackifiers and content of a fatty oil. Formulations A and A' contain a hydrocarbon resin, B and B' a customary rosin derivative, together with about 0.1% (A;B) and 2% (w/w) (A';B') of fatty oil as an additional liquid plasticizer. The tackifier of formulations B and B' is characterized by an enhanced dissolving power for nitroglycerin due to alcoholic groups of its main component—hydroabietyl alcohol—leading to higher release rates in vitro in comparison to the corresponding formulations of A and A'.

The galenic variants with the higher content (2%) of fatty oil (A';B') show a clearly enhanced release rate of nitroglycerin compared to the corresponding formulations (A;B) containing only 0.1% of the liquid plasticizer.

These examples may demonstrate that it may be possible to vary the drug release rates from PIB-based adhesives of identical structure to a remarkable extent by minor modifications of the quantity and polarity of the ingredients, a higher release rate of nitroglycerin being achievable by enhancing the drug solubility in the adhesive film and lowering the microviscosity of the polymeric system (3,4).

C. Drug Concentration

Figure 5 shows the in vitro drug release from three nitroglycerin-loaded adhesive films of identical structure and composition, but containing different amounts of drug and lactose as absorbents for the amount of nitroglycerin that was not soluble in the base patch.

The range of 0.8–1.2 mg of nitroglycerin per square centimeter, corresponding to a range of 29–38 mg of nitroglycerin per cubic centimeter, led to a 24-hr release rate of about 0.38–0.43 mg/cm^2, increasing with increased content of nitroglycerin/lactose. So a difference of 0.4 mg of nitroglycerin per square centimeter of these systems has changed the 24-hr release rate by only 0.05 mg/cm^2.

In the case of the samples tested, there was a linear relation between the square root of nitroglycerin volume concentration and the cumulative nitroglycerin release corresponding to equations derived by Higuchi (5) for the situation of the drug being in suspension.

D. Drug Concentration Profile

With increasing distance between the nitroglycerin/lactose-containing reservoir layers and the release area, a decreasing drug delivery is

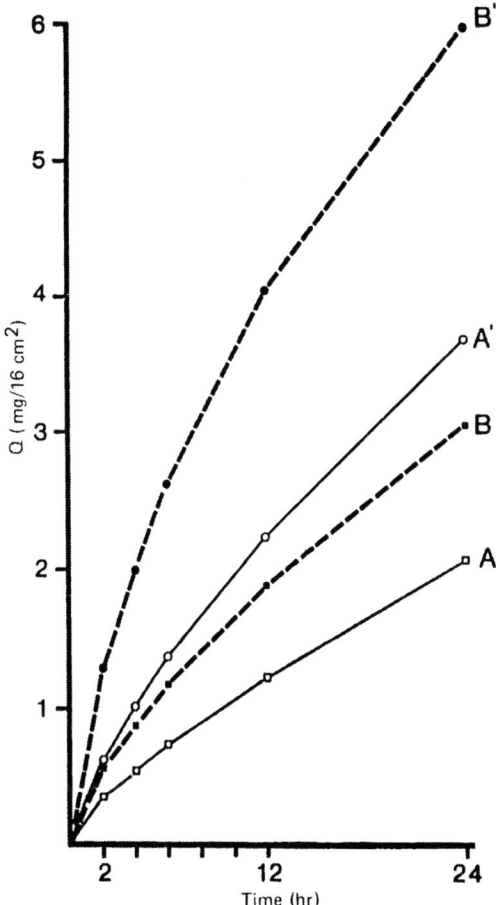

Figure 4   Comparative mean release profiles (n ~ 2) of nitroglycerin from various water-insoluble adhesive films with a modified galenical composition. In comparison to systems A and A' the pair B/B' contains a more polar tackifier; the systems A/B and A'/B' are characterized by their differing contents of fatty oil (0.1 and 2.0% w/w). The drug concentration by volume is equal for all four systems (ca. 36 mg/cm^3).

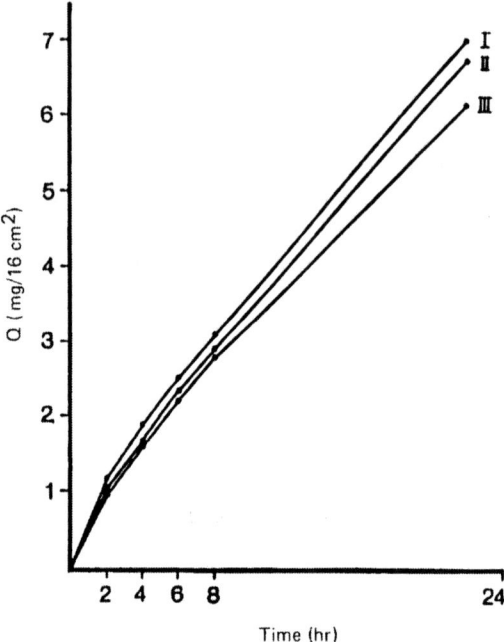

Time (hr)

Figure 5   Comparative mean release profiles (n = 2) of nitroglycerin from three adhesive-type transdermal systems of identical structure but containing different amounts of drug. The nitroglycerin concentrations for curves I–III are 38, 34, and 29 mg/cm^3, respectively. The corresponding cumulative release rates Q are in approximate linear correlation with the square root of the drug concentration; the experimental results for Q for curves I–III were: 6.99, 6.71, and 6.12 $mg/16 \ cm^2/24$ hr, respectively.

to be expected.   This can be demonstrated by insertion of adhesive layers that are free of nitroglycerin/lactose adsorbent.

Figure 6 illustrates the change of the release rates for two pairs of adhesive-type TTS (A/C; B/D) containing adhesive layers about 10 and 50 μm thick, set between the reservoir layers and the receptor medium.   The lowering of nitroglycerin release caused by the thicker adhesive layer can be compensated to a remarkable extent by reducing the amount of adhesive components in the reservoir layers and enhancing the drug concentration therein.   On the other hand, by lowering the thickness of the non-drug-loaded adhesive layer and enhancing the drug concentration in the reservoir layers, a significant increase of nitroglycerin release rates is achievable.

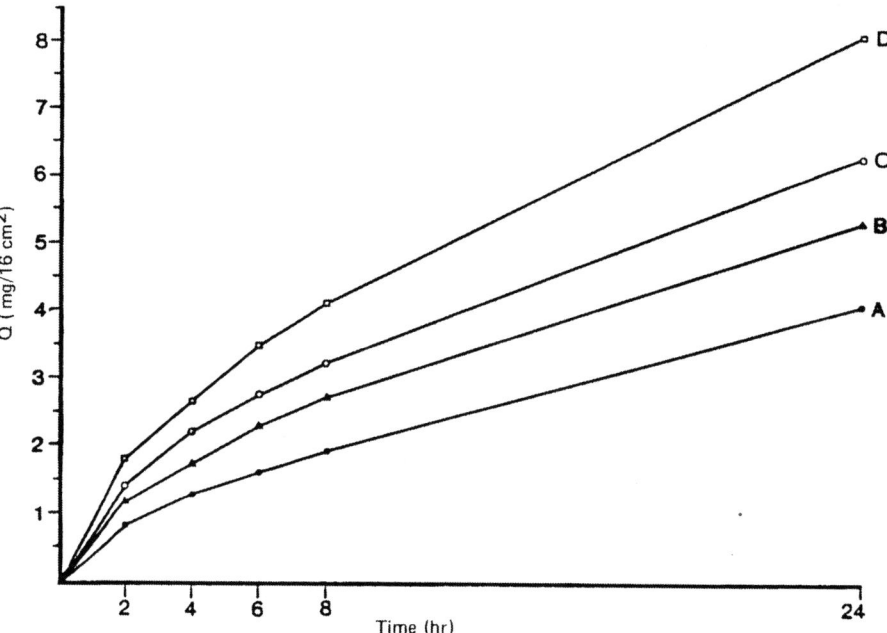

Figure 6 Influence of the distance between drug reservoir and receptor medium (isotonic saline) on nitroglycerin release rate Q from four adhesive films with the same total drug content (16 mg/ 16 cm^2). Between the drug reservoir (DR) and the receptor liquid, the systems contain a layer (L) 10 µm thick (C, D) or 50 µm thick (A, B), which is manufactured without addition of nitroglycerin/ lactose. Expressed in parts of weight, the adhesive mass is distributed between L and DR as follows:

Curve	L/DR
A	25/100
B	25/75
C	5/100
D	5/70

So the amount of nitroglycerin released over a 24-hr period was doubled for formulation D in comparison to A (Fig. 6) without any further galenical manipulations.

E. Manufacturing Method

The incorporation of drug into adhesive films is naturally limited by requirements relating to the cohesion and adhesion of the drug-loaded adhesive. An insufficient drug loading cannot be compensated in any case by a larger patch size, because the system may be then depleted too fast. The adhesive-type transdermal therapeutic system described here overcomes this problem of dosing by combining several reservoir layers, each being supersaturated with the therapeutically active agent.

An unwanted decrease of nitroglycerin release rates is avoided in the case of the Deponit system because the drug concentration profile described takes into consideration the growing of a drug-depleted layer between the skin and the reservoir zones. Furthermore, local skin irritations, quite often caused by too high a concentration of active agent, are avoided because the first individual layer closest to the skin of the patient is separated from the skin by an adhesive layer that is maximally saturated with the drug.

Since Deponit needs neither lateral walls nor covers nor edge tightening, it may be produced deliberately as large as necessary and in a form appropriate to the therapeutical requirements. This is of particular importance when the treatment is started with a minimum dosage that is slowly increased, or when a treatment is finished with a slowly decreasing dosage.

REFERENCES

1. See, for example, R. H. Guy and J. Hadgraft, *Pharm. Int.*, p. 112, May 1985.
2. M. Wolff, G. Cordes, and V. Luckow, *Pharm. Res.*, *1*: 23 (1984).
3. See, for example, J. Hadgraft, *Int. J. Pharm.*, *16*: 225 (1983).
4. K. Kehne, H. Vogt, and H. P. Merkle, *Act. Pharm. Technol.*, *27*: 17 (1981).
5. T. Higuchi, *J. Soc. Cosmet. Chem.*, *11*: 85 (1960).

15

Product Development and Technology Transfer for Transdermal Therapeutic Systems

DAVID J. BOVA, VALERIE N. AHMUTY, ROBERT L. CIRRITO,
KAREN O'TOOLE HOLMES, K. KASPER, CAROLINE LaPRADE,
R. LaPRADE, GUSTAV A. MAAG,* JUAN A. MANTELLE, JOHN A.
McCARTY, J. MIRANDA, FRANKIE A. MORTON, and STEVEN
SABLOTSKY / *Key Pharmaceuticals, Inc., Miami, Florida*

I. INTRODUCTION

Transdermal nitroglycerin delivery systems have been on the market
now for several years. Their success has stimulated other companies
to develop competitive products for the delivery of nitroglycerin and
other drugs suitable for this dosage form. This chapter presents
some of the approaches and considerations necessary for the successful development and technology transfer of transdermal delivery
systems.

Prior to discussing the product development of a transdermal
system, it is important to consider the importance of the research
phase. A good product, one that will stand the tests of time and
competition, must be founded on a sound research base. With transdermal drug delivery, as can be the case with many new technologies,
there may be a tendency to rush through the early research studies
in order to capitalize on the market potential. However, experience
in developing these dosage forms indicates that such studies are
critical in establishing a sound database, which will be used to resolve problems that inevitably arise as development and technology

*Present affiliation: Consultant, Miami Beach, Florida.

transfer progress. The following is a brief summary of the expected accomplishments of the research studies.

II. RESEARCH PHASE

The first step involving the transdermal research team is the preparation of a candidate drug proposal, outlining the feasibility of transdermal delivery for the candidate drug. A large amount of the information contained in this proposal is obtained through technical literature searches. When these sources are inadequate to determine the feasibility of this form of delivery, laboratory and marketing studies must be conducted. It is only after a proposal has been reviewed and accepted that further resources should be allocated to the project.

After a candidate drug has passed the proposal stage, a formal research team is assembled. Whereas preproposal laboratory studies may have examined initial skin flux, formal research will focus on the design of the system, raw material selection, and formula optimization.

The initial formulation research and system design can proceed via one of three primary routes: a system with an adhesive border, a system with an adhesive overlay, or a system in which the active component is incorporated directly in the adhesive (Fig. 1). All these designs have advantages and disadvantages. For example, the adhesive border system uses a nonadhesive matrix, which is considerably less complicated to formulate than an adhesive matrix. On

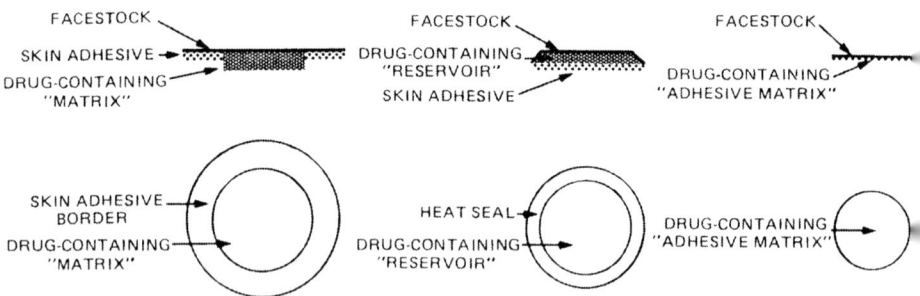

Figure 1   The three primary transdermal drug delivery system designs: *left*, adhesive border; *center*, adhesive overlay; *right*, adhesive incorporates active component directly.

the other hand, the adhesive border system is substantially larger and may require more converting operations. Once the basic system design has been chosen, selection of raw materials can proceed. All the materials must be fully compatible with the drug; in addition, they must maintain stability within the packaging components, allow for the necessary drug release, and give the matrix the desired physical properties. Preliminary formulations are prepared utilizing a range of different ingredients. Important parameters include physical appearance, processing ease, and compatibility with adhesives and packaging components. Formulations that pass the initial evaluation are tested for in vitro drug release (dissolution) and drug delivery (permeation or flux). Stability studies should be initiated with several candidate formulations.

Other critical activities in the research phase include initial skin irritation studies using animal models, and analytical methods development, including extraction of the drug from the matrix and migration of the drug and excipients into the packaging components.

The research team's responsibility does not end with the formulation. Their contribution to product design, component selection, processing, and safety continues as development proceeds. Newcomers to the field of transdermal technology should be cautious not to underestimate the long-term benefits of a strong research effort.

III. PRODUCT DEVELOPMENT AND TECHNOLOGY TRANSFER

Numerous areas could be discussed when considering the product development and technology transfer phases of transdermal dosage forms. Several areas of particular interest for these dosage forms have been selected because they represent unique considerations for a company developing its first transdermal dosage form. The sections' that follow treat the topics listed:

A. Process Development
B. Documentation
C. Methods Development
D. Packaging Development
E. Safety Testing
F. Wear Studies
G. Facilities Engineering
H. Operator Training
I. Sales and Marketing Training
J. Purchasing and Materials Handling

K. Quality Assurance and Quality Control
L. Technical Services

A. Process Development

Once a formulation and the initial processing requirements have been identified, it becomes necessary to scale up to batch size and equipment that resemble final production. The initial step is to ensure that the formulation is thoroughly characterized to determine equipment requirements for mixing, pumping, and processing.

Characterization will include a rheological evaluation of the raw materials and formulation. The rheological evaluation will give the scaleup engineer information on the viscosity behavior at various shear rates, yield point, thixotropy, and viscoelasticity. This information is then used to determine mixing and pumping requirements as well as the type and size of equipment. Next, the availability of equipment must be considered to determine the extent of custom design work and lead times.

Transdermal processing equipment is unique in many ways. Equipment usually cannot be bought off the shelf, and because the drug is being produced in unit doses, packaging equipment is normally coupled with processing equipment.

Prototype machinery design should meet certain requirements: (a) it should be versatile to provide flexibility, (b) it should be cost effective and labor efficient, (c) it should be close in design to final production machinery so that it can be used for developing initial operating instructions and training, and (d) it should be of simple design, to keep equipment maintenance, inventory of spare parts, and downtime at a minimum. Major questions that can be answered by prototype machinery involve identification of wear points, process problems, machine efficiency, service intervals, maintenance procedures, and design changes for faster and more efficient production. This information can be invaluable for design engineers involved in the selection of production equipment.

Process controls play a major role in transdermal processing equipment. Mixing speeds, pumping pressure, print registration, web tensions, and heat-sealing parameters must be maintained at optimum levels in order to run the equipment at production speeds with a minimum amount of rejected material. Transdermal unit dose packaging equipment typically produces 200 units per minute or more; thus the potential for manufacturing significant quantities of rejected product is an ever-present threat.

B. Documentation

Thorough documentation is necessary at all stages of development: research, clinical manufacturing, scaleup, and final production. The emphasis may vary at each stage, but the basic premise of all documentation is to ensure a quality product. During the research phase, documentation centers on formulation history. The overall rationale for the product is established and information concerning ingredient selection should be reported. Each raw material must be documented as appropriate for its intended use in the formulation. Since transdermal systems can often incorporate polymers or noncompendial ingredients, new materials must be characterized according to their physiochemical properties and their action in the formulation. The proportions of the excipients in the formulation should be varied to document the allowable manufacturing variations.

Some polymers used in transdermal systems may not have been used in the drug industry previously. To qualify them, studies may be required to establish their safety. Such investigations include but are not limited to tests for skin irritation and sensitization, eye irritation, and oral toxicity. Polymers may also have residual monomers or solvents, which must be characterized and quantified not only in the raw material, but in the intermediates and finished product as well.

Vendors can be very helpful in providing the information necessary to qualify materials for pharmaceutical use. Many provide Code of Federal Regulations (CFR) references on the applicability for use of their materials as direct or indirect additives in food or for food contact. It is always preferable, however, to use raw materials that have a history of use in medical devices, cosmetics, or pharmaceuticals.

Once the raw materials in the formulation and packaging components have been determined and process development has proceeded sufficiently to begin the initial clinical studies, other types of documentation are needed. Specifications for release of raw materials, intermediates, and finished goods are necessary. The minimum release requirements are the establishment of identity and purity; however, the specifications should also contain any other pertinent criteria such as pH limits, viscosity, percent solids, or blend uniformity. Master batch records in compliance with current FDA-established Good Manufacturing Practices (cGMPs) are written and approved prior to clinical manufacturing. Standard operating procedures (SOPs) and equipment operating procedures (EOPs) must be written during the process development stage. Critical defect categorization must be determined, and process controls for all phases of manufacturing should be implemented with documentation of their validity.

Transdermal manufacturing usually involves many more processing and packaging steps than other types of pharmaceutical product. Traceability and accountability can become complicated as larger batches are made. Adding drug product to web materials (common for transdermal systems) requires that the latter be treated in much the same manner as drug substances and excipients, since the drug product is often inseparable from the primary package. The intermediates and finished goods require safety testing much the same as that for raw materials. Generally, skin irritation and sensitization testing is performed in both animals and humans. Before studies may be performed on humans, an Investigational New Drug (IND) application must be filed. Much of the information collected pertaining to the safety of the materials is included in this filing.

While human studies are being conducted, stability work continues on the clinical batches. Many aspects of a transdermal stability profile are not easily determined by standard programs. Data on the wear over time are a good example of this, since wear studies of active materials on humans require clinical documentation and manufacturing procedures.

Storage conditions may affect the transdermal product in different ways. Bulk intermediates may be more sensitive to temperature differences and light exposure than bulk rollstock containing active drug. Units in primary versus secondary packaging configurations may react differently also. Reports and documentation on the stability characteristics of the product at all stages of manufacturing and packaging are necessary not only for expiration dating, but also as an indicator of possible consumer complaints and marketing problems.

Thorough documentation is the life-blood of product development for transdermal delivery systems. It is the essential tool for ensuring that high-quality product can be produced and validated. Good documentation is also very valuable for troubleshooting problems that may arise during development of these novel dosage forms.

C. Methods Development

There are many analytical tasks to be performed in the development of a transdermal drug product. The first is the determination of the identity and purity of the raw materials and intermediates used in manufacturing the drug product. Identification tests may include color tests, melting points, infrared or nuclear magnetic resonance spectrum, mass spectrum, chromatographic mobility, optical rotation, refractive index, and density.

A second task, which is normally performed concurrently with raw material analysis, is the determination of the identity and purity of the drug substance. In determining the percent purity of the drug substance or the content of the active ingredient(s) in the drug product, both absolute and relative test methods may be employed. Absolute methods may include titrations, gravimetric procedures, differential scanning calorimetry, caulometry, nuclear

magnetic resonance spectrometry, and phase solubility analysis.
Relative methods may include gas chromatography, high-performance
liquid chromatography, spectrometry (ultraviolet, visible, or infrared),
fluorometry, and polarography.
The isolation and identification of trace impurities in the drug
substance is a third analytical task, performed in an attempt to control the quantity of a specific impurity or group of impurities in the ·
drug product, such as water, solvents, metals, or trace organic
impurities. In addition to the quantitative analyses performed to
determine the percent purity of the drug, absorption atomic emission
or semiquantitative limit tests such as chromatography, spot tests,
or visual color comparisons may be employed. The chromatographic
examinations may include paper, thin-layer, gas, or high-performance
liquid chromatography.
Degradation products and the rates of their formation for the
drug substance are determined using the previously mentioned analytical methods. These assays are performed after the drug product
has been exposed to a variety of environmental conditions such as
humidity and temperature changes over time.
Analytical testing for transdermal drug products reaches beyond
the scope of excipient and active drug testing. Primary packaging
materials, because of their integral relationship in the final product,
must be tested. Extraction studies must be performed on packaging
components that come in contact with the matrix. Additionally, major
modifications of existing test procedures are necessitated by the
unique physical properties of transdermal drug systems. For example, methods must be devised to test the dissolution rate of the
drug from the matrix or adhesive, and the choice of an appropriate
solvent can often become a critical issue.

D. Packaging Development

Transdermal packaging technology is still in its infancy. This provides a challenge to the packaging engineers and the research and
development group. One challenging aspect is finding FDA-approvable
packaging components. The converting industry, the source for most
packaging components, has only recently seen the potential marketplace available to those who are willing to comply with FDA's regulations. The ability to obtain FDA approval is one of the primary considerations in packaging component selection. Other primary factors
include cost, aesthetics, and functionality. Incorporating all these
considerations into a package design that is attractive to consumers,
adaptable to large-scale production, inexpensive to produce, and
approvable by the FDA requires a tremendous effort on the part of
purchasing and product development personnel, packaging engineers,
and many others.

Two unique functional concerns of transdermal packaging components are ingredient migration and wear properties. Analyses must be performed to ensure that the ingredients of the matrix or active drug are not absorbed into the packaging components, nor should any raw materials or residuals from the packaging materials leach into the matrix. Since most transdermal systems contain drug as a solute, the potential for transfer between the drug reservoir and packaging components can be a serious concern.

A second, unique functional consideration is that of wear. Transdermal systems are designed for extended wear (up to 7 days). Additionally, drug delivery is directly related to the ability of the system to stay in contact with skin. Devices that appear to be simple at first glance can be very complicated when functionality is taken into account.

The process of selecting packaging components can be complicated and tedious. A brief summary of some of the considerations at various stages is presented here.

Various packaging materials are screened during the very early phases of a project. Small samples of potential candidates are obtained from vendors. Their physical properties are measured. Additionally, drug absorption and permeation studies are performed. If sample quantities permit, some handmade prototype patches are prepared to evaluate the feasibility of the component for the transdermal product. For example, a material to be used in the bandage should be very soft and flexible. A small wear study using a placebo system may be performed to evaluate the level of comfort of a particular packaging component.

After the initial screening process, sample rolls are obtained from the vendor so that scaleup trials can be run. The initial trials are usually performed on prototype equipment. During these trials both on-line and off-line testing are performed. Information is gathered on the material's performance during processing and also as part of the finished transdermal system. Informal stability studies on the finished product are completed to ensure the acceptability of the component before proceeding to a clinical trial.

Trial batches are manufactured to produce transdermal bandages for clinical studies on humans and for the formal stability studies required by the FDA. The trials are run on prototype equipment and provide additional information on the machinability of the components. Any problems or peculiarities with the components are carefully documented to provide historical information that is considered when drafting final specifications.

If the components successfully complete a three month formal stability study, a regulatory submissions package for that component is compiled. This package contains a specification, applicable CFR references, and the supplier's authorization to reference its Drug

Master File (if available). Any skin irritation and sensitization studies that have been performed on the components would also be included.

Artwork and copy are finalized late in development. Printing trials must be performed on bandage and secondary packaging components. Print quality and colors are evaluated and color standards are established. Some of the internal groups collaborating on these trials are marketing, quality assurance, purchasing, and R&D.

To commence with machine trials, larger lots of the packaging materials must be obtained. It is in these larger lots that the quality assurance and production groups can begin to evaluate the vendor's consistency. Vendor and material validation may also begin during this phase. As the scaleup phase progresses, the specifications go through a final revision period in R&D.

It is very important that purchasing and R&D work together closely at this point. The specifications can be designed to make the components as "generic" as possible, thus giving purchasing a good deal of latitude in acquiring goods. Custom materials should be avoided not only because of cost but also because of potential problems of availability and questionable consistency between suppliers.

Finally, prior to marketing the product, distribution studies are conducted during January and August, the months during which the most extreme weather conditions are assumed to exist in the distribution channel. Ink abrasion, heat seal, and carton integrity should be evaluated upon return of the product.

E. Safety Testing

In the selection of materials for development of transdermal products, several safety concerns must be addressed. These include worker protection, safety, and environmental concerns.

Once a particular drug has been identified as a potential candidate for a transdermal product, one of the first considerations is the safety of the laboratory personnel, as well as any others who may be exposed to the drug during research and eventual manufacturing.

Newcomers to transdermal systems should remember that most of the drugs suitable for this type of delivery permeate rapidly through the skin and have a low toxicity threshold. The first step is a literature search to determine such things as volatility, permissible exposure limits, reactivity, incompatibilities, and sensitivities. This information is combined with NIOSH and OSHA recommendations on handling, to determine the need for respirators, eye protection, and gloves, as well as type of attire. It is particularly important to determine which glove materials provide the best protection. This is accomplished by selecting different glove materials, which are tested in flux studies with saturated drug solutions. The permeation rates of the drug through these protective materials is then determined. This testing is repeated for the clinical attire, and it is determined how often the gloves and attire should be changed. When suitable gloves have been chosen, actual use tests are performed to determine the degree of dexterity provided in drug-handling situations. After the recommended exposure time, the gloves are assayed for drug absorption. The results of these tests are used as a basis for safety precautions that are incorporated into SOPs which serve as training guides for all operating and laboratory personnel involved with handling the drug product.

Other safety concerns revolve around material handling and disposal practices. "Right to know" federal and state regulations require that material safety data sheets (MSDSs) for all chemicals be available to workers involved in sampling, testing, and processing operations. Environmental impact statements are required by federal law. Their content includes primary and secondary consequences, unavoidable adverse environmental effects, alternatives, and benefit versus risk analysis.

Safety testing varies greatly depending on the nature of the active ingredient. One of the most challenging compounds for a transdermal system is nitroglycerin because of its potential for detonation. As an indication of the safety testing that must be considered, the following basic series of tests is used for development of a nitroglycerin system. These tests may not be applicable to other drugs.

1. The solubility of nitroglycerin in the polymeric system must be characterized over a range of temperatures. Nitroglycerin that has settled out of solution greatly increases the potential for explosion. Once the solubility of the system has been identified, and the range of acceptable temperatures determined, the actual sensitivity testing may commence.

2. The *card gap test with no cards* measures the ability of a nitroglycerin formulation to withstand strong shock waves from a detonating explosive booster charge. The strength of the shock wave is varied by interspersing cellulose acetate cards between the booster and the test substance. The most severe test case is that in which no cellulose acetate cards are present.

3. The *drop weight impact test* measures the ability of a nitroglycerin transdermal unit to withstand detonation after impact. A 5-kg weight is dropped from a specified height directly onto the sample such that the sample receives the full impact energy.

4. The *electrostatic discharge test* submits the sample to a high-voltage electrostatic potential stored in a 0.1-F capacitor. Any arcing or other unexpected reactions are recorded as positive results.

5. The *confined detonation test* sandwiches 6 mm of sample polymeric mixture between two steel plates. Initiation is attempted with a

commercial no 6 detonator and a 0.3-g tetryl pellet pressed through a hole in the top plate. The remains from the resulting explosion are compared to a standard to determine whether any additional reactions occurred.

The results from the sensitivity testing must demonstrate clearly that the nitroglycerin transdermal device will be safe not only during patient use but also during manufacture, shipping, and storage (where large quantities may be confined to small areas). Safety testing must also be considered for raw materials and intermediates.

F. Wear Studies

Wear tests are essential for the development of transdermal systems. Since there is no known artificial surface that behaves like the human skin, the testing of physical properties of the adhesive (tack, shear, adhesion to steel, etc.) can be used only as guidelines. A product optimized on the basis of physical testing must eventually be wear-tested.

A previously characterized panel of at least 30–40 subjects may be considered adequate to obtain a representative sample of variation in skin properties. The panelists are asked to wear placebo patches for the appropriate time frame. No skin preparation other than wiping off excess moisture with a paper towel or hair clipping (if necessary) is performed. The subjects are instructed to engage in all normal activities, including physical exercise and showering. After wear, the panelists return to have the patches examined, removed, and graded. Notes are taken on the skin condition at the wear sites, including data on the following topics:

1. Patch appearance after wear
   a. Degree of adhesion to skin
   b. Aesthetics
   c. Legibility of printed information on the patch
2. Skin appearance after wear
   a. Presence of adhesive residue
   b. Irritation on skin
3. Environmental factors: a weather report on the midday temperature, relative humidity, and amount of precipitation during the test period.

Wear studies utilizing placebo units can provide a great deal of information on the feasibility of certain components under consideration for transdermal systems. If properly designed, they can point out potential problems while the product is still under development.

G. Facilities Engineering

Facilities engineering for transdermal drug products can proceed along a number of different routes. It may be possible to begin actual production in the pilot plant. There are many advantages to this approach. The operations group has the opportunity to work closely with the development group, thus gaining "hands-on" experience and a sound understanding of the process. The risk to the company is lessened because large sums of money required for full-scale production equipment, facilities, and personnel are not committed prior to product approval and positive market acceptance. This approach requires sound preliminary market analysis to minimize the risk of building a pilot operation not capable of meeting initial market demand. When the company has enough information on product acceptance, the decision can be made to finance a full-scale, dedicated manufacturing plant run by an operations group that is well versed with the product, process, and equipment requirements.

A second option is to begin operations in a pilot plant, and to begin the design and fabrication of a full-scale production operation at the same time. This approach increases the risk of either overdesigning or underdesigning the production operation.

Another option is contract manufacturing. Depending on the unique requirements of the product and process, contract manufacturing may be considered to meet interim needs between the pilot-plant stage and in-house production. Some products will be best suited for continued contract manufacturing, even though there may be added cost.

Cost, space, personnel, expertise, and degree of operational control are some factors to consider in selecting a manufacturing option. A company must also evaluate its short-term and long-term transdermal commitment. Contract manufacturing may be very attractive to a company wishing to develop a transdermal product with minimal capital investment. Companies with long-term commitments to transdermal technology may, however, prefer to acquire in-house capability, to permit rapid capitalization on new developments.

H. Operator Training

To transfer technology from R&D to production, one must first transfer an understanding of the process. Foremen cannot manage and supervise workers on a manufacturing line unless they themselves have an understanding of the process from start to finish. This means a hands-on working relationship with all the equipment and machinery, not just theoretical knowledge. Once supervisory management has acquired a complete understanding of each phase of manufacturing and each piece of machinery involved in the process, the training of operators can begin.

Along with an understanding of the total process, an understanding of the final product is also critical. Operators will be much more efficient and conscientious if they can mentally fit their own operations into the overall scheme of the total process and end product. Each operation in the process is much like a piece in a jigsaw puzzle. A person who knows where his or her piece fits can see the full picture.

Hand in hand with education and understanding is safety. Operators who do not know their machinery cannot run it safely. Even though today's machinery is fitted with the latest in safety devices, safe operation of machinery cannot be overstressed.

Once the orientation, education, understanding, and safety aspects have been covered thoroughly, experience under operational conditions can commence. Potential operators must first observe the procedures. After an observation period including documentation and record keeping, selected minor operations are gradually turned over to the operator trainees. As the trainees gain experience in the actual operation of the machinery, more operations become their responsibility. After a sufficient amount of machine time, the new operators are gradually eased into equipment startup and shutdown. Even after the manufacturing personnel have become proficient at machine operation, it is generally necessary to retain the development staff for consultation purposes. Several months of machine operation are normally required for technology transfer. Machine and process variables can contribute to problems that require skilled troubleshooting during this period.

When training operators, it should be noted that throughout the training process, maintenance personnel should be included. Like the operators, the maintenance personnel must have an overview and an understanding of the process and product in order to perform their functions.

Actual machine operation is only part of operator training. Numerous other supportive aspects must be included in technology transfer. In a totally new process, there are custom-made parts, components, and assemblies that are expensive and can have long lead times. An inventory of spare parts must be maintained, and communication between development and manufacturing personnel regarding frequency and duration of downtime is critical. Training and equipment manuals written by the development group must be given to production. Copies of process development procedures (PDPs) are provided and transposed into SOPs.

Maintenance personnel, while learning the idiosyncrasies of new process equipment, must also learn the preventive maintenance requirements as well as calibration information. Any device that measures and/or controls volume, pressure, temperature, speed, etc., must be calibrated, with traceability to the National Bureau of Standards.

The development staff should also be involved in initial contact between production engineers and equipment vendors. Through the lengthy period of developing a new process, personal contacts are made that can minimize delays and confusion in the purchase of full-scale manufacturing equipment.

I. Sales and Marketing Training

Transdermal delivery systems offer unique opportunities and challenges in the areas of sales and marketing. These dosage forms, perhaps more than any other delivery system, are specifically designed with aesthetic appeal to the patient in mind. This facet opens new doors in the sales and marketing of ethical drugs. Transdermal systems have pushed ethical drug companies into questions and issues that focus heavily on consumer acceptance. These systems are designed to be worn for extended periods, and it is inevitable that the sales group will be concerned about the aesthetic appeal their system will have versus the competitor's. Of particular concern are decisions involving size, shape, color, flexibility, and unit labeling. Decisions on these issues must be made very early on and require extensive interaction between the product development and marketing groups. Tradeoffs are inevitable. For example, selection of barrier materials will involve balancing stability (stiffer, more rigid materials are generally better barriers) with comfort during wear (flexible films are generally poor barriers but wear well). Other examples include tradeoffs between size/shape and cost. Because of the need for long-term stability, stresses will arise between time dedicated to research, both laboratory and marketing, and the push to progress with the project. It is the responsibility of the product development staff to determine and explain the tradeoffs between aesthetics, cost, manufacturing, and functionality.

A second unique aspect of transdermal systems is the need for broader training programs for the sales force. The decisions discussed above will lead to perceived competitive advantages or disadvantages. The sales training team should include several members of the product development group for initial training programs. Training efforts should also include responses to negative perceptions in the physician's mind regarding aesthetic qualities. Finally, all training programs should include a discussion on skin physiology and adhesive wear.

J. Purchasing and Material Management

Transdermal technology creates new dimensions for those involved in purchasing and materials management. Transdermal packaging involves more than a standard bottle and closure. Although blister packaging introduced the pharmaceutical industry to flexible packaging materials, transdermal technology has expanded into more diverse areas of the converting industry. Purchasing and materials management must have knowledge of plastic films, pressure-sensitive adhesives, release liners, coextrusions, laminations, and coatings. Because few purchasing staffs in the pharmaceutical industry have such converting experience, it is important to begin the technology transfer process in the early stages of product development.

Slide presentations and visits to observe pilot operations act as an introduction to the transdermal manufacturing process. Raw materials and packaging components are interrelated to the process. An appreciation and understanding of how and why materials were selected is necessary.

Because most pharmaceutical operations do not require interaction with the types of vendor required by transdermal manufacturing, most vendors are initially sought by R&D personnel. However it is very beneficial to invite purchasing representatives to attend even the first vendor meetings. This not only allows the purchasing group to keep current on the project, but also exposes them to the industry. By learning the converting language and by finding out what is available from industry, the purchasing agent is more quality conscious and cost effective in seeking additional vendor sources.

Prior to scaleup, it is very beneficial to form a materials committee as a means of transferring technology from the R&D group to the operational level. The committee should consist of representatives from areas including R&D, purchasing, materials management, scheduling, quality assurance, and marketing.

R&D specifications should be presented to this committee, and the material requirements can be clarified and discussed. Not only can material specifications be addressed, but such special considerations as packaging and material handling procedures can be covered. It is most likely that a pharmaceutical company will require much more stringent packaging procedures than a converter is accustomed to providing its customers. For example, special overwraps and labeling may be required.

Because transdermal packaging involves the use of materials in rollstock form, special roll-handling equipment is necessary to maneuver rolls that may weigh as much as 350 lb. It is not possible to move such materials with a hand truck as in the case of bottles or folding cartons. Employee safety and undamaged rolls are the main concerns for material handlers.

The materials committee should continue to meet throughout scaleup and into the early stages of production startup. As scaleup progresses, R&D and operations can work as a team in addressing on-line problems and relating these problems to the material supplier.

As production startup nears, concerns of the committee tend to focus on scheduling, ordering, and delivery of raw materials and packaging components. At this point, the technology transfer phase is at its final stage and the R&D representatives find little need to continue as committee members.

K. Quality Assurance and Quality Control

The design and implementation of quality control checks and a thorough quality assurance program for the new product are integral to product development and consist of a major portion of the documentation required for the subsequent transfer of a new transdermal system to the production phase.

Specifications, sampling plans, pilot validation protocols, test methodologies, master batch records, standard operating procedures, equipment operating procedures, and many other quality-oriented documents have been designed by R&D during product development. At the point of technology transfer, a document package is prepared by R&D for distribution to the quality assurance, manufacturing, and regulatory affairs groups (Table 1).

Quality assurance assumes the responsibility for ensuring that specifications for each new raw material, component, process intermediate, and the final product are in place and approved by R&D, manufacturing, and regulatory affairs. Quality assurance reviews and approves validation protocols, and ensures that appropriate checks and controls are documented at appropriate stages of the manufacturing process. Quality assurance is also responsible for ensuring that validation of tests methods is conducted by the quality control group.

L. Technical Services

One group having a particular interest in the technology transfer is technical services. This group is responsible for product maintenance problem solving, and cost reductions. Technology transfer should start early, allowing for interaction with product development personnel. This provides familiarity with the product's developmental problems. Many times problem areas in the development phase are similar to difficulties encountered in production. Having prior experience with the problem and hopefully the solution will help to expedite resolution of problems that arise in production.

The usual transfer of information starts with the process. It is important that each phase of manufacturing be understood. Machine variables, process variables, and manufacturing limits as they specifically pertain to the operation must be understood. Raw material and component performance must be examined to gain sufficient

Table 1   Technology Transfer Documentation Package

I. Product Rationale/Design Characteristics Statement

II. Formula: Statement of Allowable Variability

Generally wt/wt % of raw material in a finished dosage form, and amount per unit of each raw material in a finished dosage form.

III. Raw Material Section

List of raw materials and their function in formulation

A. Compendial name
B. Trade name
C. Vendor name and address
D. Material Safety Data Sheets (MSDS)
E. Technical bulletin
F. Drug Master File (DMF) letters or toxicology information
G. Specifications—historical presentation
H. Test methods
I. Data presentation for each lot received
J. Storage, handling, and expiration dating statement

IV. Process and Product Section

A. Historical presentation of master batch records
B. Historical presentation of specifications
C. Test methods
D. Data presentation for each lot manufactured
E. Process development procedures (SOPs generated specifically for product)
F. Summary/highlights of R&D manufacturing experience
G. Toxicology information as applicable
H. Stability data

V. Component/Packaging Section

A. List of materials and suppliers
B. Specifications and technical data
C. Test methods
D. DMF references as applicable
E. Data presentation for each lot received
F. Special testing reports (if applicable)

VI. Reference Investigational New Drug (IND) Documents

knowledge to be competent working in a support function. Intermediate, work in progress, and finished goods must similarly be considered.

As part of this support function, it is necessary to cooperate with other departments to answer requests and resolve problems. Many times, internal requests demand the support of outside vendors. Problem areas associated with the process, raw materials, or components require that a close relationship be developed and fostered. This experience with the process and relationship with the vendors makes it possible to troubleshoot on a routine basis, provided a foundation was laid in the transfer phase.

IV. CONCLUSION

Transdermal drug delivery technology is a new and exciting field in the pharmaceutical industry. The challenges presented by this technology require that many functional groups venture into new areas. Companies that are able to reorient their employees, particularly those in the research and development group, can benefit from the market potential of these new dosage forms. Successful technology transfer of transdermal technologies requires close and open communications between a variety of groups. It is only in this atmosphere that transfer programs will proceed smoothly.

ACKNOWLEDGMENT

The authors would like to acknowledge the excellent assistance of Jan Bushman and Kevin Murphy in the preparation of this chapter.

REGULATORY REQUIREMENTS AMONG
INTERNATIONAL HEALTH AUTHORITIES

16

Regulatory Considerations in Transdermal Drug Delivery Systems in the United States

VINOD P. SHAH and JEROME P. SKELLY / *Division of Biopharma-*
ceutics, Center for Drugs and Biologics, Food and Drug
Administration, Rockville, Maryland

I. INTRODUCTION

Reproducible drug delivery through intact skin for the purpose of
providing systemic therapeutic efficacy represents a major challenge
to pharmaceutical scientsts and manufacturers. The recent introduction of Transderm-Scop, Transderm-Nitro, Nitrodisc, Nitro-Dur,
and Catapres-TTS patches into the marketplace are examples of the
extent of interest in this area of drug development.

There are probably many reasons for this interest, among them:

Avoidance of first pass elimination in liver or gastrointestinal tract.
Avoidance of gastrointestinal incompatibility.
Minimization of the inter-/intrapatient variation associated with oral
    therapy.
Drug delivery can approximate zero-order kinetics.
Reduction of side effects by avoiding toxic plasma levels.

Part of the chapter was presented by Vinod P. Shah at the symposium
entitled Developmental Aspects of Transdermal Delivery Systems, at
APhA, 39th National Meeting of Academy of Pharmaceutical Sciences,
Minneapolis, October 1985.

Maintenance of steady drug concentration.
Provision for minimal drug exposure by significant dose reduction.
Provision for long-term therapy from a single dose.
Enhancement of therapeutic efficacy.
Improvement of patient compliance.
Allowance for rapid termination of drug input.

The aims of developing a transdermal drug delivery (TDD) system, also referred to as a transdermal therapeutic system (TTS), are to maximize bioavailability, optimize therapeutic efficacy, and minimize side effects. Until recently, human skin was considered to be an inert, nonpermeable membrane that provides a protective surface for the body. However, studies have now shown that intact human skin can serve as an effective route of administration for drugs.

For the purposes of clarification, topically applied drug products should be categorized into the following classes of drug products:

1. *Dermal or topical drug products* may be defined as those that are applied onto the surface of the skin for the purpose of delivering drugs with localized pharmacological action. Drug molecules may penetrate through the stratum corneum, diffusing to a target tissue in the vicinity of the drug application site to produce a therapeutic effect. Depending on the extent of drug–skin interaction, some drug molecules may be absorbed into the systemic blood circulation.

2. *Transdermal drug products* may be defined as those that are intended for delivering drugs with systemic activity. Although they are also applied topically, the drug molecules delivered undergo percutaneous absorption; that is, they are absorbed through the skin, then taken up by the microcirculation network in the dermal papillary layer, and finally transported to target tissues via the systemic circulation to achieve the intended therapeutic effect. The terms "percutaneous absorption" and "transdermal penetration" are used interchangeably.

Before a topically applied drug can act either locally or systemically, it must penetrate through the stratum corneum. Percutaneous absorption can be visualized as consisting of a series of sequential steps: adsorption onto the surface of the stratum corneum, followed by diffusion through the stratum corneum, viable epidermis, and papillary dermis into the microcirculation.

It is not the intention of this chapter to discuss at length the toxicological or clinical requirements for TDD systems. These are mandated by the drug entity itself and its intended medical use. Rather, we want to emphasize the biopharmaceutical regulatory aspects of transdermal drug delivery systems. The examples referred to herein are employed to illustrate specific biopharmaceutic issues concerning the development of new drug delivery systems. In order not to hinder any creative innovation in this area, we have taken a flexible approach in establishing the biopharmaceutic requirements as a basis of drug approval. Therefore, with the purpose of encouraging innovation, we will discuss the biopharmaceutic considerations applied in the recently approved transdermal drug delivery systems, namely, Transderm-Scop patches (for the prevention/treatment of motion sickness); Nitrodisc, Nitro-Dur, and Transderm-Nitro patches (for the treatment of angina and conjestive heart failure); and Catapres-TTS patches (for the treatment of hypertension).

II. BIOPHARMACEUTIC CONSIDERATIONS

Biopharmaceutic considerations are pivotal for transdermal drug delivery systems because they determine specific kinds of clinical and/or toxicological studies that will need to be performed. There is an absolute need to define:

1. The dosage form delivery system, in terms of the rate and extent of drug delivery
2. The pharmacokinetics and metabolism of the active therapeutic moiety itself, where such information is lacking
3. Reproducibility of the drug delivery system

It should be stressed that the pharmacokinetics and metabolism of a drug delivered from a transdermal drug delivery system may differ significantly from that administered orally, due to the bypassing of liver and/or gastrointestinal metabolism. In such instances, the pharmacokinetic profile of the drug should parallel an intravenous infusion, which delivers the drug by a zero-order mechanism. In evaluating transdermal drug delivery systems, there is a need to:

1. Evaluate the site of drug administration, in order to optimize drug delivery.
2. Consider parameters such as optimal skin area for drug administration and blood flow at that site.
3. Assess the role of the skin in controlling (and, in some instances, sustaining) drug delivery to the systemic circulation.

For most drugs, the bioavailability and pharmacokinetic parameters are often defined using oral and/or intravenous administration. The TDD systems, in general, deliver the drug at a rate comparable to an intravenous infusion rate. Therefore, ideally, the bioavailability and pharmacokinetics of a transdermal drug delivery system should be defined in comparison to an intravenous dose. When intravenous dosing is not available, oral and/or intramuscular administration may be employed.

Transdermal delivery of scopolamine was evaluated in comparison with oral and intramuscular drug administrations as well as an intravenous infusion. The study demonstrated that scopolamine is delivered transdermally at a rate comparable to a zero-order infusion over a 3-day treatment period. The rate of transdermal drug delivery for scopolamine was designed to maintain the low plasma levels necessary for its antiemetic effect (for motion sickness), while at the same time avoiding its side effects such as drowsiness and tachycardia, which are associated with the higher plasma levels attained with oral dosing.

In considering a systemically effective drug delivery system that uses an absorptive surface other than the gastrointestinal tract, one cannot ignore the likelihood that such a dosage form will generate metabolites and pharmacokinetic profiles significantly different from those obtained from oral dosage forms. For examples, where a first-pass effect is associated with oral drug delivery it would be necessary to demonstrate that the systemically effective transdermal drug delivery system developed is capable of avoiding the hepatic first-pass metabolism associated with oral administration. In addition, the transdermal drug delivery system is likely to deliver the drug over a longer period of time. These differences in pharmacokinetic profile have been demonstrated in the comparison of two systemically effective nitroglycerin products (sublingual tablets and transdermal patches). The data showed that percutaneous absorption of nitroglycerin from a transdermal drug delivery system results in detectable plasma levels for 24 hr, in contrast to the maintenance of detectable plasma levels for only 15 min following a sublingual administration (Fig. 1). In the case of transdermal clonidine, steady-state blood levels and urinary recovery data were compared with oral administration. The transdermal patch was applied on the upper, outer arm and worn for 7 days, whereas oral drug was administered twice a day for 4 consecutive days. The steady-state blood levels (Fig. 2) and urinary excretion data from the patch were found to be comparable to results obtained with oral dosage form.

In addition to defining the pharmacokinetic profile of a new drug delivery system, it is necessary to demonstrate brand-to-brand and batch-to-batch (within a brand) reproducibility in drug release. This can be achieved by comparing different batches of the drug delivery system in the same group of subjects/patients or by development of suitable in vitro testing. In the case of scopolamine, batch-to-batch reproducibility was demonstrated by in vivo bioavailability studies on two nonsequentially manufactured batches (Fig. 3).

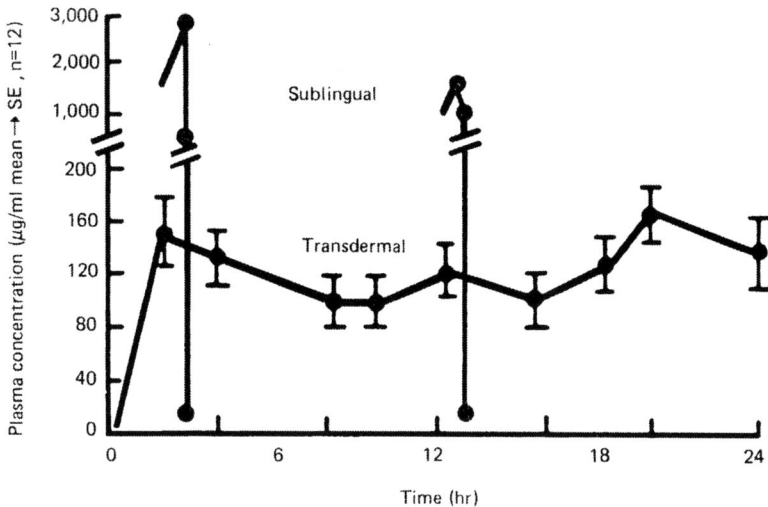

Figure 1 Comparison of plasma nitroglycerin levels produced by Transderm-Nitro 5 and sublingual tablet. (Courtesy of Dr. John W. Fara, Alza Corporation, Palo Alto, CA.)

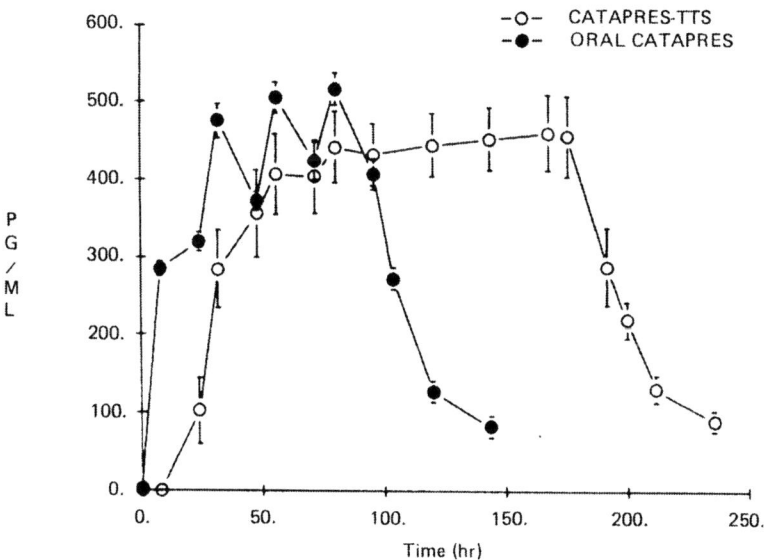

Figure 2 Comparison of plasma level profiles of clonidine after twice-daily administration of 0.1-mg clonidine tablets for 4 days and application of Catapres-TTS 5-cm^2 patches for 7 days.

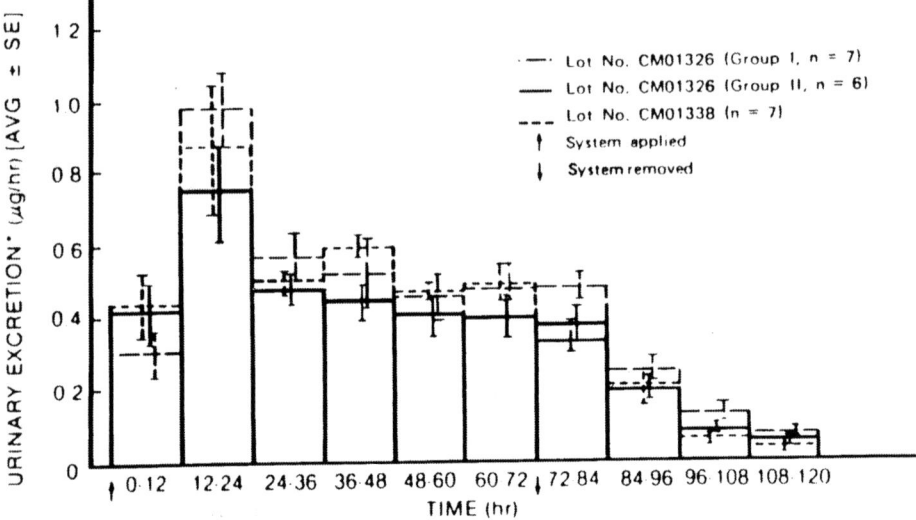

Figure 3 Urinary excretion profiles of free scopolamine following transdermal administration of two different batches of Transderm-Scop systems. (Courtesy of Dr. J. Shaw, Alza Corporation, Palo Alto, CA.)

Following our success in the development of in vitro dissolution methods for assuring lot-to-lot bioequivalency of solid oral dosage forms, we explored the feasibility of adapting the FDA paddle method (USP Apparatus 2) to enable development of a reproducible in vitro dissolution test for transdermal drug delivery systems. The method was modified by placement of a watchglass, to which the TDD system was affixed, in the bottom of the dissolution flask. The TDD system (e.g., a nitroglycerin patch) was held in position by sandwiching it between the watchglass and an aluminum wire screen (Fig. 4). The drug release profile from the TDD patch was then determined in water with the paddle speed of 50 rpm over a 24-hr period. The results are shown in Figures 5 and 6. The release patterns of nitroglycerin from the TDD patches produced by the same firm, but with different dose strengths (i.e., Ciba or Key with four strengths and Searle with two strengths) exhibited dose proportionality, and when the drug release data were plotted as percent label claim release, a virtually superimposable release pattern was observed among all strengths. These results indicate that the in vitro method developed is reproducible and can be used for the determination of drug release characteristics to assure the batch-to-batch uniformity

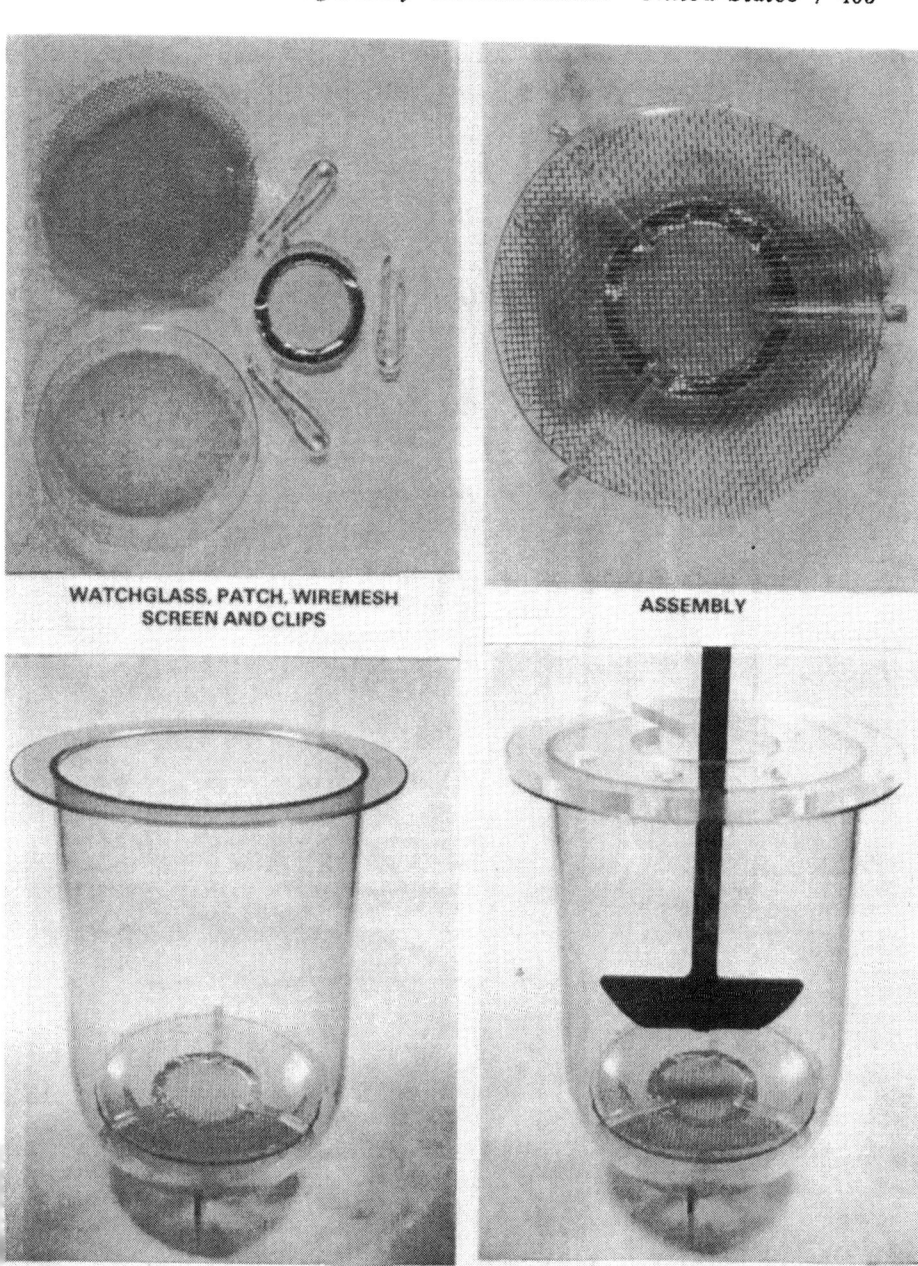

WATCHGLASS, PATCH, WIREMESH
SCREEN AND CLIPS

ASSEMBLY

ASSEMBLY IN DISSOLUTION FLASK

FINAL SET UP WITH PADDLE
APPARATUS

Figure 4   Experimental setup for transdermal patch dissolution
studies.

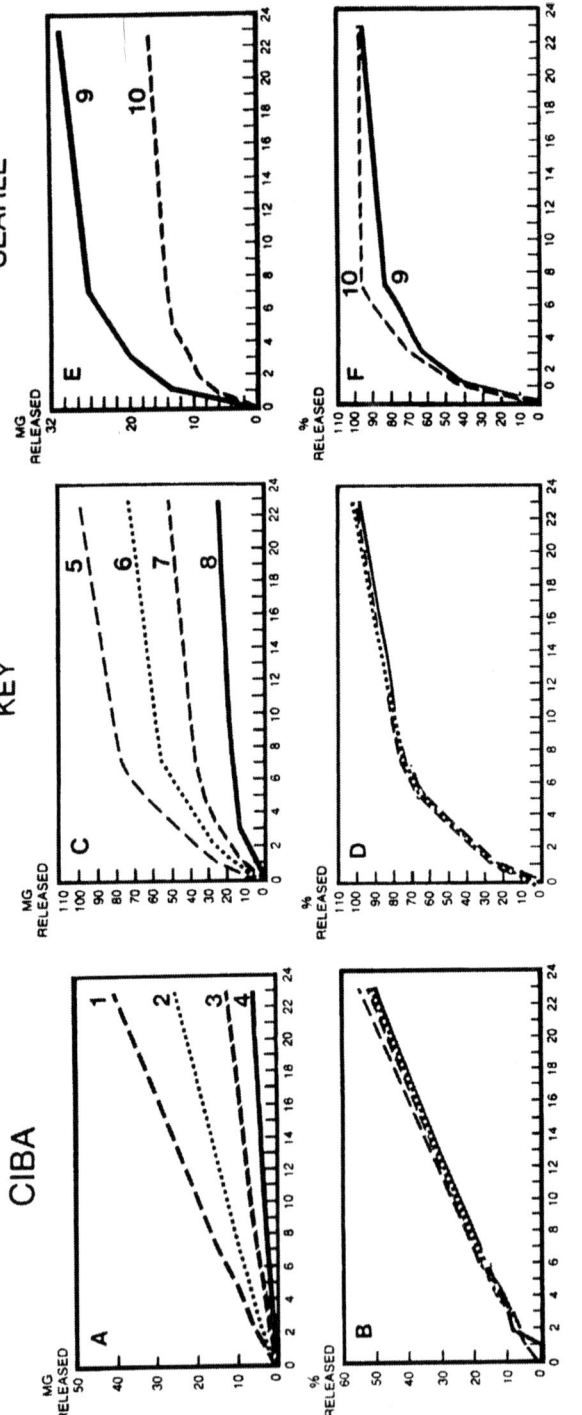

Figure 5 Comparison of in vitro release profiles of nitroglycerin from transdermal patches, given as milligrams per patch (A, C, and E) and as % label claim release (B, D, and F). A and B: curve 1, 15 mg (30 cm^2); curve 2, 10 mg (20 cm^2); curve 3, 5 mg (10 cm^2); and curve 4, 2.5 mg (5 cm^2). C and D: curve 5, 10 mg (20 cm^2); curve 6, 7.5 mg (15 cm^2); curve 7, 5 mg (10 cm^2); and curve 8, 2.5 mg (5 cm^2). E and F: curve 9, 10 mg (16 cm^2); and curve 10, 5 mg (8 cm^2).

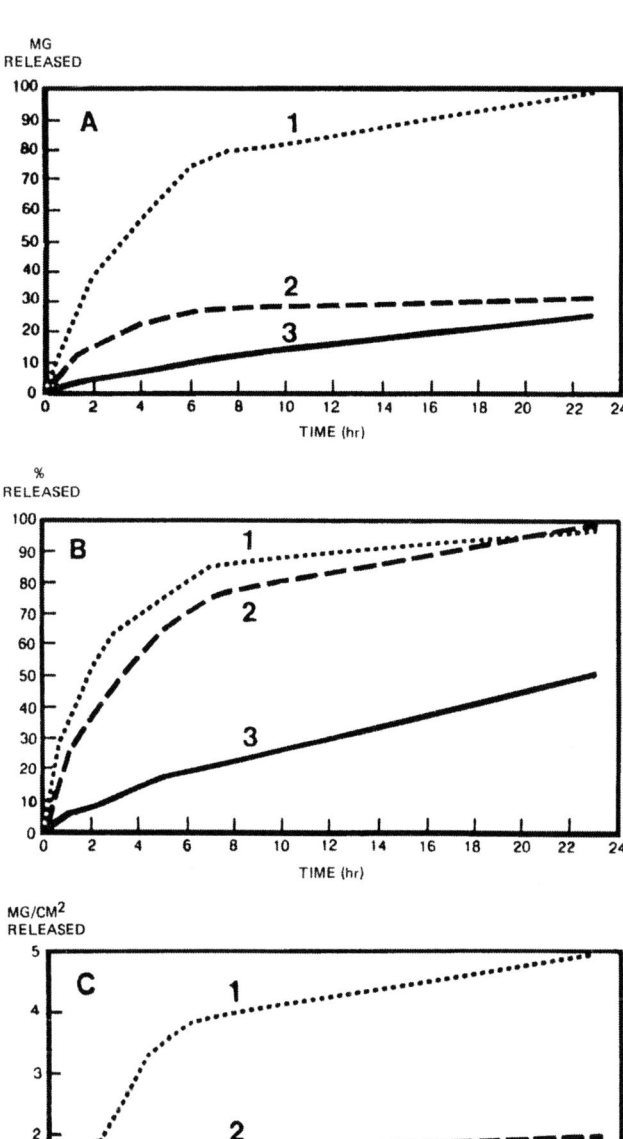

Figure 6   Comparative dissolution data of nitroglycerin (milligrams of drug released, % label claim released, and milligrams of drug released per square centimeter) from three marketed transdermal patches: curves 1, Key patch (10 mg/20 cm^2); curves 2, Searle patch (10 mg/16 cm^2); curves 3, Ciba patch (10 mg/20 cm^2).

of transdermal patches. The comparative in vitro dissolution results shown in Figure 6 illustrate the difference in drug release profiles of three brands of nitroglycerin patches. This is expected, since the three manufacturers use different drug release technologies for the manufacture of their transdermal drug delivery systems. It is, therefore, anticipated that the specifications for assuring batch-to-batch equivalence (after approving bioavailability data) will vary from one brand to another.

The horny layer, especially the deeper horny layers, can sometimes act as a drug depot and modify the transdermal permeation characteristics of some drugs. Therefore, at the time of evaluating TDD systems, the protocol should be designed to allow for a determination of whether the tissue serves as a drug depot. In the case of transdermal scopolamine, the skin has been found to have a depot effect, whereas in the case of transdermal nitroglycerin, it does not. This determination can be made by monitoring blood and/ or urinary drug levels after the patch is removed.

The basis for the approval of TDD systems from a biopharmaceutic standpoint consists of:

1. Demonstration that the plasma concentrations of the active moiety are comparable to those achieved by an approved dosage from. (If the metabolite profile is different, some clinical studies may be required.)
2. Demonstration of lot-to-lot reproducibility.
3. Determination of pharmacokinetic parameters to support drug labeling.

It may not always be feasible or desirable to define the bioavailability profile of a transdermal drug delivery system relative to an intravenous dose (bolus or zero-order infusion). The use of other routes of drug administration, which provides additional pharmacokinetic data, may be desirable to permit appropriate labeling.

III. REGULATORY REQUIREMENTS

Bioavailability studies are not required for topical drugs intended for only local effect, e.g., calamine lotion, zinc oxide, etc. Transdermal drug delivery systems intended for the treatment or prevention of a systemic disease (regardless of the type of active therapeutic moiety employed) are regarded as "new drugs" within the meaning of the federal Food, Drug and Cosmetic Act, Section 200.31, and as such require submission of scientific data to substantiate their clinical safety and efficacy. Furthermore, all such drugs are controlled-release dosage forms and, therefore, must demonstrate their controlled-release characteristics to support drug labeling in accordance with FDA requirements.

Transdermal drug delivery systems require demonstration of safety, both in terms of local irritations and systemic toxicity. In the event that the systemic toxicity of an active therapeutic moiety is defined in the scientific literature (e.g., nitroglycerin and scopolamine, etc.), the FDA may waive the demonstration of animal systemic toxicity, but it may require additional clinical testing for safety in human subjects. Where blood level comparisons of the transdermal medication to an already established systemic route of administration of the same drug (e.g., intravenous, intramuscular, oral) is available, the systemic safety issues may be ruled out, if the blood levels generated are comparable to those obtained in the patients treated with the currently approved label dosages.

Clinical testing for efficacy is required for transdermal drug delivery systems delivering new drug entities and may also be required to support new efficacy claims on drugs already marketed. Biopharmaceutic considerations can play an immense role in the case of marketed drugs, since the FDA may rely on blood-level comparisons alone if the pharmacodynamic effects of the drug have been well defined using a systemic route of administration.

Clinical efficacy data should be submitted to support a new medical claim or any claim of superior efficacy. Any claim to enhanced or superior reproducibility or prolonged therapy will require appropriate bioavailability/pharmacokinetic studies to support drug labeling.

In certain instances, additional metabolism studies in man may be required to define the cutaneous metabolism of the drug where significant alteration in metabolic pathways is suspected due to different hepatic-portal elimination or gastrointestinal metabolism.

The types of studies required as the basis of approval of a new drug application need to be customized and are largely dictated by the following considerations:

1. Critical nature of the active drug
2. Availability of marketed systemic dosage form of the same drug
3. Medical and biopharmaceutic rationale
4. Literature data on the drug entity
5. Agency experience with the drug and/or drug delivery system

It should be stressed that these novel drug delivery systems require careful scientific evaluation based on the pharmacological and pharmacokinetic properties of the drug and drug delivery system. Critical drugs (drugs with a narrow therapeutic index) or drugs that require titration may need additional specialized studies to define the safety, efficacy, and labeling requirements. Such studies, in our opinion, need to be customized. In most instances where systemic toxicity of the drug entity is well known, the need for further animal toxicity testing is obviated. Where toxicity data are required, such requirements should parallel other systemic drugs of the same pharmacological class.

IV. GENERIC VERSIONS OF TRANSDERMAL DRUG PRODUCTS

The passage of the "Drug Price Competition and Patent Term Restoration Act" in September, 1984 (commonly referred to as Waxman-Hatch bill) enacted certain requirements for the approval of generic drug products. For generic transdermal products, additional concerns should be addressed. These can be summarized as follows:

1. Demonstration of bioequivalence to the innovator product using blood levels and/or urinary recovery data.
2. Employment of a drug release mechanism similar to the approved products. If it is different, safety and efficacy data on the new TDD system may be needed.
3. Use of the approved adhesive materials. If different, skin irritation data may be needed.
4. Use of the approved inactive ingredients. If different, safety data may be needed.
5. Use of the approved patch material. If different, safety data may be needed.

17

Regulatory Approval of Transdermal Therapeutic Systems in the United Kingdom

PAUL ADAMS / Department of Health and Social Security, London, England

I. INTRODUCTION

In the United Kingdom, transdermal drug delivery systems are regarded as medicinal products. They need to go through the same regulatory procedures and experience the same official scrutiny as more conventional preparations.

Drug regulation in the United Kingdom is based on the Medicines Act of 1968. This Act of Parliament requires that the quality, safety, and efficacy of a medicinal preparation be demonstrated to be satisfactory in the context of therapeutic indications and dosage schedule, and that the professions and patients are informed by relevant facts, which are required to appear on the data sheet, packaging, or label according to the method of sale and advertising.

Each new product, whether it is a new chemical entity or a new presentation of a known drug, is assessed on its own merits. This assessment by the Licensing Authority and its advisory committees is in the light of contemporary medical and scientific knowledge and seeks to evaluate the claims of the applicant as well as to discern the likely safety hazards that may be associated with the product in use.

Two main areas of regulation are encountered before a product is available for sale in the United Kingdom: clinical trial certificates and product licenses. A clinical trial certificate or an exemption from holding such a certificate needs to be obtained before clinical trials can be undertaken. Comprehensive guidelines are available in the Medicines Act 1968—Guidance Notes for Applications for Clinical Trial Certificates and Clinical Trial Exemptions (MAL 4). It is also possible for an investigator who initiates a clinical trial to obtain materials under a doctors' and dentists' exemption, which is explained in Medicines Act Leaflet Number 31 (MAL 31).

II. PRODUCT LICENSE APPLICATIONS

The normal requirements for product license applications are given in the general guidelines previously known as MAL 2 (now called "Guidance Notes on Applications for Product Licences"). While these guidelines are comprehensive and cover all types of application, they are sufficiently flexible to indicate the need for particular studies where special routes of administration are proposed, as in the case of transdermal delivery.

At the present time there are no specific regulatory demands published in relation to transdermal drug delivery; there is no set series of regulatory hurdles the product must pass. Neither is it the intention of the Licensing Authority to enforce a uniformity of products in relation to their dose, dosage schedule, pharmacokinetics, or mechanisms of action. Since the Medicines Act of 1968 demands neither that a product fulfill a particular need in the marketplace nor that it be equivalent to any other product, each drug application is weighed on its own merits. The fact that a similar product may have received a license is no warrant for automatic licensing of a similar but different product subsequently, and data will need to be presented to demonstrate that the new preparation is of satisfactory and consistent quality and is efficacious in the population, having a satisfactory safety profile.

It is the concern of the Licensing Authority that the applications for product license, with their data sheets, should at the time of licensing reflect the "best state of the art," without prejudice to previous or subsequent licenses. There is no demand for novelty for its own sake, neither is there any automatic advantage to be gained by new systems.

III. ABRIDGED APPLICATIONS

When a transdermal system contains an active medicament that is a new chemical entity, clearly all the criteria for new chemical entities must be met. These are displayed in full in the guideline booklets mentioned. However, when the active medicament is a known chemical entity, which has previous clinical experience and scientific data, an abridged application may be submitted. The abridged application presupposes that the drug has already been submitted to satisfactory preclinical animal studies, including toxicity testing in two mammalian species (rodent and nonrodent).

Systemic and local toxic effects should be known, and specific local tests such as skin irritation in the rabbit and sensitivity in the guinea pig are required, as is eye irritation for substances likely to be applied to the face or neck. Photosensitivity testing may also be appropriate.

A full pharmacokinetic profile of the drug and metabolites in the species used for toxicity studies is required.

The foregoing data will support the human efficacy data but primarily will validate the animal toxicology in comparison with man.

Depending on the nature of the chemical entity, its pharmacology, and pharmacokinetics, carcinogenicity, and reproduction studies, may also be required. Then the safety profile of the product must be demonstrated in animals and supported by human volunteer and clinical data, including skin irritation and sensitization studies, using the product to be marketed.

Efficacy must be demonstrated in clinical studies. Although plasma levels in volunteers may give a guide to the potential efficacy, these data need to be validated in long-term clinical experience, which will confirm the suitable dose-duration-effect relationships of the drug in the transdermal form and will take tolerance into account.

So, before an abridged application is to be submitted, the applicant must be quite clear as to the extent of preclinical knowledge that may be assumed. Since the United Kingdom has no "freedom of information" act, applicants may normally assume only what is in the published literature—all data supplied by previous applicants are confidential to the Licensing Authority and cannot be divulged.

It is, I think, most helpful in preparing an abridged application, or indeed at an early stage in development, to consider the scientific and medical questions that will be asked by the regulatory authority and its advisory committees as they seek to determine the safety and efficacy of the product in use. Each new transdermal system, or each new combination of a system with a drug, will present a new series of safety hazards and questions of efficacy. The company applying for a product license or clinical trial certificate should address these questions specifically, rather than just seeking to identify a minimum series of hurdle exercises to be accomplished.

I intend, therefore, to remark on examples of scientific and medical questions that will be asked during the regulatory assessment, particularly relating to transdermal drug delivery. (It is taken for granted that in a presentation of the chemistry and pharmacy of the system, a rationale for its development and its formulation will be given to satisfy the pharmaceutical assessors that the quality of the product is consistent and satisfactory for the intended purpose.)

Transdermal drug delivery poses particular problems in relation to: (a) the determination of clinical efficacy, (b) dose variability within and between patients, (c) systemic toxicity and adverse reactions, (d) local toxicity and mechanical trauma, (e) instructions to prescribers and pharmacists, and (f) instructions for patient use. Each of these areas is discussed in turn.

A. The Determination of Clinical Efficacy

In conditions such as hypertension or hypercalcemia, in which clinical efficacy is synonymous with the physical or biochemical measurement, that measurement will suffice to demonstrate the efficacy. Other drugs such as theophylline appear to have a close relationship between plasma levels and clinical effect. Where this can be validated, that measurement may also be taken by itself to show efficacy, provided long-term tolerance does not occur. But for the majority of drugs, such a close relationship is not consistent. And even where it may have been thought to be consistent, during intermittent therapy such as twice- or thrice-daily tablet administration, we may be unaware of the possibility of tolerance, especially when the plasma and tissue levels remain uniform over a long period of time.

Thus, it is not certain to what extent comparability of drug plasma levels with another preparation may assist in demonstrating efficacy. Although this has been widely accepted for conventional generic forms of branded products, the wide variability of response for prolonged-release transdermal preparations, even when using subjects as their own controls, effectively precludes such data from serving as the sole determinant of efficacy.

The variety of transdermal systems now emerging in development demands an independent assessment of each product. Although transdermal drug delivery avoids a hepatic first-pass effect, the skin has its own metabolic function and is probably an intrinsically much more variable site of absorption than the gut; hence there is a need for a large, varied population of patients. Volunteer data alone therefore are unlikely to be sufficient, but such data are useful in confirming the populations and conditions of use in which the drug will have an optimum risk/benefit ratio.

Likewise, the animal and in vitro model systems, although useful for screening and quality control procedures, only point to efficacy; they do not prove it. However such data should be included to demonstrate the consistency of the company's case.

For the majority of products, the double-blind, placebo-controlled clinical study, preferably against placebo, is the prime evidence of efficacy. For a drug in long-term use, minimum exposure of 100 patients for 1 year is required. Where massive early patient exposure is likely after marketing approval has been granted, companies may wish to detail plans for a postmarketing surveillance study in the application.

While efficacy in short-term studies must be demonstrated, long-term maintenance of efficacy may be sought to determine the extent of tolerance. Comparative data against established therapies will establish a relative risk/benefit ratio to place the new product into therapeutic perspective.

B. Dose Variability

It is essential that individual batches of the product have reproducible release characteristics that may be demonstrated on in vitro systems. Despite the sophistication of some systems, the controlled-release characteristic is regarded as evidence of quality rather than an automatic predictor of absorption at a particular rate. Certainly the drug dose flux in vitro and patch surface area must be standardized, but the biological variables of skin thickness, site, sex, age, race, hydration, lipid content, vascularity, and temperature may result in widely different absorption and metabolism kinetics across the population, or even within one individual's experience of the drug. Where a particular system is designed to minimize the effect of these biological variables, the efficiency of the design will need to be demonstrated in clinical experience.

Data should also be presented to show the variations caused by defatting the skin (by soap, detergents, or solvent cleaners that may be used to remove adhesive residues, etc.), and by repeated applications to the same site or on an area previously stripped by adhesive. Variability can also be caused by applications at different sites, and the differences between smooth and shaved hairy skin might be investigated.

If the system delivers a bolus dose followed by a slower rate of release, repeat dose characteristics to steady state should be performed. The sites of application (i.e., new or repeat site) should be stated.

Absorption enhancers may be used with some products, and this combination with the product will need to be tested under a variety of conditions to show the influence of the biological variables. It is also important to note that the toxicity profile of the absorption enhancer should also be clearly defined. If the enhancer is a new chemical entity, a full range of tests is needed, and the system must be assessed as a new drug with a full application.

These studies show the conditions under which the product will be effective, and they identify potential safety problems. It is not expected that products with similar drug content, rate of release, and surface area will be equally efficacious, but it is expected that each product will perform reliably according to the prescribing instructions, and such instructions would be based on the data above. At the present time it is considered that products should not be regarded as interchangeable and should not be prescribed on a generic basis.

C. Systemic Toxicity and Adverse Reactions

The design or review of animal toxicity studies should take account of the lack of hepatic first-pass metabolism but should also note the skin metabolism by using the transdermal route. This may well affect the interpretation of chronic toxicity and reproduction studies performed by oral administration. Human adverse reaction data from long-term studies should be presented, including any evidence of the product's inefficacy or development of tolerance.

D. Local Toxicity and Mechanical Trauma

Toxicity may be due to the drug or its vehicle, the adhesive compound, or physical trauma resulting from the adhesive system.

The drug substance itself should be tested for irritation, sensitivity, and photosensitivity in animals and man; likewise, such tests should be performed on the adhesive compound and vehicle. The product should be applied to animals, but the differences in skin type and the problems of size will make human volunteer studies more definitive.

The trauma of an adhesive device is often seen after removal, either as skin stripping, bullae formation, or intraepidermal bleeding. Damage may occur though during use, as a result of the differential movement of the skin and device, which results in sheer forces separating epidermal or subepidermal cells with the appearance of bullae and striae. The more rigid the device—in the lateral plane— and the more powerful the adhesive, the more likely are traumatic effects: the epidermis becomes the weakest mechanical structure, and normal skin movement due to muscle and joint activity may cause tearing of the skin. Thus, a local adverse reaction may be chemical, immunological, or physical in origin. Potential problems should be identified in volunteer and clinical trials, and suitable instructions provided to avoid these adverse effects.

The implications of such local damage to diabetics, the elderly, those with steroid-affected skin, and those with psoriasis or rare conditions such as epidermolysis bullosa, should be addressed in the

application. Also, potential hazards associated with electrical de-
fibrillation should be identified.

E. Instructions to Prescribers and Pharmacists

The technical data will permit a statement of the content of the drug
contained within the device, the rate of release of drug in vitro,
and the surface area of release. However, this information will not
define the dosage instruction, which should be described in terms
of the number of applications of the device per day or per week,
and will clarify whether repeat applications should be on the same or
a different area of skin.

However, it is advisable to make the dose contained within the
device available in the product information to assist in cases of
overdose by product abuse or inappropriate ingestion.

Prescribing information stated on the data sheet should identify
the dose range through which the patient may safely be titrated and
the precise manner and site of application and reapplication. It
should identify circumstances likely to lead to hazard or inefficacy,
and it should state any subpopulations that need particular care.

F. Instructions for Use

The patient needs a clear introduction to the appliance and medication, and consideration should be given to a package insert explaining the use of the product and stating the circumstances in which
the user should seek medical advice. This information may be given
pictorially, bearing in mind that an unfamiliar product may be prescribed for patients who do not have English as their first language.

IV. CONCLUSION

Marketing approval for all named products in the United Kingdom
depends on the applicant company satisfactorily addressing all the
relevant issues with regard to safety, quality, and efficacy. The
company must present a coherent argument for the product based
on animal and human data that identify appropriate dosage and safe
conditions for use.

ACKNOWLEDGMENT

I wish to thank Prof. M. Rawlins, Prof. B. Barry, and Dr. G. Jones,
who have made their comments on this chapter. The above views
are those of the author and do not necessarily represent the official
policy of the DHSS or its advisory committees.

18

Regulatory Approval of Transdermal Therapeutic Systems in Japan

TSUNEJI NAGAI and YOSHIHARU MACHIDA / *Hoshi University, Shinagawa, Tokyo, Japan*

I. INTRODUCTION

The regulations regarding the approval of applications for new drugs often cause distressing problems not only for manufacturers or importers in Japan but also for foreign pharmaceutical companies who wish to export their products to Japan. We have often heard that troubles arise in understanding the Japanese regulatory system of approval between the staff of non-Japanese parent companies headquartered overseas and their branch offices in Japan. These misunderstandings may have been due not only to linguistic difficulties hampering communication but also to failure to understand the differences in the systems.

In the past, before the Japanese government established its Good Laboratory and Good Manufacturing Practices (GLP, GMP), the regulating authorities did not accept data compiled in foreign countries. We personally believe that this was reasonable from both scientific and political viewpoints, and was not enforced to protect domestic Japanese pharmaceutical companies in competition with foreign ones. Considering the circumstances surrounding Japan, dual attitudes prevailed. The idea that we should be fair in accepting foreign data even if such material was compiled abroad was countered with the thought that we should be fair in not accepting it, too.

This duality created dissatisfaction among the staff and management of foreign companies, especially from advanced nations. However, the situation has greatly changed since the GLP and other related guidelines were established to assure first of all the safety of drugs, and in part to help solve the problems of international trade between Japan and other nations, especially the United States. Now, almost all data (except for clinical trials) are said to be accepted, if they are compiled following the above-mentioned Japanese guidelines. These circumstances may expand to those of clinical trials when the so-called GCP, (a guideline for practice in clinical trials), is established in the near future.

Dr. Nagai's past experience (serving the Ministry of Health and Welfare as a member of both the Subcommittee on New Drugs and the Subcommittee on Combination Drugs), prompts him to say that even data that have been compiled without following the Japanese guidelines exactly might be accepted, assuming that there are no problems in the reasoning logic, if equivalency to data compiled following the above-mentioned guidelines can be indicated. However, many companies have preferred to recompile data following the Japanese guidelines.

A better understanding of the Japanese regulatory system for approval of pharmaceuticals might be helpful in solving potential problems businesses might face in Japan. We will attempt to show the approval process as clearly as we can from our own experience. Here we would like to emphasize that we are not representing any Japanese regulatory authority but are participants from the academic side. Therefore, readers should query the Japanese authorities concerning matters not explained here.

First, we will explain the general matters concerning the approval of pharmaceuticals; second, we will discuss the approval of external preparations including transdermal therapeutic systems (TTS).

II. APPLICATION REQUIREMENTS FOR APPROVAL OF NEW PRESCRIPTION DRUGS IN JAPAN (1)

All applications for approval to manufacture or import new prescription drugs in Japan are examined with regard to their usefulness based on efficacy and safety by the Committee on Drugs on the Central Pharmaceutical Affairs Council under the Ministry of Health and Welfare. The new drugs are examined according to eight classes, as follows (1):

1. New active ingredients
2. New fixed combination
3. New route of administration
4. New indications

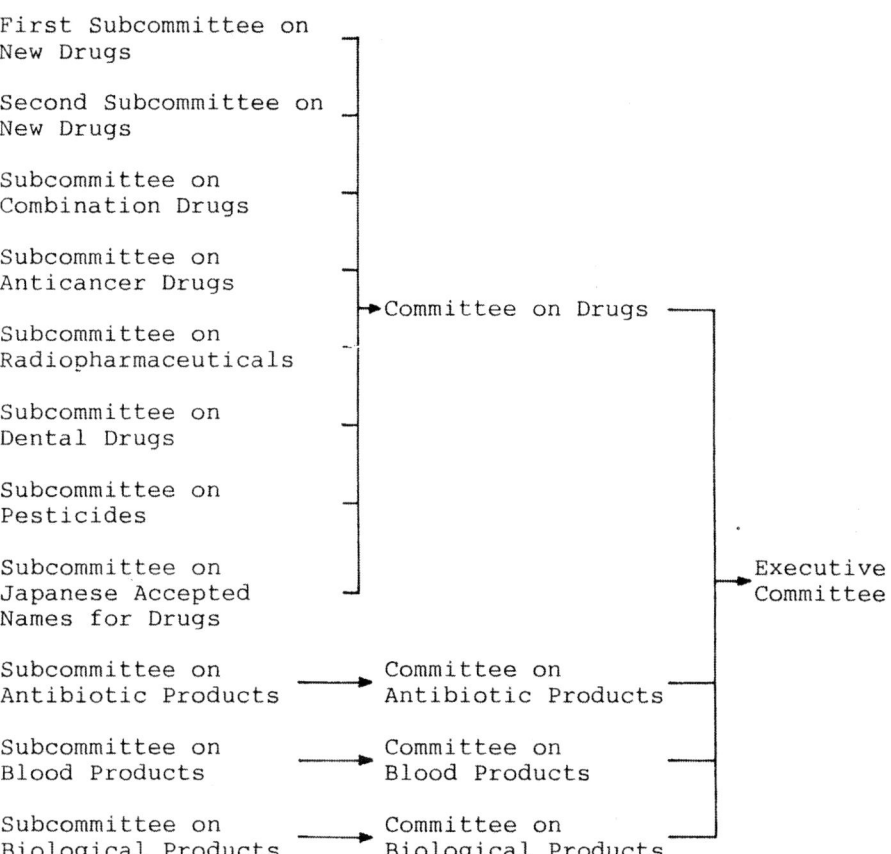

Figure 1   Committees and subcommittees of the Central Pharmaceutical Affairs Council engaged in examination for new drug approval. (From Ref. 1.)

5. Pharmaceutically new dosage forms
6. New dosage (content)
7. Additional dosage forms
8. Miscellaneous

Figure 1 shows the Committees and Subcommittees of the Central Pharmaceutical Affairs Council (CPAC) engaged in the examination of new drug approvals.

The drugs listed above are examined at the various subcommittees as follows: class 1 by the First Subcommittee on New Drugs, class 2

Table 1   Details of Data by Category and Number[a]

Category	Number
A. Data on origin, details of discovery, use in foreign countries, etc.	1. Data on origin and details of discovery 2. Data on use in foreign countries 3. Data on characteristics and comparison with other drugs
B. Data on physical and chemical properties, specifications, test methods, etc.	1. Data on determination of structure 2. Data on physical and chemical properties, etc. 3. Data on specifications and test methods
C. Data on stability	1. Data on long-term storage testing 2. Data on severe-conditions testing 3. Data on accelerated testing
D. Data on acute toxicity, subacute toxicity, chronic toxicity, teratogenicity, and other toxicity	1. Data on acute toxicity 2. Data on subacute toxicity 3. Data on chronic toxicity 4. Data on influence on reproduction 5. Data on dependence 6. Data on antigenicity 7. Data on mutagenicity 8. Data on carcinogenicity 9. Data on local irritation
E. Data on pharmacological action	1. Data on test endorsing effectiveness 2. Data on general pharmacology
F. Data on absorption, distribution, metabolism, and excretion	1. Data on absorption 2. Data on distribution 3. Data on metabolism 4. Data on excretion 5. Data on bioequivalence
G. Data on results of clinical trials	Data on results of clinical trials

[a]As used in the classification of Table 2.
Source: from Ref. 1.

by the Subcommittee on Combination Drugs, classes 3–6 by Second Subcommittee on New Drugs. The drugs in classes 7 and 8 are examined only at the Ministry of Health and Welfare without examination by a subcommittee.

Drugs for special use such as dental drugs and anticancer drugs, shall be examined by the other subcommittee shown in Figure 1, even if they can be classified into the eight classes above.

The members of the CPAC committees and subcommittees are composed of medical and pharmaceutical specialists. Generally, meetings are held once or twice a month in the First and Second Subcommittees on New Drugs, and once every one to three months in the other committees and subcommittees.

The number of items of data required for application of prescription drugs depends on the classification of drugs. Table 1 shows the details of data by category and number, and Table 2 shows the data required for a drug in each class. For example, at least 19 items of data are required for drugs containing active new ingredients, but only 16 items are required for drugs introducing a new method of administration, and merely 3 items for "me-too" drugs. Details concerning each datum will be described in the following section.

III. SCIENTIFIC DATA REQUIRED FOR APPROVAL OF TRANSDERMAL THERAPEUTIC SYSTEMS

At present, no special regulatory class or category for "transdermal therapeutic system (TTS)" is fixed in Japan; TTS is included in the category of "external preparations" such as cataplasms, ointments, or plasters. Usually, most TTS products in general have been classified as class 3 or 5 in Table 2 and will be examined by the Second Subcommittee on New Drugs.

Recently, tape-type preparations of nitroglycerin and isosorbide dinitrate (ISN tape) were approved, and they are the only TTS preparations on the market in Japan.

We will discuss the approval of ISN tape as an example. As is known, the drug ISN receives a serious first-pass effect. Thus, the bioavailability in peroral dosage forms has been said to be 10% or less. For this reason, ISN tape was developed as a preparation that has a high bioavailability and prolonged action compared with peroral sustained-release dosage forms.

This preparation is composed of three parts: a backing made of plastic film, an ISN-containing adhesive layer that functions as the drug reservoir, and a protective peel strip. The composition seems to be nearly identical to the TTS preparations containing nitroglycerin or scopolamine developed in the United States. The dosage of the ISN tape can be adjusted easily by cutting the tape to an

Table 2 Data by Class of Prescription Drugs

Class of drugs	A 1	A 2	A 3	B 1	B 2
(1) Drugs containing new active ingredients	○	○	○	○	○
(2) New fixed combination prescription drugs (combination prescription drugs that differ in active ingredients or their composition from Japanese Pharmacopoeia combination drugs and from existing drugs approved for manufacture or import as prescription drugs, excluding multidigestive enzyme preparations and cataplasms with a mild action, if their novelty is denies after their synthetic evaluation)[d]	○	○	○	×	×
(3) Drugs in new route of administration	○	○	○	×	×
(4) Drugs providing new indications	○	○	○	×	×
(5) Drugs in new dosage forms (drugs that are common to already approved drugs in active ingredient, route of administration, and indications, but different, in principle, in dosage and administration as a result of pharmaceutical changes to, for example, sustained-release preparations)	○	○	○	×	×
(6) Drugs in new dosage	○	○	○	×	×
(7) Drugs in additional dosage forms (drugs) that are common to already approved drugs in active ingredient, route of administration, indications, and dosage and administration, but different in dosage form and composition, excluding drugs in class 5)	○	○	○	×	×
(8) Miscellaneous drugs[g]	×	×	×	×	×

[a]Corresponding to category and number of data in Table 1: ○ = Data s be submitted; × = data may be submitted but are not required; Δ = da submission shall be determined depending on the conditions of drugs.
[b]Not less than 150 cases in not fewer than five institutions. For each indication, not fewer than two institutions with not less than 20 cases i each institution.
[c]Not less than 150 cases in not fewer than five institutions.
[d]Data shall include data providing ground of reason for combination. S data shall, in principle, be those collected from clinical or animal tests.

Category and number of data[a]

C	D	E	F	G	Cases and institutions
1 2 3	1 2 3 4 5 6 7 8 9	1 2	1 2 3 4 5		
o o x	o o o o Δ Δ Δ Δ Δ	o o	o o o o x	o	b
o o x	o o o x x x x x Δ	o o	o o o o x	o	c
o o x	o o o o x x x x Δ	o x	o o o o x	o	c
x ˅ o	x x x x x x x x x	o x	o o o o x	o	e
o o x	x x x x x x x x x	x x	o o o o x	o	c
x x o	x x x x x x x x x	o x	o o o o x	o	c
x x o	x x x x x x x x x	x x	x x x x o	o	f
x x o	x x x x x x x x x	x x	x x x x o	x	

The data may be omitted if the applied drug is deemed almost equivalent to already approved drugs and if the significance of combination of ingredients is scientifically established.
[e]For each main indication, no fewer than two institutions with not less than 20 cases in each.
[f]No fewer than two institutions, with not less than 20 cases in each institution.
[g]Data shall include list(s) of references to toxicity, pharmacological action, absorption, distribution, metabolism, excretion, and clinical evaluation, as well as outlines of the evaluation and the results of efficacy reevaluation.
Source: From Ref. 1.

appropriate size. The plastic backing part covers the skin surface
as it administers an occlusive dressing therapy (ODT) effect, producing better transdermal absorption of ISN.

A. General Matters

In relation to the fact that the above-mentioned ISN tape has been
approved, the following important points, which are required for an
application of approval for similar types of adhesive preparation, are
considered:

1. The usefulness of the preparation shall be clearly described
   on the basis of the data with regard to prolongation of action,
   improvement of bioavailability, and safety.
2. The clinical necessity of the preparation and also the technical
   or pharmaceutical merits shall be cleared. Convenience for use
   as a sole merit shall not be recognized as a condition for
   acceptance.
3. Topical and transdermal toxicological properties of the preparation shall be cleared.
4. A well-grounded description shall be done in determination of
   the dose.

B. Details of Data Required

Detailed data that may be required for an application of drugs in
class 3 (new administration routes), such as ISN tape, are considered as follows:

1. Data on origin and details of discovery or development, use in
   foreign countries, etc.
2. Data on physical and chemical properties, specifications, test
   methods, etc. Especially for this type of preparation, tests
   of shape and of adhesiveness (e.g., ball-tack test) shall be
   included. Moreover, specifications on the adhesive agent and
   the backing material also shall be described. If there is no
   existing instance for usage of these materials in pharmaceutical
   preparations, data on their safety shall be submitted as well.
3. Data on stability.
   a. In addition, data on long-term storage tests that have been
      conducted under room temperature conditions (25°C) for
      more than 3 years, and at 75% RH for more than 2 years,
      shall be submitted in accordance with the general stability
      test guideline for pharmaceutical preparations.
   b. Data on severe-conditions testing with respect to light,
      temperature, and humidity shall be submitted.

4. Data on safety.
    a. Animal tests.
        i. Acute toxicity test in transdermal and subcutaneous administrations
        ii. Acute toxicity test in application to the skin
        iii. Primary irritant test (by patch test)
        iv. Repeated-insult irritation test
        v. Phototoxicity test
        vi. Sensitization test
    b. Testing on human subjects: primary irritant test (by patch test).
    c. Data on irritation after storage: in cases in which the safety of the preparation after storage (which may be related not only to the degradation of components in the preparation but also to the alteration of the preparation in the total system), is not confirmed, data from irritation testing on the sample after long-term storage or severe conditions testing shall be required.
5. Data on pharmacological action: in principle, test data endorsing the drug's effectiveness shall be taken in an administration route similar to that used in clinical application. Additionally, the effectiveness shall be investigated in comparison with existing preparations (e.g., peroral ones), and the mechanism at the onset of an effect shall be discussed in the investigations.
    a. Animal tests: in comparison with the peroral dosage form, the relationship between the effect (e.g., on hemodynamics in the case of ISN tape, such as systolic blood pressure, diastolic blood pressure, average blood pressure, heart rate, and pulse pressure) and drug disposition shall be investigated with the proper time lapse(s) after administration.
    b. Testing in human subjects: the relationship between the effect (e.g., on hemodynamics and capability against exercise tests) and the plasma drug level shall be discussed in the investigations.
6. Data on absorption, distribution, metabolism, and excretion: in comparison with another route of administration (peroral dosage form, if an existing product is available), drug disposition shall be investigated after a single and/or repeated administrations by topical application(s) in both animal and human subjects. In the experiments, plasma level, urinary excretion, and concentration in organs shall be determined after the proper lapse of time. As for the metabolites, the identification, determination, general pharmacological action, toxicity, and metabolic pathway shall be discussed in the investigations. If necessary, labeled drug also shall be used in the experiment.
    a. Animal testing: to compare with peroral administration, the drug time lapse disposition after transdermal administration and peroral administration shall be investigated.

b. Testing in human subjects (healthy and patient volunteers): in comparison with peroral administration, plasma drug levels and urinary excretion after transdermal administration shall be investigated.

7. Data on results of clinical trials: in principle, the clinical trials of a drug shall be made with a total of not less than 150 cases in not fewer than five institutions, consisting of not less than 20 cases in each institution. However, this could be modified depending on the type and properties of the test drug. Especially in external preparations, double-blind clinical trials present many difficulties in guaranteeing the impossibility of discrimination between the test drug and the control. In other words, a trial with the control preparation, which is made containing the control active ingredient in the same dosage form as the test sample, may be very often nonsensical, because the usefulness of the preparation usually depends not only on the active ingredient but also strongly on the total system in the dosage form. It is recommended that an impartial, unbiased comparative clinical trial be designed, since the double-blind test is considered to be the most desirable. Regarding the double-blind test, which shall be done in part at least, fairness is essential. As a control drug for the test, a commercially available product, which has been confirmed clinically to have no problem with regard to efficacy and safety, shall be used. If the dosage form of test drug is different from that of the control one, a combination with such a preparation as a double dummy shall be applied.

a. Practice of clinical tests shall be as follows:

   i. Double-blind crossover comparative test (in comparison with the existing oral preparation, especially a sustained-release one, if commercially available)

   ii. General clinical tests:
Clinical testing at different institutions
Long-term-administration test

b. The clinical effect shall be investigated on basis of the results in the above-mentioned tests with regard to the following items:

   i. Clinical effects tested at different institutions and on different diseases

   ii. Clinical effects tested on different items for evaluation

   iii. Clinical effects tested on different directions for use and different doses

   iv. Clinical effects tested on different background factors

c. Side effects shall be observed in relation to:

   i. Different directions for use and different doses

   ii. Systemic symptoms

iii. Topical symptoms, such as those that can be observed topically on the skin after an application of the test drug.

IV. PROCEDURE AND TIME NEEDED FOR APPROVAL

The procedure for approval may be understood from our explánation at the beginning of Section III.A. The time necessary for approval has seemed to be very important for the applicants. Although we have no formal data available, it appears to take about 2 years on the average for approval, according to information given by manufacturers. The time necessary may depend on the quality of the data documents submitted. If there are mistakes in the documents submitted, the applicant is requested to revise them or to make an additional investigation; then, of course, the time required for approval is lengthened. On the regulatory side, the Japanese authorities have made efforts to shorten the time for the examination of new drug applications. Recently, an additional division was established for the evaluation and registration of new drugs in the Ministry of Health and Welfare. Accordingly, we expect that the time needed for approval will be shortened. Nevertheless, it is recommended that applicants acquaint themselves with the Japanese regulatory system for approval of new drugs and achieve a good understanding of it.

V. REGULATORY POLICY IN OTHER ASIAN COUNTRIES

It is quite difficult to get precise information concerning the regulatory policies of countries elsewhere in Asia. It seems that Asian countries have usually followed the administration standards of their respective former colonial rulers, partly due to convenience in communication in a common language. Regulatory policy for approval of drugs in these countries emphasizes essential drugs and drugs that are introduced from foreign countries where they are already widely available, having been confirmed to be useful clinically. Therefore, we understand that in many Asian countries the regulations are not as strict as those of North American and European countries and Japan. We have heard that drugs approved in Japan are accepted easily in some Asian countries, because there is no noticeable difference racially among Asian people.

Recently, technical cooperation among the countries of the Association of Southeast Asian Nations (ASEAN: Indonesia, Malaysia, Philippines, Singapore, and Thailand) regarding pharmaceuticals has increased as these nations have become quite active and involved with help from the Western Pacific Regional Office of the World Health Organization. They exchange information concerning pharmaceutical regulatory affairs to find a manner suitable to the above-mentioned specialty, and they work to the common good as much as possible.

The Japanese government invited about 15 regulatory specialists from ASEAN countries to Japan in the 1985 financial year for training in the field of pharmaceutical regulation, as a part of Japan's International Cooperation for Welfare Services projects. Because of the circumstances outlined in this chapter, there was quite a lot to discuss regarding the regulatory approval of TTS devices during this symposium.

REFERENCE

1. *Requirements for the Registration of Drugs in Japan*, Yakuji Nippo, Ltd., Tokyo, 1982.

Index